SEARCHING FOR MEDICAL TRUTHS

By Oliver E. Owen, M.D.

Copyright © 2006 by Oliver E. Owen

ISBN 978-0-7414-3009-0

Published by:

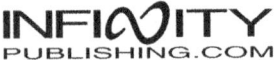
PUBLISHING.COM

Info@buybooksontheweb.com
www.buybooksontheweb.com
Toll-free (877) BUY BOOK
Local Phone (610) 941-9999
Fax (610) 941-9959

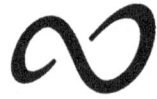

Printed in the United States of America

Published November 2012

For Paula, Michele, Rodney and Lydia

Contents

Foreword

This book is a personal story of an individual engaged in clinical research at a time when investigator-initiated research on humans was at its zenith.

Oliver E. Owen, M.D. was born in Roswell, New Mexico, located in the high plains of the southeastern part of the state. In 1941, Roswell became the home of Walker Army Air Force Base. During the Second World War, there was an influx of people who generated excitement and enthusiasm in the Roswell village. Many of the schoolteachers were wives of army air force personnel stationed at the Base. The local and immigrant teachers were talented and devoted individuals who encouraged students to pursue higher education. The Roswell villagers created a nurturing community.

After World War II, rationing of food was discontinued and an epidemic of obesity was begun in North America. Clinical professors at medical schools were the primary individuals who dominated advances made in health care. This book tells the story of Dr. Owen's personal quest from 1962-2005 as he strived to gain medical insight as a clinical investigator. Work was initiated at Johns Hopkins Hospital and carried on at the Harvard University Peter Bent Brigham Hospital and Temple University Medical School and Hospital. The book describes his development and experiences as a dedicated medical scientist who had eye-to-eye contact with both normal and patient volunteers while uncovering the mysteries of human body metabolism. He and his colleagues defined the mechanisms that promoted survival during starvation and discovered disturbances that led to death when overall metabolism went awry. The book also includes background information regarding the organizational aspects of how clinical research is conducted.

As obesity was on the rise in North America, the threat from diseases that accompanied the excessive accumulation of body fat were becoming widely recognized. While starvation was a sure way to lose weight, a few clinical investigators thought that if prolonged starvation was going to be employed to reduce body fat, individuals subjected to fasting should be studied to detect impending dangers as well as the benefits of starvation. The metabolic mechanisms that came into play that allowed survival needed to be discovered. The source of fuel consumed by the brain during starvation was a peculiar enigma. Dr. Owen and his colleagues defined brain metabolism during starvation, discovering that ketone bodies (formerly thought to be toxic byproducts of fat metabolism) were in reality vital fuels for brain metabolism, and their consumption by this master organ of the body was essential for survival during starvation. This insightful finding triggered a reversal in the perception of ketone bodies by physician-scientists. Ketone body utilization as fuel by the brain spared the need of the body to mobilize proteins (amino acids) from muscle and other lean body tissues to synthesize glucose for brain energy needs.

Subsequent studies on obese volunteers undergoing lengthy starvation revealed that intricate orchestrated interplay exists among individual organs (brain, liver, kidney, muscle and adipose tissue), essential to support life during prolonged periods of starvation.

In addition to describing mechanisms employed during starvation, two other prominent disease conditions in the United States, alcoholic cirrhosis and diabetic ketoacidosis, were studied in detail. How excessive consumption of alcoholic beverages destroys the ability of the liver to provide glucose and ketone bodies for fuel to meet the body's energy requirements, and how the rest of the body comes to the aid of the dysfunctional liver of alcoholic patients, were detected and described.

Dr. Owen's research group's studies revealed how the catastrophic and simultaneous dumping of glucose, ketone bodies and free fatty acids into the bloodstream results in flooding the body with an overabundance of fuels during diabetic ketoacidosis. His team of clinical investigators gradually accumulated data regarding body composition (fat mass and fat-free mass) of lean to morbidly obese individuals with a five-fold difference in body weight. Body compositional variables were contrasted with energy requirements. From their data the principles of energy requirements for adult humans were developed. These studies showed that as the body size increases, the resting metabolic requirements increase. However, there is a wide range of energy requirements of people of identical age, sex and body weight. In addition, Owen and colleagues published data showing that humans can consume food at a rate of 150 times their resting metabolic requirements. Further, walking uphill at a rate of about 3 miles per hour increases energy requirements only five-fold. If you want to lose weight, cut caloric intake!

During his time as a clinical investigator, it became evident that the drug industries were sponsoring more and more clinical studies. This activity was designed for profit. Investigator-initiated clinical research sponsored mostly by federal grants was disappearing from the American medical scene. Furthermore, litigation induced a fear among clinical investigators which restricted the enthusiasm to search for causes and cures of medical diseases.

In spite of all the miraculous tools that are now available, today's population is still dealing with the heartbreak and misery associated with medical problems, such as Alzheimer's disease, because sufficient numbers of well-trained clinical investigators are no longer available or able to discover cures for this dementia and other human maladies. This shortage of clinical investigators is preventing timely medical breakthroughs to improve health care in America and worldwide. This situation will undoubtedly result in a critical healthcare delivery deficit.

Dr. Owen hopes this book will help shed light on the critical shortage of clinical researchers and funding, and stimulate a resurgence of interest in and awareness of the importance of medical research in which medical doctors have eye-to-eye contact with normal and patient volunteers.

Prologue

I started writing this book after retiring from the practice and teaching of medicine. Most of the data presented in the book are derived from scientific articles written by coworkers and me and published in top peer-reviewed medical journals. The scientific revelations are mixed with some homegrown philosophy and storytelling.

The theme of this book revolves around clinical investigation as seen through my eyes. It portrays my thoughts as a clinical investigator/medical doctor who has searched for the mechanisms underlying health and disease states and responded to a "calling" to serve people for four decades. It provides data and conclusions about research done on normal and patient volunteers. The book is a story of how body functions, some deranged by diseases, can be defined using information gathered through studying and comparing normal and patient volunteers. Teams of physician-scientists and volunteers shared responsibilities in our search for scientific evidence needed to understand normal and abnormal metabolism, centered around the production and use of fuels by organs for maintaining life.

This book was written for the intellectually curious. It should help to bridge the gap between lay people and the medical professionals. Part of the book is focused around energy requirements, body composition and obesity. Other parts of the book contain more scientific information and may please those who are interested in grasping the specific metabolism of the larger organs like the brain, liver, kidney, adipose tissue and muscle. Fuel for energy is a theme that traverses the book. The cardinal role of all organs is to maintain a constant supply of energy so life can be maintained.

In the mid-1960's, the time was right to make significant clinical advances in knowledge pertaining to metabolism in normal people and patients with medical diseases. Accurate techniques for measuring the nature and quantities of fuels needed to support the body's energy requirements became available. Changes in the concentrations of factors that modified metabolism, hormones, could also be measured in body fluids.

The intent of this book is to entertain and inform the reading audience. If an individual poring over the data encounters facts he/she cannot understand, continue to read. The information intended should come forth eventually. The book contains some personal stories; some relate to studies of adult humans. The data were collected from volunteers and analyzed between 1965 and 2004. The results from studies came in a piecemeal fashion. A reappraisal of data sometimes provided a slightly different interpretation than that perceived at the time the studies were done. An overview from the data provided a wholesomeness that was not always envisioned when some of the early studies were done and reported.

A clinical investigator is usually a physician or surgeon who is part of a team that uses scientific methods to discover medical truths. Accomplishments are commonly the result of group rather than individual efforts. Some member(s) of every team must have eye-to-eye contact with normal (healthy) and patient (diseased) volunteers.

Groups of clinical investigators and coworkers, which varied over the lifetime of my research efforts, conducted studies on normal individuals and compared their findings with patients suffering from diseases like morbid obesity, alcoholic cirrhosis of the liver, and diabetic patients during the severely decompensated state of ketoacidosis.

The majority of the research efforts were done at or near the General Clinical Research Center in Temple University Hospital. Volunteers, patients and staff developed a "team spirit" of trying to contribute knowledge needed to understand human body metabolism: sum of processes of life support, and especially the processes by which a substance (food, fuel, hormone) is mobilized and either assimilated or eliminated by the body, or both.

Willing and cooperative patients, volunteers, and their families are key to successful clinical research. They all need to be deeply committed to finding a cure or treatment for diseases afflicting people. In essence, clinical research is the interaction among people to uncover the mysteries that promote life or cause death.

After the Second World War, when food became abundant in the United States, the American citizens began to gain weight, and too many became morbidly obese. This was the natural consequence of living in a society where foods of high caloric content were readily available. Self-denial of food with some degree of tolerance to hunger is mandatory to prevent or treat obesity. Hunger, like obesity, is a natural state of humans. People who live in an environment where nutrients are available in overabundance must learn to avoid overeating.

A lot of the cost associated with medical care is related to obesity. Because obesity was on the rise among the American population and was associated with diabetes, hypertension, renal failure, heart attacks, strokes, and with some cancers, insurance companies in the1960's would pay to have grossly obese individuals hospitalized and subjected to starvation for weight reduction. Starvation was a sure way to lose weight. A few clinical investigators thought that if such drastic measures were going to be taken, those starving obese patients should be studied. Very little useful information on body metabolism during starvation was available. What mechanisms came into play that permitted people to survive prolonged periods of starvation? Lurking on the sidelines were questions regarding how to maintain the life of an astronaut lost in space, circling the earth, or going to the moon. Other than water, what were the bare essentials needed to prolong survival?

The National Institutes of Health sponsored clinical facilities in selected hospitals where normal and patient volunteers could be studied. It was generally recognized that excessive food consumption created an imbalance between energy requirements and energy expenditure that resulted in obesity. However, the accumulation of fat was viewed as an extremely complex disorder. Although practically everyone has the potential to become obese if an excessive quantity of food is consumed, some individuals display a genetic predisposition to develop gross obesity. A sure way to shed body weight and reduce the incidence of diabetes mellitus and probably heart disease and strokes is to decrease body weight by losing body fat. The safety of undergoing starvation, and how the body maintained its overall energy requirements and individual organ metabolism were unknown.

When we began studying humans, the scheme of overall body metabolism (the sum of all physical and chemical processes by which energy is made available for use by humans) had not been developed. We took on the task of defining energy requirements of humans with enormous variation in body size during rest, exercise and diseased states. In addition, we defined the role body organs played in providing and consuming energy to maintain metabolism, the process of "homeostasis."

Throughout the book, data are presented regarding total body energy requirements as they relate to body size and body composition of lean and obese individuals. The basic laws of weight gain and weight loss are simply stated. Caloric balance vs imbalance dictates changes in body size.

Our first research effort, published in 1967, showed that obese patients undergoing 5-6 weeks of starvation maintained normal energy requirements for their body size. Unlike the results reported by others, we found no "metabolic efficiency" developing in obese starving adults. However, we solidified the suggestions that starving humans provided with water developed a low excretion rate of urinary nitrogen and a high concentration of blood ketone bodies. Ketone bodies were thought to be toxic waste products associated with diabetes mellitus. Instead, we showed that ketone bodies replaced glucose as the primary fuel for providing the brain with energy during starvation. This finding triggered a reversal in our way of thinking about the importance of ketone bodies in the bloodstream during fasting states. We went on to show that glucose production was depressed during starvation, and the kidney shared the role with the liver in producing the small quantity of glucose. Further, the liver produced enough ketone bodies to supply the body with these water-soluble fuels that could replace glucose as a source of energy. We subsequently showed that, after prolonged starvation, the largest organ of the body, muscle, preferentially extracted free fatty acids for energy, thus sparing the consumption of both glucose and ketone bodies. In addition, we learned that the kidneys filtered ketone bodies from the bloodstream but reabsorbed the vast majority and, thus, maintained a high concentration of ketone bodies in the bloodstream so they could be used by the brain. Urinary nitrogen excretion in the form of ammonium during starvation was coupled to the loss of ketone bodies in the urine and concurrent synthesis of glucose by the kidney. Nonetheless, a small loss of ketone bodies in the urine during starvation seemed to be necessary to promote the kidney's ability to synthesize some of the essential glucose needed to maintain life.

We characterized fuel mobilization and oxidation using scientific methods. In patients with alcoholic cirrhosis, when the liver fails to deliver an adequate amount of water-soluble fuels (glucose and ketone bodies) for the rest of the body, the adipose tissue compensates the liver's shortfall by releasing more fat into the bloodstream. When one organ fails, another organ tries to pick up the deficit. This compensatory behavior among organs is not present when insulin secretion from the pancreas is inadequate. Diabetes mellitus is a clinical situation which is the antithesis of the normal balance between production and utilization of fuels. In the most severe diabetic state, diabetic ketoacidosis, there is a lack of integration between the production rate of fuels by the liver and the release of fat into the bloodstream from adipose tissue. Catastrophic tissue breakdown occurs, producing body fuels in overabundance that flood the bloodstream, inducing large losses of urine containing glucose and ketone bodies. Subsequent dehydration develops, and vascular collapse and death occur.

Throughout my clinical investigations I oversaw studies in which we measured energy requirements of "healthy" human beings during rest, after eating, and during physical activity. We also measured body compositions of adults with body size varying over a 5-fold range. We accumulated data from over a thousand adults, ranging from very lean to morbidly obese. The most important results showed that the greater the body size the greater the energy requirements. There, however, are many exceptions to this axiom. The range of energy requirements related either to total body weight or to fat-free mass (lean body weight) is huge. Individuals of similar sex, age and body weight (or lean body mass) have a range of resting metabolic requirements that varies almost 2-fold. Thus, although a generalization can be made, that the more you weigh, the greater your resting energy requirements, the range of energy requirements for a given sex, age or body weight is enormous.

From the clinical studies of normal and patient volunteers, there emerges a fundamental truth regarding life. The continuous provision of fuels to provide energy requirements for the body may be the most fundamental physical aspect of life. The various organs of the body work in an orchestrated manner to supply, conserve, select and convert the body stores of usable fuel into sources for generating energy to maintain life. In some disease states, when an organ becomes defective, other organs try to compensate for its shortfall. However, in other disease states these compensatory mechanisms fail.

The United States was a nation that produced great clinical investigators between 1955 and 1980, but the research environment in America changed. The promulgation of clinical investigation initiated by biomedical scientists at research-intense medical institutions diminished. Much of the current biomedical information produced by basic science at academic medical centers is derived from animal fragments. Clinical investigators, as a species of individual medical scientists who search for the cause and cure of diseases, have progressively disappeared in the United States. Administrative micromanagement techniques and regulations, inadequate federal funding, and insecurities of would-be clinical investigators at academic medical centers have sucked the enthusiasm out of studying humans. Trial lawyers have not helped the spirit of individuals who could advance knowledge if not conquer diabetes mellitus, cancer, Alzheimer's disease, etc. Currently, clinical research is primarily driven by the pharmaceutical industry, designed for profit. There is preciously little "free-wheeling" in research endeavors.

Diabetes mellitus, obesity, congestive heart failure, Alzheimer's dementia and AIDS are examples of diseases that are becoming more prevalent and threatening human lives. Attempts to resolve the disorders may take on heroic proportions. It should always be the intent of clinical investigators to put forth a proposition (a clinical study) that has a minimum risk and maximum benefit. Although quests for scientific medical knowledge have risks of inducing harm to humans, clinical investigators must push for new knowledge to correct disease processes that plague humans.

There was a time when a partnership developed between a clinical investigator and a patient-volunteer. Both benefited from their endeavors. The clinical investigator was rewarded by appreciation, and the patient-volunteer's prize was better health care for self and/or someone else. I wonder if this partnership can ever be revived. Nonetheless, future prospects do not detract from the glorious feeling of bygone days.

Acknowledgments

A diverse group of individuals provided the help needed to collect the data presented in this monograph. Patient-volunteers gave of themselves and encouraged others to serve as experimental subjects. Most of the financial aid to conduct the research studies was provided by the National Institutes of Health. An occasional source of funds to tide us over came from private donations, Smith Kline and French (1968) and Wilkie Buick/GMC Truck/Subaru (1987). Harvard, Johns Hopkins and Temple universities provided the facilities needed to conduct the research protocols and gave the oversight necessary to protect the welfare of humans. Investigator-initiated research grants and General Clinical Research Center grants sponsored by the federal government were key to executing our studies on healthy and diseased people. After 1996, my personal resources were used to continue analyzing and writing articles, and summarizing and publishing data included in this book, which had accumulated from clinical research over the preceding 3-4 decades.

Physician-scientists, surgeons, basic scientists, medical research fellows, medical residents and medical students along with nurses, dieticians, technical assistants and administrators all made significant contributions.

My deep appreciation is extended to Drs. George F. Cahill, Jr. and Richard W. Hanson for editorial reviews and advice, and to Dr. George A. Reichard, Jr. who counseled me on numerous occasions. Ms. Andrea Elovson provided helpful advice and edited several chapters in this book. My daughter, Lydia, also gave me editorial assistance. I am grateful to my former colleague, Karl J. Smalley, for his persistent aid in computer assistance and his clever humor that spurred me on while completing this book. Finally, I could not have written and assembled this monograph without the unusual devotion and dedication of my wife, Paula.

Chapter I. Development of a Medical Doctor and Clinical Investigator

The educational system in the United States of America had the elasticity needed for me, a young man of modest means from New Mexico, to attend college, receive a medical degree from the University of Colorado School of Medicine, complete three years of residency training at Johns Hopkins Hospital, and then become a research fellow at the Joslin Research Laboratories of Harvard Medical School. With my mentor at Harvard, Dr. Cahill, we defined brain metabolism during starvation, demonstrating that ketone bodies (formerly thought of as toxic byproducts of fat metabolism) were in reality vital fuels for brain metabolism and essential for survival during prolonged starvation. This insightful finding triggered a reversal in the perception of ketone bodies by physician-scientists and started me on an academic medical career as a physician and clinical investigator.

Youthful Background

Ordinary people have chances to live free and productive lives in this great country, the USA. This chapter is about an average guy who was given a chance to become a medical doctor and clinical investigator.

The general practitioner declared that he had never delivered a baby in such a cold environment. An unheated screened-in back porch of the home where my parents were living in Roswell, New Mexico, was the place of my birth on Christmas Eve, 1934. The birth certificate lists my father's occupation as cattle rancher and my mother's as housewife.

My great-grandfather had been the sheriff of Lincoln County shortly after the heyday of Billy the Kid. The Lincoln County courthouse also housed the jail. Bullet pock marks made by Billy the Kid during his escape in 1881 still adorn the walls of that old courthouse/jail. Pictures of my great-grandfather with his handlebar mustache, standing beside various deputies, outlaws and a hanging gallows, used to be on the walls of the courthouse/jail in Lincoln.

1

However, by now, most of those photographs have disappeared.

My dad grew up on his father's ranch just east of Capitan, New Mexico, a small town not far from Lincoln. Because one of his responsibilities was to break horses, he became a good bronc rider. He had a 10th grade education and, after leaving the ranch, developed and owned the Ever-Ready Motor Company in Roswell. From approximately the age of 50 until his death at age 66, he worked for the civil service.

During the mid 1940's he threw his old saddle in the trunk of the car and took the family (wife and three sons) to the regional rodeo, held the Fourth of July on grounds between Capitan and Lincoln. My dad had not been on a horse in 10 years. He entered the rodeo as a bronc rider. When the chute's gate opened, Dad leaned back in his saddle and gave the horse full reins. When the horse started bucking, Dad scraped the wild devil from its shoulders to its flanks with his spurs, waving his hat all the time. Dad "rode that son-of-a-bitch to the ground," to use local vernacular. The old ranchers in the crowd from the area called my dad "Blackie" because of his coal black hair. They sat or stood in the stands and screamed and shouted with glee at Blackie's performance. He won first prize. It was delightful to see him ride and later for me to reminisce about that rodeo.

My mother grew up on a ranch not far from my father's. She completed the 8th grade in a one-room schoolhouse. As a mother, she stressed cleanliness. In addition to being protective of her three children, she pushed them to do their best. She would prepare meals and welcome young and old friends to join with us to eat. She sewed many tailored shirts for her boys. She was a proud woman, and as she aged, she tried to maintain a good physical appearance. She was innately intelligent but poorly educated. She worked in my father's business overseeing availability of parts for auto repair and keeping books on financial matters. After my dad closed the garage and sold the property, Mother went to school to become a practical nurse. She had great respect for the Catholic sisters who taught her nursing techniques and was gratified during her years of serving and caring for others.

About every 5-10 years I get a hankering to drive across the United States. That desire usually fades and I travel by air. However, occasionally I make the trip by car. The last time I drove between Lincoln and Capitan, there was not a single wooden board or post marking the place of the old regional rodeo grounds. The chutes, corral and bleachers had all disappeared. I'm not entirely sure why I look forward to returning to that once hallowed area for the old ranchers and cowboys of New Mexico. Nonetheless, I make the trip and experience reverence.

When I was born, the United States was recovering from the Great Depression and Americans were able to have enough food, keep warm and be reasonably clean. The future was brighter than the immediate past. Life for most Americans was improving.

I was one of three brothers and became relatively independent at a young age. Roswell was a prosperous town during 1941-1945 and after World War II. The social programs in the schools were expanding, and I had the opportunity to learn from school classes and to participate in extracurricular activities like sports, drama and politics. For some, the band offered musical opportunities. Social events were frequent and easy to attend. The spirit of the young people in the community was exuberant. I started boxing in the eighth grade and was awarded a varsity letter. I continued the boxing sport through the 12th grade and became a state champion. Thereafter, I fought in the Golden Gloves Tournament of Champions held in Chicago in 1953. The pressure put on a boxer to win is more than in most other sports. A boxer comes face to face with an opponent in a ring that is clearly defined and well lit. All actions are visible. Not only the pounding fists, but the mental toughness and the heart are fully exposed. A champion gives his all every single second in the fight. After the grueling battle, win, lose or draw, the decision for that fight is final.

Good fortune smiled on me when I was selected to serve as the Senior Class President. I didn't ask for this honor. The nomination was made from the floor during an assembly hour; a vote was called, and I was elected. Unexpectedly, after the election I became acutely aware of new responsibilities. I was expected to lead in a manner that benefited the welfare of the entire senior class. I had to rise to the occasion and try to express attitudes that improved the environment for my classmates. This leadership role process brought additional meaning to my life.

Most of the boys and girls dated frequently and had joyous and healthy relationships that promoted civility and maturity. We were a happy bunch of kids.

Having grown up listening to the great and late Lefty Frizzell playing his guitar and singing the songs he wrote in our home in Roswell, New Mexico, left me with an indelible love for country-western music. My dad owned a small automobile repair garage. He, my uncles with their boot shop, and the Castle Drugstore hired Lefty, the young Pecos Valley troubadour, to sing on the KGFL radio station and to advertise their businesses from 11:30 a.m. to 12:00 noon. This program became a popular hit for the area. Everywhere you went between 11:30 and 12:00 you could hear Lefty singing over the radio. He was also well received in the local dance halls and saloons. His blemished morals ultimately became more evident. Lefty was arrested for statutory rape and confined in the Chavez County jail. During his jail time he used a nail to scratch the words, "I love you; I'll prove it a thousand ways," on the jailhouse wall. It was a song dedicated to his wife, Alice. My dad "went his bail" after about six months. Lefty subsequently signed a contract with Columbia and recorded "I Love You, I'll Prove it a Thousand Ways." This song and record shortly thereafter became the number one country-western recording in America. Lefty subsequently had a series of hits and became a legend as a country-western singer and songwriter.

Neither of my parents had gone to college, not because they weren't bright enough but because they never really had the chance. My ancestors on both sides were ranchers, not doctors or scientists.

When I graduated from Roswell High School in 1953 a teacher told me that the average vocabulary of students consisted of only 800 words. Most of the high school boys could say "uh huh" and "uh uh," and "can I help you, buddy?" This description of their lack of verbal talents fails to characterize their virtue. What the townsfolk lacked in verbal artistry they more than made up for in genuine character. The people of the Roswell village were straightforward, honest, industrious and good people. It also undermines the talented and devoted schoolteachers. Many of them were well educated, and several were the wives of army-air force personnel stationed at Walker Army-Air Force Base. The airplane, Enola Gay, flew out of Roswell carrying the atomic bomb that was dropped in Japan in 1945.

In July 1947 an unidentified flying object crashed on a ranch outside of Roswell. If the government wanted to limit the spread of information, it is hard to imagine how anyplace in the USA could be more easily silenced than an event that happened in the non-verbal high plains of southeastern New Mexico in 1947.

So what does any of this have to do with my becoming a clinical researcher, an individual who looks for the causes and searches for therapies for diseases? Well, everything really. Had I not grown up in such a friendly and supportive community, I might have led a very different life. Some of my luckiest breaks were more than just luck. They were the result of the hard work and ingenuity of people who cared -- my parents, teachers and friends.

Take my winning a Ford Foundation Scholarship, for example. The scholarship covered my tuition, room and board at the University of New Mexico. What were the odds that a kid from Roswell would hear about, no less win a scholarship to college? If it hadn't been for the tireless efforts of a very special teacher, Mr. Arthur Gaddis, it would never have happened. And I wasn't the only one who benefited from his dedication. This teacher made it his

5

mission to find college money for many of the students at Roswell High. I felt proud and profoundly fortunate.

In September of 1953 I started at the University of New Mexico. I remember the students eating at the cafeteria in Mesa Vista dormitory complaining about all the carbohydrates served for meals. I did not know what carbohydrates were, but I liked the food. It tasted better than what I was used to eating. The scholarship to UNM was a most fortunate award for me. In retrospect, I recognize that my reading and writing abilities were abominable and my spelling skills were worse. Therefore, my first two years of college at the University of New Mexico were difficult for me. I was one of those high plains New Mexicans with a limited vocabulary, and I did not know how to study effectively. In addition, I was financially broke.

Like a lot of young men, my extracurricular activities were sometimes misdirected. I took part in a spontaneously developed panty-raid. Someone took pictures of the rowdy boys outside the girls' dormitory. I was wearing a white sailor's cap that was easily recognized in most of the photos. When the Dean of Students called me into his office with the photographs spread out in front of him and asked me if I participated in the panty-raid, what could I say?

During the summer after my sophomore year, my luck ran out. I received a letter from the Dean of Students informing me that my scholarship had been revoked and that I was no longer eligible to participate in any extracurricular activities, including football.

After that second year at the University of New Mexico, I went to Farmington, New Mexico, to work in the oil and gas fields. Individuals working on oil rigs used for drilling the wells were called "roughnecks." These hardy devils were, indeed, "rough necks." Most would have a fistfight over any quarrel. They were tougher than hell. Most followed the work from one field or state to another, moving into towns and converting the villages into boomtowns. They worked, fought, loved and left, usually owing the landlords money. They had their own code of ethics.

6

An oil rig functioned 24 hours a day 7 days a week. Five men composed a crew and 3 crews worked 8 hours daily keeping the drilling rig running continuously. A toolpusher oversaw the operations of several rigs drilling in reasonably close proximity to each other.

I went to the oil fields with John Cox, a huge muscular man and outstanding tackle who played for the New Mexico University Lobos in the Skyline Football Conference. During the hiring process John told the "boss" I could work anything from the "derrick on down." I hardly knew what the derrick was, let alone how to handle the lead tongs, back-up tongs, be the motorman or work the derrick. I immediately recognized that the driller was the "boss." During a boom period, the rigs needed men to operate and the driller hired me. Fifteen minutes after I arrived at the rig site, he recognized that I knew nothing about an oil drilling rig. With practically no patience, he started barking orders. I listened, learned quickly, and survived.

The five men on a drilling team consisted of the driller, the boss of the crew; adding drilling pipe to extend the depth of the drilling bit requires two men working the lead and backup tongs for firmly grasping the pipe at the joints needed to loosen and tighten the joint; a motorman to place the slip around the drill pipe below the collar to prevent it from falling into the hole; and a derrick man to work the top of the rig to remove or add a length of drilling pipe from pipe stem. The driller commands the actions and runs the power train of the machinery. Periodically the entire stem of massive drill pipe has to be removed from the "hole" and the drilling bit on the bottom of the first drill pipe replaced with a new, sharp, drilling bit. In the 1950's the hole was often more than 5,000 feet deep. They are much deeper today. Great care must be exercised to not drop an object down the hole which would interfere with drilling to the depth needed to obtain oil. When the drilling pipe is removed from the hole to replace the drilling bit, a metal plate is quickly slapped over the hole to cover it. Unfortunately, on one occasion before the cover was in place, one of the crew members nicknamed Rathole accidentally kicked a metal hammer which shot across the deck floor and fell into the hole. Any relatively large hard metal object lying in the center and on the bottom of the hole has to be removed before drilling can continue. The removal process is called "going fishing." It may take crews several days using special equipment to remove a large, metal hammer. Nonetheless, we succeeded. Rathole threw his arms around the tool pusher and thanked everyone for their grueling effort to remove the hammer. At that point the tool pusher said, "Rathole, you are fired." Rathole calmly picked up the hammer, dropped it back down the hole and walked off the rig.

There are many stories centered in the oil fields. The combined stress of the job and the penchant for brawling resulted in fights. One day when I arrived at the drilling rig to begin my shift, a muscular character was wearing my gloves. I had previously asked him not to borrow my gloves, as they were essential equipment for protecting the hands of a roughneck and quickly wore out. This big burly man would frequently demonstrate his might by holding the handle of a large sledgehammer in his hand with an upper extremity extended in front of him. He would slowly lower the head of the heavy hammer to his lips and kiss it to show his extraordinary strength. I told him again to stop using and wearing out my gloves. He looked at me, flexed his muscles and said, "What are you going to do about it?" Without bothering to answer, I lay into him. My fists became "punishing weapons." I pounded and pulverized that cocky son-of-a-bitch into total submission. He lay limp on the ground unable to utter a word. The driller and tool pusher were shocked by my flurry. I had a baby face and they called me the college kid. After that sudden display of violence the tool pusher called me aside and said he would buy me a new coat to wear to college if I would beat the hell out of the rancher who complained constantly about the oil rig on his property and the crews driving over his land. Thereafter he and the crew called me "Mean Ass." Needless to say, I never had to go looking for my gloves again.

Sleeping quarters were limited in the Farmington-Bloomfield-Aztec area. My trusted friend and oil field mentor, John Cox, and I rented half of a room in a boarding house in Aztec, New Mexico. John and I sometimes worked different shifts. One night I awoke to meet the man who rented the other half of the room with another bed. As I raised out of bed he crossed the room, stuck out his hand and said, "My name is Brown." He had recently been released from prison after serving 20 years. He was incarcerated because he had killed a man who had sexual relations with his wife. He told me that while in prison he studied the Bible. He said it was written in the Bible that "Thou shalt not take what thou cannot give." He quickly stated that he "had taken the life of a man but he could give life in the belly of any whore." I found his rationalization interesting but grotesque, and I went back to sleep.

Once we drilled for oil/gas on the Bistai Indian Reservation. Alcoholic drinks were not sold on the reservation. Just before entering the reservation there was the ElVacito bar and dance hall. In this establishment tables and chairs were placed around the dance floor. A chicken wire fence separated the seating area from the dancing area. You had to stoop down to get under the wire to enter the dance floor. This barrier was in place to prevent patrons from throwing beer bottles at the dancing couples when jealousy and anger erupted.

One evening, when driving from the oil field to town, we stopped at the ElVacito for a beer. The jukebox was blaring honky-tonk tunes. A woman, probably 30 years of age and who appeared old to me at the time, was a known stripper from Texas. She was one of the women that followed roughnecks from town to town. She walked to the center of the dance floor and began dancing and undressing. One of the crew members joined her as she frolicked across the floor teasing off her clothes until she became nude. He mimicked her piece for piece of clothes before he fell to his hands and knees and began crawling across the floor. He had drunk too much beer to be civil. She jumped on his bare back, skin to skin, and pretended she was riding a horse,

9

which he was. Suddenly someone screamed, "The cops are on their way here." John and I ran out through the kitchen and drove away.

Working in the oil fields paid good money. After working 40 hours a week, a worker got time and a half payment. I learned how to work everything from the "derricks on down." A derrick hand works about 85 feet up in the derrick and receives incentive pay for taking a risk. There comes a time when the drill bit has to be changed about once every 24 hours. Our crew would remove the mile of drill pipe and the next crew had to change the drill bit, replace the pipe down the hole, and restart the drilling. It took two crews about 4 hours each to do their share of the work. There was a shortage of derrick hands, and if I stayed on to replace the drill pipe after removing it, I got paid for a full shift of work. Thus, I worked 56 hours a week on one shift and, depending on the bit changing circumstances, several additional shifts most weeks. I made a lot of money needed to return to college. However, this brought up a serious conflict. I was making as much money as a college professor. I wondered if I should return to school. Still and in spite of a rare flash of physical altercations, I wanted to do something I thought was good for people, like the accomplishments of a medical doctor. I decided to follow my boyhood dreams of becoming a physician.

As the summer ended and it was time to return to school, John and I decided to play a "good-bye" trick on one of our bosses. When he drove up to the rig near Ignacio, Colorado, we gently picked him up and carried him to the edge of a cliff along a river. We threw him over the edge. He landed in the cold water in the river below, screaming, "You bastards will never work for Great Western Drilling Company again." So what! John was returning to the University of New Mexico and I had been admitted to Central State College in Oklahoma to complete my college education.

By the time I transferred to Central State College in Oklahoma, I had met the love of my life. Her name was Paula Merrell. This was before my scholarship at the

University of New Mexico was revoked and I was still trying out for the football team. Paula happened to live next door to a friend of mine. He and I were passing a football back and forth one afternoon when Paula showed up. Joyfully, I threw her the ball and she easily caught the pass. At the time, I had a girlfriend and Paula was engaged to a paratrooper stationed in Korea. But we both liked to dance, and over the summer we went out on a few dates. By the time my job on the oil rig was over, I knew I had met someone very special. But there was little I could do. Not only was Paula engaged to someone else, her family were devout Mormons, and they did not approve of dating a non-Mormon.

Paula's ancestors migrated across America to Utah. One of the great-grandparents' families pulled a handcart from Iowa City to Salt Lake City, suffering severe hardships. After polygamy was outlawed in the United States, some ancestors were among those who moved to Mexico with their families and established the community of Colonia Diaz. Grandfather Fenly Merrell was an acquaintance of Pancho Villa. When the Mexican Revolutionary War broke out, Pancho Villa needed a new wagon for transporting ammunition. Villa took Fenly's new wagon and gave Fenly an old one (saying it was good enough for farm work) plus one-hundred pesos. Pancho's brother, Ipolito, along with six other Mexicans, shortly thereafter came and demanded the money, which Fenly had hidden. In Fenly's words: "I told them I didn't have any money for them so they jabbed me with their guns and knives. I still did not give up or get scared. They then got a line from the harness and hung me up to a tree north of the barn. The first time they let me down I was just strangled. They gave me a chance to give up the money but I didn't, so they lifted me up again. That time when I came down I was weak and couldn't stand alone but still would not give up. Up I went again, and that time when I came down I was out. When I came to I was lying on the ground with my head on a man's knee, and he was saying 'wake up' and slapping me on the face. That time I told them they could have the money." Many years later while

11

visiting Paula I observed the smooth scar around Fenly's neck from that trauma he received when he was a younger man.

As the war activity increased, some of the Mormon families in Mexico quickly packed up some of their belongings and crossed the Rio Grande River at El Paso, Texas, where Paula's father was born. A few years later, a group of families that had returned to the USA developed a small but thriving community along the Gila River at Virden, New Mexico. In 1915, Paula's mother was the first child born in the newly established village. She was one of 13 children in the highly verbal and musically talented Mortensen family.

Paula was born in Miami, Arizona, where her father worked for a brief period of time for a copper mining company before moving back to Virden, New Mexico. Paula's early years of schooling were in Virden, where each classroom consisted of two grades, both of which were taught by the same teacher. During first grade, there were a few Mexican children who could speak very little English, along with those who were in first grade for the second year, having learned English the previous year in school.

When Paula was in high school, her family settled in Farmington, New Mexico. She was a popular girl who participated in choir, served as cheerleader, and was selected homecoming queen during those relatively innocent and idealistic 1950's.

We had only three or four dates during that summer, but I realized she was something special. She had an engaging smile and progressively became unafraid to let her feelings show. She believed the game of life was good and had the courage to go forward with her convictions.

At summer's end, I transferred from the University of New Mexico to Central State College in Oklahoma, and Paula entered Brigham Young University in Utah. We corresponded by letters. When her fiancée returned from Korea later in the fall, Paula broke their engagement, and I made plans to visit her in Farmington over the Christmas holidays. My love for her grew. I believed we could be partners and lovers. With her at my side, I could continue to be a near straight-A pre-med student, plan for medical school, and work 42 hours a week in St. Anthony's Hospital as a laboratory technician.

I returned to Oklahoma after the Christmas holidays a very happy man. Paula and I corresponded through letters and over the telephone. We decided to get married. I was looking forward to our planned wedding in March. But within weeks before the scheduled wedding, I began to lose weight. I developed an excessive thirst and had to get up several times a night to urinate. I had learned about diabetes in one of my courses and thought I recognized the signs. So I asked one of the other lab technicians at work to draw a sample of my blood. I analyzed it for glucose and, sure enough, the results were well within the range for diabetes mellitus. Damn! I began taking daily insulin injections and following a strict diabetic diet. I contacted Paula with the news and advised her not to marry me. But in her usual, positive fashion, she assured me that, together, we would make it. On March 31, 1956 we were married and Paula transferred from BYU to Central State College.

Some people are complemented by a partner and/or spouse who helps them accomplish their goals, missions or callings. I had such a person who facilitated my every effort. Our love promoted a revolutionary process leading to success. Together, we got through our time at Central State College. Paula stood up to the challenges encountered. She not only supported my endeavors, but she was also an unabashed critic. Loving Paula was the easiest thing I ever did.

As a laboratory technician at St. Anthony's Hospital in Oklahoma City, I drew patients' blood for preoperative laboratory studies. I also learned how to count red and white blood cells, differentiate between types of white blood cells and evaluate blood-clotting platelets off a slide specimen. In addition, I analyzed specimens of urine and a few blood chemistries. My teachers at the lab were Catholic nuns whose diagnostic accuracy and dedication could not be surpassed. The nuns would frequently get up in the middle

13

of the night to perform emergency lab work. When necessary they would repeat measurements countless times until they were sure the results were sound. It was the nuns at St. Anthony's who taught me the importance of compassion and accepting responsibility for a patient's welfare. I credit them, and Sister Mary Joseph in particular, for strengthening my commitment to serving others.

While Paula and I were still in college, a beautiful daughter, Michele, was born at St. Anthony's Hospital. Sister Mary Joseph was again influential; she helped us select her name. Michele's exposure to college life began at two weeks of age when I took her with me to a physics lecture while Paula was taking a final exam. The baby was cooperative, sleeping soundly through the ordeal.

I applied for admission to the University of Oklahoma Medical School. I soon learned, however, that I was not eligible as an in-state resident. Although I had worked full time, the Dean informed me that my two years in Oklahoma as an employee and undergraduate student did not count toward my state residency requirements. Technically, I was still a resident of New Mexico. Oklahoma Medical School was not accepting out-of-state residents that year. Unfortunately, New Mexico did not then have a medical school. The state did, however, participate in the Western Interstate Commission for Higher Education. This organization paid the difference between in-state and out-of-state tuition for five students admitted each year to the University of Colorado School of Medicine.

To be considered for the Commission's program, prospective students needed to attend an interview in Denver, Colorado. I hitchhiked during the winter to Denver for an interview. Paula bought me a new pair of warm leather gloves for Christmas to protect my hands during the travels. After attending the interview, I rode a public transportation bus to the city limits of Denver where a man in a car heading east to Limon picked me up. By the time we got there it was snowing. I can still hear the wind howling as I waited by the side of the road in Limon for another lift. I stood there in the blistering cold for more than an hour before I turned my coat up around my ears and just started walking. By the time a trucker stopped and pulled me in, I was half frozen. The trucker was a considerate man and took me all the way back to Edmond, Oklahoma, where Central State College was located.

The insulin I had injected that morning continued lowering my blood glucose. Although I always carried candy to eat in case my blood glucose fell too low, somehow it was dangerously low and my memory at this point failed me. I managed to walk into our home where Paula met me and gave me orange juice, and a new life began.

Several weeks later, I received a letter of acceptance, welcoming me to the University of Colorado Medical School. Finally, support, opportunity, luck and hard work had come together. Paula, Michele and I were on our way to medical school.

Medical School and Residency Training

I was accepted to the University of Colorado School of Medicine! What a lucky break! When support, opportunity and willingness came together, I began a journey that led to a career as a doctor, teacher, clinical investigator and, later, an administrator. I remember telling Paula that if I could pass medical school courses with a C grade I would be pleased. Somehow, I made straight A's for my first year and was among only three junior students elected to the Alpha Omega Alpha National Honorary Society. In the end, a terrible speller of English words (but good in spelling Latin and Greek words) from a dusty town in New Mexico graduated *Summa Cum Laude*.

Our son, Rodney, was born during the second year of medical school. From the start he was a large, strong boy. His sister, Michele, was very motherly and protective of him. We were a tightly knitted family.

During my sophomore year, a professor of biochemistry told me that I should go to Johns Hopkins for further training. This was the first time I had ever heard of Johns Hopkins University Hospital and School of Medicine.

As the years passed, I learned a lot about this majestic university hospital and its noble physicians/scientists.

Once again, good fortune intervened in the form of a wonderful mentor. Dr. Robert J. Glaser, Dean of the University of Colorado Medical School, helped me get a coveted residency position on the Osler housestaff at Johns Hopkins Hospital. Starting my residency training at Hopkins meant moving to Baltimore, Maryland. So in the early summer of '62, Paula and I packed up our belongings and, with Michele and Rodney, headed East. Needless to say, Baltimore, Md. wasn't exactly like Roswell, New Mex., Oklahoma City, Okla., or Denver, Colo. The illustrious Johns Hopkins Hospital in 1962 was surrounded by a degenerative ghetto neighborhood. A telephone extension ran from the hospital into the home of each resident. When it rang, we were expected to answer the call and come in, regardless of what time it was or what we were doing. We all lived close to the hospital and worked six and one-half days and six nights per week. Residents on the Osler service were relieved from duty on Saturday afternoon and night or Sunday afternoon and night, providing no patient was too sick to leave his/her care in the hands of another resident. The patient population was usually critically ill. I had the combined off-service time of Saturday afternoon, Saturday night, Sunday and Sunday night only one month in three years. Admittedly, all residents had annual vacations.

Working seven days a week with an occasional double shift in the oil fields was nothing compared to my medical residency. On a rig, I busted my ass each shift, but when work was done, it was done. On shift – off shift was delineated by sleep and recreational time. During my residency, the days, weeks and months bled into each other with no discernible end in sight. I got sleep when I could, not necessarily when I needed it most. If working on an oil rig was a 50-meter dash, I liken my residency at Johns Hopkins to a cross-country marathon. There were nights when I would drag myself home at three o'clock in the morning wondering, "is this all worth it?" Methodically I would reflect upon my chosen career. No one had forced me to do this. I chose this career pathway. Nonetheless, sometimes in my despair, I forgot why I went to medical school and drug Paula and the children through this downtrodden realism.

Living in the rough ghettoes next to the Johns Hopkins Hospital in the 1960's was trying. One Saturday or Sunday evening I heard my 4 year old son, Rodney, crying from pain. I ran out in the alley as he was coming home from the next door neighbor's house where he had been playing with his friend, Joey. Apparently Joey's mother became angry and struck Rodney in the face with a toy car. I stood still as I watched a fracas unfold. Joey's father came tearing out of the house, reeking with the smell of alcohol and screaming at me. A remembrance flashed through my mind. When I was about 5-6 years old my parents sent me to the next door grocery store to get a quart of milk. A man known to my father as John had been drinking alcohol. Unprovoked, he grabbed me and began choking me. I broke free and ran home. Dad asked me what happened; I told him John choked me. Dad got up from his chair. Without a word he walked to the store and pulverized John. When Joey's father ran toward me, I set my feet like a boxer, clinched my fist, and slugged him on the chin. He went sprawling across the alley. I jumped on top of him with both feet and knees and kicked and kneed the hell out of him. Then I picked him up and threw him in a large trashcan. A few of my colleagues saw this unusual display of physical activity and referred to me as the "Hammer" after that one-minute encounter. Unfortunately, I was a man who grew up in a physical environment where fist-fighting was not unusual. In fact, during an uncivilized period during the late 1800's two quarrelling ranchers gathered their cowhands, rode their horses to town, met, and had a fistfight. The winner became mayor of Albuquerque, New Mexico.

The influence of the southwestern gun and fist fighting behavior unfortunately had left an undesirable imprint on me. However, the civility and equanimity of the Johns Hopkins University community began to enlighten me. A willingness to back up, give ground, and employ thought rather than bodily actions began to emerge. My evolution can be likened to another southwesterner, President Bush.

At Johns Hopkins it was my patients' gratitude and kindness that kept me going. One night a middle-aged, muscular black man came to the emergency room complaining of severe chest pain. He was suffering from a heart attack, and he was in a critical state. Coronary units had not been developed at Johns Hopkins Hospital in 1962. The patient was admitted for me to give him care. He stopped breathing. We placed a tube down his windpipe, and I used a self-inflating rubber bag to pump air into his lungs. I squeezed that bag until my hands were red and tender because of the friction created from compressing the bag. He had maintained a heartbeat and eventually he began to breathe on his own. I was totally exhausted. At about 3-4 a.m. he appeared to have reasonably stable heart and breathing rates. I left his bedside to sleep. When I returned early the next morning, he looked at me and said, "Thank you, white man, for saving my life." I knew immediately what medicine was all about.

It was late in the night, and I was dead tired when a lady in her 40's was admitted to the Osler medical service. It was my turn to provide care for this patient. She was suffering from acute abdominal pain, maybe a gallstone. After I obtained a medical history I began doing a physical examination. After evaluating the head, eyes, ear, nose, neck, chest and heart, I began examining the abdomen. Her head was slightly elevated on pillows. After carefully feeling for her liver and gall bladder through her abdominal wall, I pulled a chair alongside the bed and sat down as I continued the examination. I placed my stethoscope in my ears and on her abdomen to begin listening for bowel sounds. Unbeknown to me, I rested my head on her abdomen. Suddenly, I raised my head a little and looked across the room. There stood the chief medical resident who oversaw the performances of his more junior housestaff. I never said a word; just kept moving the stethoscope around her belly listening for bowel sounds. When the chief resident walked out of the room I asked the patient why she let me fall asleep

18

on her abdomen. She replied, "Because you were tired." It has been these humanistic moments and heartfelt appreciations that have endeared me to medicine. Many more remembrances filled my brain through the years, but it was these early experiences that made me realize that I had made the right decision to be a doctor. It was the incalculable gratification that comes from helping other people that kept me on course during those trying years at Hopkins. Of course I wanted to finish my training and share a good life with my wife and children. I wanted to be able to pay the bills and afford some of the finer things. I also wanted my family to be proud that I was a doctor, worthy to serve the suffering.

During my residency training years, Paula worked as a medical secretary for Dr. Maumenee, Director of the Wilmer Eye Institute of Johns Hopkins. Michele and Rodney spent their days in the on-site nursery school until Michele entered first grade when she was bused daily to an outlying school for her education. At the end of each school day, the bus would let her off at the hospital entrance, and she would weave her way through corridors to check in with Paula at work before going on downstairs to the nursery school. But not before she stopped in to say hello to some of the physicians and researchers whose offices were located on the floor. Michele didn't care how busy or famous these men were. She'd dance right up to them and they loved it. When I learned about Michele's routine, I apologized to the pre-eminent neuro-ophthalmologist, Dr. Walsh, who told me that her daily visits were among the highlights of his day.

During my residency training I was assigned a rotation on a National Institutes of Health sponsored General Clinical Research Center (GCRC). The Center was a defined space in the hospital with its own nursing and technical staff, bedrooms and bathrooms for a specified number of patients, dieticians and kitchen, and laboratory technicians and laboratories. It was intended to be a place where clinicians and basic scientists from different disciplines could work together in a carefully controlled environment. Coordinated and concerted research effort could be directed toward solving some of the more common diseases that plague humans. Research protocols had to be approved by a committee that protects the rights and welfare of patients. Another committee ranked the proposed studies for scientific merit.

Clinical research was a new venue for me. I found the interdepartmental sciences of diverse research interests and physicians of various medical disciplines working in close collaboration doing studies fascinating. Man, this was a great environment for adventure into the unknown. Patients were grateful for the resources put forth on their behalf, and physician-scientists were excited about gathering useful information to advance patient care.

It was not unusual for patients to present to the Johns Hopkins Hospital emergency room with bizarre or freakish disorders. One such patient was an 800-pound man who was brought to the ER by the police. This patient had gotten into a pay telephone booth and could not get out. He remained trapped standing upright for a day or two. He was filthy with excrement on the lower half of his body. His smell was grossly offensive. His legs were swollen, red and leaking fluid through skin blisters. Great effort was needed to cleanse him. He was hospitalized and treated for his acute ailments and for heart failure. Large quantities of urine were lost from the body. His health state stabilized. He was housed on the General Clinical Research Center and an investigative study was initiated to learn how a morbidly obese patient tolerated prolonged caloric deprivation. He was intermittently starved and semi-starved over a period of about 14 months. He tolerated periods of food deprivation and lost about 400 pounds of weight. His pants would then wrap around him with grossly excessive material. Although this was not the first time a patient was subjected to prolonged starvation, it attracted national attention because of the length of the study. Nonetheless, it was known that morbidly obese patients could fast or semi-starve for long periods of time and undergo major loss of weight if they were provided water to drink. Being one of the residents that oversaw the welfare of this patient did not generate the enthusiasm in me that it should have. However, it generated a little curiosity. As he lost a huge amount of weight, daily urine collections were done during his starvation or near-starvation periods. He was intelligent and listened to the comments made by his physicians. Unfortunately, he would occasionally claim that he needed "sugar" for his brain to function and would drink beverages containing carbohydrates. None of the senior investigators or residents knew that the brain derived energy from sources other than glucose (sugar) during starvation. Further, no one knew how sensitive the urinary excretion rates (of nitrogen and ketone bodies) were to the ingestion of small amounts of carbohydrates (glucose). Previous studies on brain metabolism after an overnight fast when glucose is readily available showed that the only energy-yielding substrate consistently extracted from the blood by the human brain was glucose. Further, newly synthesized glucose for terminal oxidation (consumption) during starvation was known to be derived from protein breakdown (amino acids), primarily from muscle. If protein is broken down to synthesize glucose for the brain, the byproducts of protein breakdown generate nitrogen compounds that are excreted in the urine. It was reasonably well established that the by-product of one gram of urinary nitrogen was equal to 3-4 grams of glucose synthesis. The urinary excretion of nitrogen, which reflected protein breakdown (proteolysis) was much too low to generate 100-125 grams of glucose thought to be necessary for running the brain. However, this fact escaped recognition by the clinical investigators studying this morbidly obese patient-volunteer.

In the spring of 1965, near the end of my three-year residency program at Hopkins, our third child, Lydia, was born. Paula had worked up through the day of delivery, and was told that if she would like, she could set up a bassinette in the office and continue working with the new baby by her side. She declined, but Dr. Maumenee sent one of his employees each day with dictations which Paula transcribed at home.

Fellowship Training

After completing my specialty training in internal medicine at Hopkins, I wanted to return to the University of Colorado Hospital and Medical School for fellowship training in metabolism and endocrinology. However, the chief of endocrinology and metabolism, Dr. Dalton Jenkins, thought I should go to Boston to train under the direction of Dr. George F. Cahill, Jr. at Harvard. Dr. Cahill, a creative, colorful and insightful physician-scientist acknowledged that whole body metabolism during starvation needed to be re-investigated. (He may have recognized the paradox of the brain's dependency for glucose and the low urinary nitrogen excretion.) I followed the advice of Dr. Jenkins, and in 1965 was accepted for a Harvard fellowship training position under the guidance of Dr. Cahill.

Paula and I packed our belongings, rented a U-Haul truck and drove to a new environment, the metropolitan Boston area. Dr. Cahill and his family were leaving for Nantucket for a vacation. The Cahill family let us stay at their magnificent home in Needham, located on the upper Charles River. We would get out of bed in the morning, throw open the French doors to the second floor balcony, and feel as though "we had died and gone to heaven." We lived in the Cahill home for about a month while searching the Boston suburbs for a place to rent. We found a lovely small house in Wellesley and began a new and better kind of life. Paula stopped working as a medical secretary and became a stay-at-home mom. Our three children found wonderful playmates, and the neighbors and schools were outstanding. Somebody was watching over us.

I started my fellowship training at the Harvard affiliated Joslin Research Laboratory. The Peter Bent Brigham was one of the affiliated Harvard teaching hospitals, and it had a General Clinical Research Center. Next door to the Harvard University School of Medicine and the Peter Bent Brigham Hospital was the majestic Countway Medical Library.

I asked Dr. Cahill what he wanted me to do. He said, "Do what you want to do." I spent a month or so in the Countway Library reading articles on body metabolism, biochemistry and physiology. I developed a "rested body and mind" and began to rethink overall body metabolism. Preciously little information was available regarding survival mechanisms during prolonged starvation.

After I arrived at the Joslin Research Laboratories as Cahill's fellow in 1965, a series of systematic studies were initiated to understand metabolism during starvation. Following the first year of my fellowship another individual, Dr. Philip Felig, joined the group. He was the former chief medical resident at Yale University Hospital. We all became friends and developed a phenomenal team that solved some of the mysteries of survival during starvation. I left Boston after a 3-year fellowship program and continued my clinical investigations on the General Clinical Research Center at Temple University Hospital in Philadelphia. My research at Temple lasted for an additional 2-3 decades. For more than a decade after leaving Temple I intermittently returned to analyzing and reporting data that accumulated there during my tenure between 1968 and 1988.

I was recruited to be Professor and Chair of Medicine at Southern Illinois University School of Medicine in 1988. Our children were grown, so my wife and I picked up and moved to Springfield, Illinois. This small school was much different than those located in the northeastern corridor of the USA. After serving the school for about 8 years, I left academic medicine to become a private practitioner of endocrinology and metabolism. I again was blessed. One of my former medical students at Temple had become the leader of a group of private cardiologists. The group took me into their practice and allowed me the privilege to be a quasi partner until I retired at 66 years of age. During this stint, I learned about the gap between academic medicine and private practice. Since retiring from practice, I have published articles in peer-reviewed journals, written several chapters for textbooks, and reviewed articles submitted by other authors for publication. But my most fervent activity has been devoted to writing this book which offers insight into health and disease states, specifically obesity. Maybe I have contributed something worthwhile to help my fellow human beings gain knowledge about organs of the body and overall metabolism in health and disease states.

This chapter has portrayed educational and training opportunities available to an average USA citizen. I took advantage of those options.

Chapter II. A Glimpse at Clinical Research and Practice

It is human nature to want to be together, to share hope and happiness, to sympathize with those in distress, to extend a hand to those who need help. It is human nature, on balance, to want to improve the welfare of family, friends and society.

Historical Background

"The National Institutes of Health started modestly in a small attic room in the Marine Hospital in the village of Stapleton on Staten Island, New York, in August, 1887. There, 27-year old Dr. Joseph Kinyoun set up his one-person Laboratory of Hygiene as the federal government's first research institution for identifying and searching for cures for the infectious diseases that were ravaging its citizens. In 1891, after 4 years of intensive investigation into the origin and causes of such epidemic diseases as cholera, diphtheria, typhoid, smallpox, typhus, plague and tuberculosis, the Laboratory of Hygiene needed more space, was moved to Washington, D.C. and was renamed the Hygienic Laboratory. In Washington, members of the Hygienic Laboratory continued to tackle public health problems. In order to investigate Rocky Mountain spotted fever, researchers were sent to the Bitterroot Valley in Montana, the region where the disease was first observed. Working conditions were quite primitive, with researchers occupying tents and mountain cabins. During 45 years of research, the disease was defined, its cause discovered, its carriers identified, and its distribution understood. In the course of the work five scientists contracted the disease and succumbed to it.

During this period, Dr. Joseph Goldberger of the Hygienic Laboratory also initiated the first long-term epidemiological investigation of a chronic, noncommunicable disease – pellagra – epidemic in the southern United States in the early 1900's. This foray into nutritional research marked an expansion of the research frontiers to be addressed by the laboratory.

Further change came to the Hygienic Laboratory in 1930 when its continued progress and success convinced Senator Joseph E. Ransdell of Louisiana that fundamental research could lead to cures for disease. Thus, the Ransdell Act was passed by the Congress, reorganizing and expanding the Hygienic Laboratory and changing its name to the National Institute of Health. Eight years later, in 1938, a continually growing National Institute of Health began its move from Washington, D.C. to suburban Bethesda, Maryland.

World War II marked a change in the basic research conducted by the National Institute of Health. The scope of investigation was broadened to include fundamental medical research on major chronic diseases such as cancer, cardiovascular disease, arthritis and mental illness. In 1948 four institutes were created to support work on cardiac disease, dental disorders, infectious diseases, and experimental biology and medicine. In that same year construction was begun on the Clinical Center, a hospital with over 500 beds, where promising therapies would be developed. This was also the year when the National Institute of Health (singular) officially became the National Institutes of Health (plural)." (Taken verbatim from the History of the NIH, U.S. Department of Health and Human Services.)

On June 22, 1944, President Roosevelt signed into law the GI Bill of Rights that entitled veterans to financial support for education and training. With the investment of billions of dollars for millions of veterans, the nation has in return earned many times its investment in increased taxes and a dramatically changed society. These newly educated individuals became industry leaders in manufacturing, music, literature, broadcasting, entertainment and medicine. Their contributions were critical to America's economic and spiritual development after World War II.

Equally responsible for the surge in biomedical sciences by the USA were the increased sponsorship and financial support of the National Institutes of Health (NIH) Centers and Offices. These magnanimous institutes were eventually comprised of 19 Institutes, 7 Centers, and the National Library of Medicine, located in Bethesda, Maryland.

The center at NIH that gave me the opportunity to remain involved in medical research after leaving Harvard was developed in 1959 and became a subdivision of the National Centers for Research Resources in 1962. This center oversaw the operations of the General Clinical Research Centers (GCRCs). This component of the National Institutes of Health Centers and Offices burgeoned into a network of 80 GCRCs located across the USA. The majority of GCRCs were affiliated with large academic medical centers and teaching hospitals. The GCRCs are currently evolving into Institutional Clinical and Translational Science Awards (Centers).

The GCRC at Temple University Hospital

Temple University was founded in 1891 by Dr. Russell Conwell, and its medical school was started in 1901. Temple University's Health Sciences Center was established in 1960 with the expressed purpose for providing an organizational framework under which the goals and objectives of the separate institutions (namely, Schools of Medicine, Dentistry, and Pharmacy; the College of Allied Health Professions; and Temple University Hospital) could be coordinated.

The late Dr. Sol Sherry, a pioneer in thrombolytic therapy (dissolving blood clots) for acute myocardial infarctions (heart attacks) and for dissolving blood clots in peripheral (leg) veins, was a professor of medicine at Washington University School of Medicine in 1959. He was one of the founding committee members of the special subsection of NIH that became the NIH's General Clinical Research Centers. Before the GCRCs were conceptualized and put into development, clinical research activities were scattered throughout the general hospitals. A dedicated and sophisticated nursing, dietary and technical staff was not available to conduct the highest caliber of clinical investigations.

Between 1961 and 1963 Dr. Sherry served as chairman of the GCRC committee at the NIH. He and his committee members formulated the objectives of the country's GCRCs. As a group they emphasized augmenting clinical research that resulted in improved patient care. A distinctive area in a hospital was to be designated the site for a GCRC. The awarding of federal funds for the proposed centers was based on competitive grants. Centers were to be located in metropolitan areas throughout the nation. The first grant to Temple for a GCRC was awarded in 1965. The Temple start-up unit was a small, fledgling, rudimentary hospital unit without sufficient organizational structure. Expansion was essential. Grant support would not have been renewed in 1968 if the newly recruited Professor and Chair of Medicine, Dr. Sherry, had not encouraged the NIH site visit team to provide support until he could revitalize the clinical faculty at Temple.

It was Sherry who recruited me to Temple University in 1968 and appointed me Director of the General Clinical Research Center. The money Temple received from NIH went towards hiring highly trained nurses, dieticians, research technicians and a medical director. Before 1968, Temple University Hospital had not been a site of intense research activity. Communication and collaboration between the basic scientists and practicing physicians and surgeons were poor. My goal as director was to make the GCRC an accessible resource for the entire university and to promote interdisciplinary research of the highest quality.

The antiquated physical structure of the GCRC was improved when a new cardiac catheterization laboratory was updated and located adjacent to components of the GCRC. In addition, a branch pharmacy was established between the research kitchen and the research laboratories. These developments augmented the research activities among the cardiologists and pharmacologists with the GCRC staff.

From the beginning of my career at Temple, Dr. G. A. Reichard, Jr. (past President of Lankenau Medical Research Center), then a research scientist working for Smith-Kline and French, helped to energize research conducted on the GCRC. He became an adjunct professor of medicine at Temple who developed methods for measuring the production and utilization rates of radioactive fuels circulating in the body, radioactive carbon dioxide exhaled in the breath, and radioactive glucose and ketone bodies excreted in the urine. Top notch research activities began to take off at Temple's GCRC. Throughout most of my tenure as the GCRC's director (and subsequent co-principal investigator), I was joined by Dr. Guenther Boden who became an internationally renowned clinical investigator focusing on the interplay between hormones and metabolism. He subsequently became one of the key figures in metabolism regarding fatty acid metabolism and diabetes mellitus. [This German born academician worked diligently to improve my English writings. An outsider once commented on the Owen-Boden collaboration that "one can't speak it (English) and the other can't write it, but as a pair they do all right."]

With the progression of time a secretary's job was upgraded to an administrative manager who became an integral part of overseeing the complexities of the GCRC. Ms. Rachelle Browndorf (later Ms. Little) assumed this responsibility on the Temple GCRC. Her exorbitant work ethic and strong personality led to her involvement on the national scene for GCRC administration. She continued her educational activities and was subsequently awarded MBA and JD degrees. Ms. Little went on to hold prestigious administrative jobs at three other major medical institutions. The nurses working in the GCRCs were the cream of the hospital's nursing crop. They were familiar with every active research protocol and provided exemplary nursing care. The late Ms. Isabel Carson became the head nurse on

Temple's GCRC, and her superb oversight of nursing activities was one of the primary reasons that the GCRC delivered such outstanding health care and executed research protocols. The GCRCs had their own highly qualified laboratory technicians. Temple's GCRC team had an unusually gifted laboratory technician, Ms. Maria Mozzoli, whose analytical skills were complemented by her extraordinary ability to maintain impeccable laboratory records. Several highly committed research dieticians served at Temple's GCRC. They were among the first center personnel to become engaged in outpatient activities, primarily focused around patients ailing from obesity and diabetes. By the late 1970's the GCRCs across the nation underwent a philosophical shift from inpatient to include more outpatient research activities. This change from inpatient to outpatient activities was a cost-containing effort. The research laboratories associated with the GCRCs became more diversified for measurements for both inpatients and outpatients. In Temple's GCRC, most of the readily identifiable fuels and hormones that circulate in the bloodstream were measured. Radioactive compounds in the blood associated with research studies were measured. In addition, urinary excretory products were quantitated, and the energy requirements and body composition of human beings in various clinical circumstances were determined.

After I took over the directorship of the GCRC, I got a board member of Temple University Hospital, Mr. Daniel Polett, to become involved in the activities ongoing on the research center and to participate in NIH site visits for funding the GCRC.

By the beginning of the 1970's, the Departments of Medicine, Dermatology, Surgery, and OB/GYN at Temple had interphased with the Department of Biochemistry, the Fels Research Institute, the Department of Physiology and the Thrombosis Center. Dr. Lawrence Lundy of the Department of OB/GYN, had developed an intense and special interest in a group of women who were unable to become pregnant. He and his colleague deciphered the cause of their infertility. They suffered from the aftermath of

30

taking "birth control pills" early in their life. The pill induced the suppression of ovulation that lasted for an extended period of time after they stopped taking the birth control medications. Collaboration developed between investigators using the GCRC and other components of the university, namely body compositional determinations made by Dr. Zebulon V. Kendrick, Department of Physical Education.

By the late 1970's computers were revolutionizing the way researchers collected and analyzed data. Data accumulated faster than they could be properly analyzed. The combination of word processors and statistical components of computerized data offered us the possibility to be more accurate in assessing and publishing the data from our studies. However, it should be noted that computers and word processors improved the accuracy of our data but did not speed up the reporting of our data. We were better at data analysis, but more work and expertise were required to execute our technical advances.

As Program Director I realized that we needed someone to develop and manage the information we were collecting and analyzing on the GCRC. First, Ms. Browndorf contacted many computer experts and visited a few GCRCs around the nation to gather the information needed regarding equipment needs and costs associated with computerizing our GCRC. In the 1980's we recruited a competent and imaginative biostatistician, Dr Marcia Polansky, who became instrumental in designing all research protocols for statistical soundness. She collaborated with investigators on the study design and implemented analysis and helped to interpret the data. Collaboration developed between investigators using the GCRC and other components of the university. As the years progressed, the sophistication of the GCRC grew, with outreach programs involving other medical institutions. Dr. Polansky helped me in recognizing the talents of Mr. Karl Smalley and in recruiting him. He was a college senior at Temple University's home campus who later graduated *Magna Cum Laude*. He clearly had as much native intelligence as anyone

31

ever recruited to the Temple GCRC. He not only helped with the informatics and data analysis connected with research projects, he also made important intellectual contributions. Mr. Smalley reanalyzed much of the classic data regarding bioenergetics. His contributions allowed researchers studying metabolic reactions after eating, starving or exercising to advance their thought processes and publications. In addition to faculty and staff, numerous students, residents and fellows studied and worked on the research projects. Their youth brought pleasure, laughter and imagination to the GCRC.

Several more departments deserve additional recognition because of their high activity on the GCRC during the years I was director. The Department of Dermatology merits special acknowledgment. Dr. Eugene VanScott and his younger faculty members and residents in dermatology were actively investigating several diseases with emphasis on psoriasis and mycosis fungoides. They worked in conjunction with Dr. Robert Gallo of the NIH, searching for a virus in the etiology of mycosis fungoides, a cancer of the skin. Dr. VanScotts's success in treating this malignant tumor helped in his being awarded the Lasker Award 1972. An indefatigable vascular surgeon, Dr. Frederick A. Reichle, worked tirelessly to save the lives of patients with cirrhosis of the liver and suffering from esophageal and gastric hemorrhages. He also salvaged the legs and feet of many diabetic patients suffering from inadequate circulation of blood to the lower extremities. The basic science departments, especially those of Biochemistry and Physiology, were engaged in research activities. Drs. Mulchand Patel and Richard Hanson guided biochemical studies that delineated the human body's ability to use ketone bodies to synthesize myelin fat in brain tissue and lipids in the subcutaneous fat. They also measured the enzymatic activities of fragments (biopsies) obtained from livers, kidneys and adipose tissues, along with many other insightful studies.

One morning a week any clinical investigator who had a patient housed on the GCRC made bedside monitoring and teaching rounds. It was his/her responsibility to bring the group attending rounds with him up to date on the protocol and results of the study.

The GCRC, which began as a discrete inpatient unit at Temple University Hospital, changed to also providing research resources to an outpatient population. In addition, the GCRC staff made a strong conscious effort to educate medical students, residents, fellows and faculty members. They were given an opportunity to be involved in clinical research. Between 1968 and 1989, annual funding increased 10-fold. Funding was contingent upon a competitive renewal process, usually for 3-5 year intervals.

The GCRC at Temple University Hospital became the gold coast center of the hospital, largely due to the expertise and involvement of the nursing, dietary and technical staffs which complemented the physicians/surgeons/basic science investigators. This occurred in spite of the decrepit physical surroundings prior to construction of a new physical plant in 1985.

The head nurse became the glue that held together the interdisciplinary team members. She directed the ward clerks who answered the telephones, filed laboratory reports in the patients' charts, and provided information to facilitate the flow of patients and information throughout the center. The head nurse selected the other nurses who provided most of the patient care, monitored the patients' health status, and collected urine, blood, fecal, sputum and other specimens to be sent to various laboratories. The nurses assisted the physician-surgeons in doing various experiments, e.g., setting up the equipment and sterile setups needed to obtain specimens (blood, biopsy material, etc). The head nurse and her staff were the first to detect signs and symptoms of improvement or deterioration of a patient or volunteer. Talking and touching patients and walking from bed to bed or through the lounge or dining area, the nurses were first to provide valuable new insight on the medical status of each patient-volunteer. The nurses spent much more face to face time with the research subjects than did any other professional engaged in the GCRC activities.

33

A manager of nutritional research progressively became an integral part of Temple's GCRC. The incidence of malnutrition (over- and under-nutrition) in inner urban populations was becoming commonplace, ranging from gross wasting of the body with narcotic addiction, AIDS and alcoholism to morbid obesity, complicated by diabetes mellitus, high blood pressure, excessive fat in the bloodstream, and related strokes and myocardial infarctions.

Informatics (data management) became a core issue for clinical investigators collecting and managing data. NIH supported the development of computer systems which linked the various components of the GCRC with the university-wide network that could be connected to other GCRCs across the nation. The core informatics component of a GCRC enabled investigators to design research studies and interpret data with sophisticated techniques.

Extrinsic to the day-to-day management conducted by the GCRC medical director, a scientific advisory committee evaluated the merit of research proposals and awarded them priority scores. Those with the most meritorious priority award usually had first access to the resources of the GCRC. In addition, there was an Institutional Review Board (IRB) with physician-scientists, lay, clergy and legal members who oversaw the welfare of the patients. In 2001, about 12 years after I left Temple University Hospital as director and co-principal investigator of the GCRC, the National Institutes of Health required that an individual be hired to serve as the research subject advocate. (Apparently the research subject advocate developed primarily as a consequence of the death at a neighboring institution of Jesse Gelsinger, who was subjected to the transfer of genetic material via a viral vehicle that resulted in an overwhelming sepsis and death.) The research subject advocate provides an unbiased opinion regarding the safety of the patient and assurance that all individuals participating in research activities are fully informed about the risk involved in the proposed research maneuvers. The research subject advocate provides information to patients/volunteers involved in clinical trials.

34

The advocate assists the GCRC investigators in reviewing the data and monitoring safety of the protocols. The advocate assures that the studies are performed in accordance with the IRB approved protocols and monitoring plans. The advocate facilitates the reporting of any serious adverse events or conflict of interest. The total impact of having a research subject advocate cannot be determined at this time.

The GCRC at Temple University served a vital and indispensable resource for the School of Medicine and Hospital. It provided investigators of various disciplines the opportunity to increase knowledge of human health and disease states. It was a controlled environment where coordinated and concerted efforts from investigators in various disciplines, both basic and clinical sciences, could devote their efforts in a collaborative manner to advance biomedical knowledge. The GCRC represented a major attraction needed to recruit young full time faculty members into clinical departments. It facilitated the training of residents, fellows, physician/scientists and paramedical personnel. It fostered student/faculty interplay through teaching rounds, periodic research conferences and discussion of research projects. Some students were active members of research teams doing the studies. The GCRC also provided a place for curious residents, fellows and staff members to discuss clinical problems observed in the general hospital and for the development of investigative programs to delineate the cause of these ailments. It was a unit that in its entirety served as a university laboratory without boundaries for obtaining data from patients and normal volunteers on how to deliver a better form of health care to the general hospital inpatient and outpatient populations.

During my three years at Harvard as a clinical investigator we studied somewhere between 20 and 30 obese volunteers in the hospital. During the subsequent three decades at Temple, I estimated that we hospitalized and studied about 500-600 inpatient volunteers. In addition, we collaborated with Dr. Daniel G. Sapir at Johns Hopkins and studied an estimated 32 inpatients. Further, studies with Dr. George A. Reichard at the Lankenau Research Center included an additional 12 inpatients. However, the largest number of patient-volunteers my colleagues and I studied at Temple were outpatients. In this environment we did investigational studies on at least 1,000 patient-volunteers. On the inpatient studies conducted at Harvard and Temple, we concentrated on fuels in the blood; brain, liver, kidney and muscle metabolism during starvation; the effects of hormones on metabolism; and changes in energy requirements and body compositions during starvation. In the outpatient studies at Temple, our focus was primarily on overall energy requirements and body compositions of humans under various conditions.

The results of early studies on brain, liver and kidney metabolism done at Harvard influenced my subsequent research efforts done at Temple over the next two to three decades.

Examples of Significant Research Advances at Temple's GCRC

Diabetes mellitus was, and is, rampant in the overweight, aging, indigent ghetto population surrounding Temple University Hospital. In these individuals, arteries supplying blood to the lower extremities frequently become occluded. Novel surgical intervention procedures were developed by Dr. F. A. Reichle and his colleagues which salvaged many legs and feet among these suffering patients. He presented his data at international medical meetings and paved the way for many other vascular surgeons to become involved in salvaging rather than amputating extremities of patients with inadequate blood circulation.

The dermatologist, Dr. Eugene Van Scott, and his colleagues developed techniques for inducing clinical remission in many patients suffering from lymphomatous lesions of the skin. Through their effort, the GCRC became a national referral center for patients suffering from the skin cancer, lymphoma (mycosis fungoides). Their work on psoriasis continues today, but outside of Temple University Hospital.

36

Another remarkable anecdote began in 1977 when one of Temple's plastic surgeons developed fulminating rheumatoid arthritis. In the course of performing an operation, when he extended his index finger to tie a knot, the extensor tendon ruptured. The possibility that methotrexate, a drug widely used to treat cancer, could be used to control the mutilating inflammation of rheumatoid arthritis was entertained by Dr. Van Scott and his colleagues. The surgeon was given intramuscular injections of methotrexate with remarkable resolution of his rheumatoid arthritis.

Shortly thereafter, a 40 year old patient from New Mexico came to Philadelphia to be evaluated and placed on an experimental treatment program for rheumatoid arthritis. He was in severe pain with incapacitating inflammation of the cervical vertebrae, hands, elbows, knees, ankles and feet. We were worried that diseased vertebrae in the neck could collapse and his head would compress his brainstem and cause quadriplegia. He was given a test dose of methotrexate before subjecting him to an experimental regimen. In ten days his improvement was grossly evident. We had hoped that methotrexate might prevent paralysis and provide him with enough relief so he could continue to work and provide sustenance for his family. Thirty-two years later, he is still a productive real estate developer and tolerates his rheumatoid arthritis without major impediment.

We were not the first team in the nation to use methotrexate to treat rheumatoid arthritis, but we were the first to use it in Pennsylvania and specifically on the Temple University Hospital's GCRC. The benefit from methotrexate to treat devastating rheumatoid arthritis spread through the hospital staff and the community and U.S. This research effort subsequently advanced clinical medicine.

Diabetes mellitus is a devastating disorder and is the classic disease where the normal concentrations of fuels in the bloodstream are lacking. Knowledge we gained from normal adult humans regarding fuel homeostasis was applicable to the understanding of the treatment of patients with diabetes mellitus, some suffering from ketoacidotic coma, and patients suffering from liver failure.

Dr. W. Clark and colleagues developed criteria for classifying benign and malignant melanomas. His staging methods developed on the GCRC are internationally used.

Methods for modernizing nutritional assessments, specifically those relating to obesity, were revitalized and advanced. Eventually hundreds of patients were studied to determine their energy requirements and body compositions. The energy imbalance of ingested food and exercise in augmenting caloric requirements or deficits were studied in detail. This translated directly into causes of obesity and abnormalities in blood glucose, triglycerides and cholesterol.

Mechanisms for maintaining the availability of fuels in the bloodstream among patients with alcoholic cirrhosis were at one time a major thrust of the Temple GCRC. Understanding survival mechanisms in patients with alcoholic cirrhosis was important because hospitalization for alcoholism was one of the chief reasons for admission to Temple University Hospital. We initially thought the kidney in patients with alcoholic cirrhosis would complement the liver by contributing glucose to the blood and thereby supplying fuel to the body to meet its energy requirements. However, we found it was fat mobilized from the small storage depot that supplemented the liver and not the kidney. Further, we learned that patients with scarred (cirrhotic) livers had behavior likened to accelerated starvation. Their wasted bodies reflected this nutritional state.

The behavior and effects of a variety of hormones were described in great detail by Dr. G. Boden and his colleagues. He developed the immunoassay for measuring the concentration of secretin in the blood. He also characterized family members with the malignant endocrine tumor, glucagonoma, and treated them.

The metabolism of ketone bodies (acetoacetate, beta-hydroxybutyrate and acetone) was studied in great detail in healthy obese starving volunteers, alcoholic patients with hepatic cirrhosis, and diabetic patients suffering from ketoacidosis. Through combined efforts, Dr. G. A. Reichard,

Jr. at Lankenau Medical Research Center, Dr. D.G. Sapir at Johns Hopkins Hospital and I identified the abnormal mechanisms inducing diabetic ketoacidosis. This understanding of abnormal metabolism saved many lives; it augmented our understanding of how inappropriate, fulminating, tissue breakdown causes death. Further, we, and investigators at other centers, demonstrated the specific beneficial effects of rehydration, insulin, electrolytes and glucose administration during diabetic coma. These treatments clearly affected survival for patients resuscitated from devastating diabetic ketoacidosis.

Medical students, residents and fellows working on the GCRC gained important knowledge that helped them in subsequent years to provide better care for a variety of patients suffering from diseases.

Before research teams were dissolved or misdirected toward a crash, a sizeable amount of significant advances in understanding health and disease states were made at the Temple GCRC. It was team effort, not individual performance, that led to these accomplishments.

The Temple GCRC contributions added not only to the delivery but primarily to the advancement of health care for about 500,000 patients located in the immediate inner city ghetto, as well as patients living in the greater metropolitan area, the entire state of Pennsylvania, the nation, and some throughout the world.

These accomplishments were obtained through the joint efforts of professors, fellows, residents, and students, and administrative, nursing, nutritional and technical staff members. There was practically no "I did it," but instead there was, "We did it." The satisfaction that comes from understanding how to treat and save the life of a dying patient is a never-ending phenomenon of personal reward.

The Crash

A heightened ominous feeling was creeping throughout Temple's academic medical center by 1985.

The influence of research in general, and of a GCRC specifically, is regulated by a hierarchy of administrators.

39

The summed impacts of a university president, vice president of the health sciences center, deans of the health sciences center, chairpersons, faculty members, fellows, residents and students are all reflected by the administrative, educational, patient care and research activities. All regulators do not recognize that research activities promote patient care, and research and patient care promote education. The deterioration of clinical research in an academic medical environment is a prognostic hallmark of institutional decay. On the other hand, those that do realize the impact of clinical research on academic excellence may push service activities to generate financial resources because there is no other obvious method to obtain the money needed to pay for medical education. The college of medicine is unique among university colleges because it is the only school within the university that is expected to earn a large share of its expenses associated with education (and research).

Three decades ago I described the essentiality of a critical mass to maximize clinical science advances. Among a few academicians there was recognition that meaningful research is a process that moves from the bedside to the laboratory bench and back to patients. Insight starts with the patient, expands in the laboratory, and hopefully, returns to the bedside to improve clinical care. Appreciation from patients, family and friends raises the morale and heightens the goals of the clinical investigative teams. Grant support usually follows medical success. Temple University increased its rank to 33rd in the nation for NIH support. However, with a change in Temple University's president and the Health Sciences Center vice president, Temple fell to between 70th and 80th in ranking for research support. Income from the clinical practice plan was forcefully promoted by Temple's higher administration. Unfortunately, the small amount of generated income from clinical practice became a low-producing cash cow for the university. The perceived revenue fell short because the hospital and medical staff primarily served indigent patients. Eighty percent of patient care was devoted to Medicare and Medicaid patients. There is not enough profit from physician/surgeon services to these financially disadvantaged populations of patients to support a university.

Research information pertaining to cutting edge of clinical science is often passed by word of mouth at national medical conferences. These meetings are essential for top-flight clinical investigators. Schools without the financial resources to send their faculty members to meetings where new research data are presented become more poorly endowed with money and knowledge.

The loss of an interdisciplinary approach to solving medical problems encountered by the Temple patient population as well as the world's patient population could have grave consequences on health care development. This is especially true for those financially poor patients. The old clinical investigators at Temple and other universities have faded from the clinical investigators' scene and their replacements are not being developed:

Where are the NIH-sponsored 1) neuroscientists with medical degrees to advance the understanding and treatment of Alzheimer's disease; 2) clinical researchers who understand and are brave enough to direct the histo-compatibility laboratories needed for tissue transplantation; 3) medical doctors who can direct oncology drug products to eradicate widespread malignancies; 4) clinical investigators who have a grasp on stem cell transplantation and who can influence the regeneration of islet cells that will produce insulin for the treatment of type 1 diabetes; and 5) other clinicians who have a useful grasp on the application of immunity in influencing a vast array of diseases?

Without well-trained clinical investigators or sites to deliver and evaluate new methods for advancing biomedical research, care for a large proportion of the population, especially the diabetic, obese, and aging population of the USA, will be compromised.

In an academic institution, when the delicate balance between clinical research and service is tilted by administrators toward patient care in order to collect money rather than to make medical advances, the whole nation suffers. If medical school administrators develop the attitude

41

that the school cannot afford research, they slam the door on medical progress. In a state containing legislators who do not understand that research is tightly coupled to education and patient care, the welfare of the citizens is compromised.

The vistas of most academicians are limited. Their focus is too narrow. Very few fully appreciate the power that prominent state or national politicians have in providing financial support for education and research. These two components, teaching and research, cost money. There is no way the practice of medicine in current times can provide enough overage to pay for these two essential elements of a university health sciences center. Monies must come from other sources, primarily governments and philanthropies. Hard working and insightful administrators cannot generate the funds needed for an academic medical center to flourish from service (patient care) activities.

In 1985 the full time clinical faculty numbered 404 and the volunteer faculty was 1,378. In 2002 the clinical faculty had shrunk to about 300, and I am unaware of the size of the current voluntary faculty. Thus, the full time clinical faculty had shrunk in spite of the fact that the medical student population had enlarged. The medical school was placed on probation primarily because of inadequate library facilities and the lack of space for students. The GCRC lost its funding. The NIH established that the number of GCRCs throughout the nation should be 80, and Temple did not make the cut. In all fairness to Temple's hierarchal administration, clinical research has decayed across the country in spite of the fact that the NIH annual budget has increased to over 28 billion dollars. Most practicing physicians and the informed lay are questioning the benefit of the NIH-supported basic science research projects. Many of the laboratory findings have become quite esoteric, and it is virtually impossible to relate their significance to improving the health care of U.S. patients. There has been a progressive decline in physician participation in clinical research activities over the past 20 years. In April 2003 the Wall Street Journal reported that physician researchers needed to move cures out of the rat cages into suffering patients. There are, however, a limited number of physician-scientists who can bridge that gap between basic scientists and practicing physicians/surgeons.

Years ago when I was invited to talk to European medical audiences I had state-of-the-art information. However, the dominance of USA scientists in biomedicine has slipped the last decade. Relative to the USA, basic science and medical science have improved in Britain, Japan, Russia, Germany, Sweden, Switzerland, Australia, Italy and New Zealand. The slippage in U.S. physician-scientists has been documented by the scholarly publications of Leon E. Rosenberg (The physician-scientist: An essential – and fragile – link in the medical research chain. *J. Clin. Invest.* 103:1621-6, 1999.)

Dr. Rosenberg, formerly dean, Yale School of Medicine and currently in the Department of Molecular Biology, Princeton University, has published data showing that physician-scientists are progressively disappearing from the U.S. medical arena. The percent of medical students graduating between 1989 and 1996 expressing a strong interest in research as a career fell each successive year. "More disturbing are recent trends in the population of new investigators and trainees. The actual number of first time M.D. applicants for NIH research grants has plummeted in the past few years: a 31% drop from 1994 to 1997. If this progression were to continue linearly, there would be no first-time M.D. applicants by 2003." (Physician-Scientists - Endangered and Essential. *Science.* 283:331-2, 1999.) This only slightly exaggerates possible reality. However, it is virtually impossible to quantify the number of people who are presently physician-scientists or who are training to become physician-scientists because there is no definitive definition of a physician-scientist. In this book, I use the words physician-scientist as a man or woman with an advanced educational degree in medicine who has direct and persistent contact with normal or sick people who serve as volunteers or patients to discover mechanisms responsible for health and disease states. "A physician-scientist has eye to eye contact with patients." He/she employs scientific

43

rigor to delineate biomedical problems. A physician-scientist recognizes a defect in the health of an individual and seeks a resolution for the problem. Healthy humans may have to serve as control subjects so findings among patients can be contrasted with those found among normal people. For example, the blood glucose concentrations for normal people must be known before a patient can be classified as having an abnormally elevated blood glucose value which is characteristic of diabetes mellitus. Physician-scientists design research protocols to delineate the disordered biomedical conditions. They are also highly cognizant of the need to protect the welfare of all people. Their research protocols should be designed with the strongest ethical considerations in mind.

The bureaucracy of doing clinical research in the USA has become a quagmire of restrictions and regulations that have seriously impaired clinical research to the point young researchers have directed their efforts away from academic medical centers and clinical investigations. Somewhere along the way, part of the NIH administration has forgotten the teaching of one of their great directors, Dr. James A. Shannon, who stated that freewheeling research is an essential ingredient of scientific discovery. Now, it is better to have a significant (if not most) amount of research done before you submit a grant application. There is no opportunity to do any "freewheeling" research activities. Where is the window of opportunity that will allow old and younger biomedical physician-scientists to forage ahead with convictions that they can stop the decay associated with bureaucracy and transform clinical research into an effective tool to improve not only discovery for common disease but also new methods for cost-effective health care for everyone? Academicians have never been selfish with their techniques for improving the health of all people. However, there is usually a lack of knowledge on how to safely translate basic science knowledge into the clinical arena. Whose job is it to move potential health care tools into the practice of medicine?

It is disappointing that there are no comprehensive studies describing the outcome of individuals who have chosen the physician-scientist career pathways. What happened to these dedicated people? It is clear, however, that physician-scientists are no longer self-perpetuating; they are, instead, a dying breed. Their replacements are incomplete specimens, neither medical doctors nor medical basic scientists that can inter-relate or translate the fundamental biomedical discoveries to the practice of medicine. The extinction of the physician-scientist species may not be due primarily to a lack of federal funds to support clinical research endeavors. Further, there are more philosophical advisors than there are investigators. The extinction of clinical investigators is more likely due to a combination of things. For example, the years of training needed to develop the knowledge base and competency needed to be a meaningful clinical investigator are many. Also, there is a great deal of expense associated with a long training period, and the financial debt becomes enormous as the trainee ages. Once the preparatory years have been successfully completed, there is no assurance that a job opportunity in a research environment will be available. Even if a good employment opportunity is presented, job security is lacking. Currently the NIH is grossly over-committed, and although the various institutes may have to pay a tithing to gather a pool of money that can be used for young investigators, job opportunity is limited. The pay scale for most young would-be clinical investigators is inappropriately low compared to other professionals with comparable educational investments. However, the greatest compensation of all, *appreciation*, has diminished during the last two decades. Well-meaning politicians in consultation with the Institute of Medicine, American Association of Medical Colleges, American Medical Association, and other elite organizations, have carefully thought through the support needed and diligently defined the guidelines for would-be clinical investigators or the physician-scientist. However, a large segment of brain trust groups have never done very much patient-oriented research. They are unaware of the work or danger involved in the actual care of people. These huge factors have been completely overlooked by administrators and scientists who do not take care of people hospitalized on the GCRCs throughout the USA. I emphasize that there is an enormous amount of work associated with overseeing the health care of normal volunteers and patients following research protocols. Bureaucratic regulations have restricted rather than promoted clinical research into patient diseases. Research opportunities are abundant but the conversion of aggressive, idealistic young medical doctors with imagination into robotic zombies applying for grants and running the gamut of paperwork restrictions has crushed the intellectual curiosity needed and the satisfaction gained from scientific discovery. Where is the freewheeling spirit advocated by the creative and imaginative James A. Shannon? It is gone! As noted, many scientific oversight committees composed of smart verbal people have never been engaged in direct eye to eye patient care. Their trying to describe the problems of the physician-scientist is somewhat like a medical secretary trying to explain the anxiety of a neurosurgeon associated with removing a brain tumor from a child of a friend.

The financial investment the federal government makes in biomedical research ($26 billion) compared to the national healthcare budget ($1.76 trillion) for 2002-2003 should be considered. Thus, only 1-2 cents per dollar of the total medical budget is spent on biomedical research by the federal government. Further, the majority of this paltry amount supports basic science research and not clinical studies. Maybe a young medical person who owes $100,000 for his/her medical education might be forced to consider a career path other than clinical investigation.

Temple University Medical School and Hospital will survive. Its faculty members are resilient and the decline in academic standing hopefully will be transient. The faculty recognizes the causes for the decline. They are strongly committed to serving the surrounding community. They will seek a higher plane of academic accomplishments. They have a tendency to unite when under fire. They will quickly return to a favorable status. The probation was lifted. State support has become admirable. A new president has realigned the university's priorities, and a building program has started. Their recruitment has accelerated as they struggle for academic excellence. They have the heart, soul and commitment to provide outstanding health care, education and, hopefully, research.

Resuscitation

There is another component of clinical research that has been overlooked or downplayed by the medical school intelligentsia. There are a significant number of talented doctors who have left academic medical centers and settled in community hospitals. They have assumed some of the responsibility for advancing medical care that in the past has been associated with academic medical centers. Some of these practitioners are engaged in practical approaches to executing clinical treatment programs that provide a significant amount of information for the advances of the practice of medicine. Thus, due to the failure of NIH's training programs to attract young, bright, energetic physicians/surgeons, some become good medical doctors and practical clinical investigators in community hospitals. They have promoted progressive excellent health care for patients and made significant contributions needed to advance patient health care. The practicing radiologists, cardiologists, ophthalmologists, pediatricians and surgeons, to name a few, deserve special recognition for advances they have made in health care which are largely independent of academic medical centers. The pharmaceutical industry invested significantly more in research and development than the U.S. government did through NIH's entire operating budget between 1992 and 2002. The pharmaceutical industry's research budget for 2002 was $37 billion. Admittedly, industry is profit driven, but their profits are based on medical treatment advancements. They have contributed significantly to health care practices. Good examples of their contributions can be related to the discovery and therapeutic uses of 1) antimicrobial drugs, 2) stents for occlusive arterial disease, 3) cholesterol lowering drugs and other drugs in development for treating heart diseases and strokes, 4) prosthetic replacement devices for knees, hips and other joint bones, 5) drugs available and vaccines in development for HIV/AIDS, 6) new medication for neurological diseases, potentially beneficial for Alzheimer's disease, and 7) the striking improvement in cataract lens replacement therapy in the aging population. Thus, despite the failure of the NIH training programs to attract more clinical investigators, medical care has progressed.

Several obvious advances are reviewed. Before the advent of antibiotics, especially penicillin, about one-half of the patients who developed pneumoccal pneumonia died. Many of these were young, healthy people before contracting the pneumonia, which was known as the "captain of death."

More recent progress has been made in extraction and replacement of eye cataracts. In the early 1970's, patients with cataracts that obstructed vision to the point that patients could no longer read were hospitalized. Those with diabetes mellitus were treated to obtain optimal blood glucose control before eye surgery to extract the cataracts. After surgery they lay flat in bed with sandbags on each side of their neck to hold the head still with eyes facing upward. Ice packs were often placed over the eyes to diminish bleeding caused by the surgery. After several days, usually a week, the patients were discharged from the hospital. They needed thick corrective eyeglasses to see printed material. In 2004, complicated medical problems are controlled before the patient presents to an outpatient office. The cataract is excised and a prosthetic lens is replaced in the eye in less than an hour. In a short time, the patient is usually discharged from the clinic. Vision is grossly improved. Pain is controlled. Healing is usually without complications. Reading glasses may be required but they are not unattractive, thick lenses.

Current surveys suggest that 219,000 hip fractures occur annually. About 75% are women over the age of 70 years. The incidence rises with age. Mortality after a fractured hip is 12-20% in the first year. Of course, one related factor associated with death is the aging of the patient population. However, we must not forget one of the major reasons for bone replacement after hip fracture is to help with controlling pain, especially with movement. Currently, the key to successful treatment of hip fractures is early surgery, both operative and coagulation therapy (preventing blood clots from forming and migrating to the lung) and prompt ambulation.

Open heart surgery for inadequate blood supply to the heart was associated with a death rate of about 50% in the early 1960's. In 2004, it is about 2-3%, and it occurs only in the most severely compromised patients. If it were the 1950's, former President William J. Clinton and I would be dead from heart attacks.

Admittedly, healthcare costs in the U.S. are excessive. Nonetheless, it is the best in the world because of investments made to support interdisciplinary teams and hospital facilities for GCRCs, medical industry promotion of drugs and prosthetic devices, and the willingness of physicians and surgeons to be engaged in advancing health care.

It is important to recognize the fundamental difference between a clinical investigator and a pharmaceutical executive: A clinical investigator looks for the cause and a cure for a disease; a pharmaceutical executive looks for a treatment and a profit from a disease.

Two of the biggest problems currently facing American medicine are 1) how to deliver quality health care to people, in essence, the best medicine for the best price; and 2) translation of basic scientific information into clinical practice. Universities must have the financial resources to investigate and to make practical new techniques to provide patients with medical care that satisfies their needs. The gap between basic knowledge and clinical practice is currently so broad that it may be impossible to bridge the gap unless medical education is grossly changed. Such an undertaking will cost money. This financial resource should not and cannot be extracted from the practice of medicine. Currently, reading a medical article from a general medical education journal, *The New England Journal of Medicine*, for the first time may dazzle a practicing doctor. He or she may not be able to put the information into proper perspective or understand how to employ the advances. It is impossible for a general practitioner to put forth the best procedures for patients when the knowledge gap between basic science and clinical medicine is gigantic. Society must realize that the ideal practice of medicine is impossible. Tolerance must be an integral part of a physician-patient relationship. Litigation must be reevaluated. Its purpose is to protect patients from malpractice and not to force idealistic outcomes of therapy or make malpractice lawyers wealthy.

The future of American medicine will belong to the bold. Hopefully they will be leaders in academic medical centers who can reestablish pride and pleasure from medical accomplishments and promote good feelings in being physicians and surgeons. These leaders need to realign the relationships between doctors and patients. As physicians and surgeons they must once again believe in themselves. They must rediscover the joys of doctoring. The loss of confidence by patients in physicians and surgeons in the face of miraculous cures for human diseases has created a bizarre paradox. Physician-surgeon-researchers must stand up to bureaucratic and trial lawyer bullies. There must be professionals in this great country that can emerge as medical leaders and draw medical professionals together so they work in a cooperative fashion to deliver the best health care for the best price. It is just as likely that the medical students, residents and fellows will lead the fight to regain the standing of this noble profession, clinical investigation and practice of medicine.

Former President Reagan had a sense of clarity regarding purpose. I believe the practice of medicine should be at the extreme of human behavior. Medical care is the most noble of all professions. A physician-surgeon-researcher should reestablish hope, a will to thrive, a reason to regain mental and physical compensation, a return to a sturdy character. An individual of good will can transmit a spirit of healing that supercedes the natural. A research-doctor must lift any clouds of despair and replace them with a sunny horizon. The magnitude or threat imposed by well-meaning politicians and bureaucrats should not dampen the enthusiasm needed to succeed in worthy goals like curing diabetes, Alzheimer's disease, and other degenerative conditions. Aim for good health regardless of the obstacles. A clinical investigator must do bold things to conquer diseases. Transform the plague induced by trial lawyers into a better state of healthcare delivery. The job of a physician/surgeon is to heal; to remove suffering; to do the impossible when doing so is essential for compensating health. Physician-surgeon-researchers must believe in themselves; believe that they can alleviate distress; believe that their actions count; believe that their actions make a difference, a good difference. Physician-surgeon-scientists must promote kindness and humor. Learn to be firm and learn to love. He or she must convey a positive attitude by being an example of sincerity and happiness. Be in control of mental thinking and physical actions. Deploy optimistic behavior; be a doer; be a hero; be a human. Confront opposition with a positive alternative. Wear the M.D., M.D. Ph.D., and Ph.D. titles with pride. Physician-scientists should be connected with the environment, to society, to patients, and to family. The characteristics of someone who "has done good" are reflected by his/her family. Let true convictions march onward. Hopefully when a great physician-surgeon-scientist dies, his/her imprint will have immortality. Medical success should not be hidden. A medical leader should inspire others to do good for others. Lead, lead, lead! HIV, Alzheimer's disease, strokes, diabetes, depression: look forward to curing these maladies!

We are all interdependent. Give me your hand as I extend my hand to you. Let's help each other travel to a higher plane of life. Don't be self-absorbed. Reach outward, not inward!

Great leaders of American medicine have gotten other physicians-surgeons-scientists to do things that had a great impact on biomedical advances that filter down to

51

individual patients. Initiate action at the top that will continue or persist until individual patients benefit!

Turn a likely defeat into a victory. Define what needs to be done to deliver the best health care for the best price and see that it is done. We all need to develop a sense of what is appropriate and see that it is done. You have to be optimistic and hound those who need to be changed in order to promote worthy goals. Paint your dreams white, pink and blue and, if necessary, outline them in bright colors. Open your mind and welcome fresh thoughts!

Clinical investigation, whether done in an academic medical center or community environment, is in the final analysis a tool that promotes the best health care for the best price!

The foregoing aphorisms are addressed to the biomedical scientists. The following paragraphs of caution are directed to the intelligent lay.

If you develop the attitude that others are obliged to give you health care and you disregard *appreciation* for the services of others, you may be part of a move that generates a monstrous and dysfunctional healthcare system. The USA has the most advanced and comprehensive healthcare system largely because patients and their families, relatives and friends give freely to support the system. They give because they *appreciate* the effort that others put forth to help them in time of need. In essence, they give the greatest reward one can give for service, *appreciation*.

The more diverse the USA becomes as individual groups cleave into factions rather than one population, the more likely the healthcare system will rupture. Don't let democracy divide rather than unite our most noble profession, healthcare delivery. Let's maintain one identity, the best health care for the most people involved for the best price and cherish the influence of *appreciation*.

Chapter III. Fuels and Hormones

Background

This chapter is mostly a story of medical discoveries derived from studying obese volunteers over a course of two to three decades. These brave people wanted to undergo prolonged starvation for weight reduction and contribute to medical research. Our work was possible because advances had been made in techniques for measuring fuels and hormones in blood and other biological fluids. I am presenting results obtained from measuring the changes that occurred in fuels and hormones circulating in the blood after an overnight fast and periodically thereafter during prolonged starvation. We tried to measure those compounds that were widely recognized in 1965 as potential metabolic fuels (chemicals or substrates) and hormones in the blood, and to record the changes in these materials induced by starvation. We were particularly interested in changes found in the blood concentration of glucose, ketone bodies (acetoacetate and beta-hydroxybutyrate), free fatty acids, amino acids and insulin.

Our intentions grew with time and experience. Our goals enlarged to discover how the body supplied, used, converted, selected and conserved body fuels during starvation and during illness. Over the years my colleagues and I increased the numbers of fuels and hormones we measured to gauge their influence on maintaining a constant supply of energy. The accuracy of the assays used to measure insulin, free fatty acids and amino acids improved significantly.

We knew blood was a circulating medium (pool) in the body by which fuels and hormones entered and exited. We suspected that we could more accurately and reproducibly measure the production and utilization of most fuels and hormones across organs if "steady-state" conditions existed. Steady-state conditions exist in the blood when the amount of fuels and hormones entering the blood equals the amount of fuels and hormones leaving the blood.

53

Long term steady-state conditions occur when concentrations of fuels and hormones in the blood are constant from day to day. This happens when the production rate of a fuel (or hormone) equals the disappearance rate of that fuel (or hormone). We learned over time that the concentrations of fuels in the blood are also influenced by the kidney's ability to conserve (reabsorb) fuels.

We began our research project by trying to determine when the steady-state of blood fuels and hormones occurred in humans during starvation. Doing so allowed us to measure day-to-day exchange rates.

Some questions we had to answer were: How long should patient-volunteers starve before the blood fuels and hormones are relatively constant or the day-to-day changes are minimal? What are the values or concentrations of blood fuels and hormones when this steady-state develops?

As I describe changes in the blood's concentrations of fuels and hormones, the more subtle but important alterations will be stated before the gross changes in ketone bodies are presented. In subsequent chapters I will delineate between those mechanisms responsible for supplying fuels and those that remove, select and conserve fuels delivered in the blood.

Before I describe the results of our studies concerning blood fuels and hormones, I wanted to include some relevant and personal professional anecdotes.

Patient Experiences

During my college years I worked as a laboratory technician in St. Anthony's Hospital in Oklahoma City. Part of my job was to draw blood from patients prior to their admission to the hospital for elective surgery. A tourniquet was placed around the arm, and the antecubital fossa (area in front of the elbow) was cleaned with alcohol. Often, the medical staff asked the patients to pump their hand several times so the veins in the forearm would fill with blood. After the vein was punctured, the blood was drawn with a needle and syringe. This procedure was necessary prior to the modern day technique of using vacuum tubes attached to needles.

I would often draw blood from the upper extremities of about 75 patients in a day's time. However, I was not always successful. I remember a middle-aged woman who looked at me with great disgust after I tried in vain to obtain blood from her arm. She said, "Young man, maybe you would do better with a razor blade and a spoon." In spite of this sarcastic comment, I was considered an expert at sticking needles into patients' veins on the first try. Further, I never lost my sympathy for patients hurt from being stuck with a large needle. Drawing blood became a valuable asset to me during my later years as a clinical investigator because blood samples were needed to analyze fuels (substrates) and hormones periodically throughout starvation studies. Beyond the intellectual curiosity, there was the need to know if there was a signal in the blood that might warn of impending danger. Volunteers also wanted to know the results of their blood tests.

Obtaining blood from a vein of an obese patient undergoing starvation is much more difficult than obtaining blood from a healthy patient. First, the veins in an obese person's upper extremity (arm) are often submerged deeply in fat, making them difficult to feel. Some vessels readily move in the subcutaneous fat when pushed by a needle. This happens most frequently when one draws blood from a patient without the use of a tourniquet. It is especially true when you need to draw blood from an obese patient during starvation when the vessels are collapsed because the stasis (stoppage) induced by the tourniquet may alter the concentration of important electrolytes, especially bicarbonate, during some of the metabolic studies. Sometimes I had to stop my process of trying to draw blood so that the patient-volunteer and I could rest and relax before restarting the process. Of course, the patient-volunteer encountered more discomfort than I did, but it was taxing for us both.

Another important question that arose during our starvation studies was, "How much blood could be repeatedly drawn without injury to an individual who had not eaten for three to eight weeks?" Throughout the study, I had to monitor this issue very closely. We had to design a careful protocol specifying which days and at what intervals blood samples would be drawn to provide the most accurate information. Further, some of the fuels in the patients' bloodstream were fragile, requiring us to immediately place blood specimens in ice cold solution to deproteinize (remove proteins from) them. The blood was kept in an ice bath to prevent decomposition or changes in a particularly delicate fuel (or hormone). This was especially critical for pyruvate, a fragile 3-carbon compound usually derived from glucose.

The resources offered by the GCRC-sponsored program were invaluable to my work as a fledgling clinical investigator. The program provided me the opportunity to contribute to a better understanding of how the human body tolerated starvation and to evaluate whether or not such drastic course of weight reduction was beneficial to people.

My work at a clinical research center started during my senior year of medical school at the University of Colorado. I resumed my clinical activities at a GCRC as a second and third year resident in internal medicine at Johns Hopkins Hospital. One of my first encounters observing a patient during prolonged semi-starvation was the obese man who had become stuck in the phone booth and brought into the Johns Hopkins Medical Emergency Room.

After becoming a fellow in metabolism under the direction of Dr. George F. Cahill, Jr., my colleagues and I began to investigate the mechanisms that allowed the body to survive during prolonged caloric deprivation. Our initial intent was to relate changes in blood fuels and hormones to urinary excretion of nitrogenous compounds and ketone bodies, to the total energy requirements of the body, and possibly the consumption of ketone bodies by the brain after 5-6 weeks of total starvation. Many other preparatory studies and observations were ongoing simultaneously in the patient-volunteers hospitalized on the Clinical Research Center. One of these was an evaluation of brain metabolism after prolonged starvation. We closely monitored the volunteers' salt and water intake, quantity of urine, changes in body weight, blood pressure, pulse, temperature and blood electrolytes and fuels and hormones. I made a point to observe the volunteers' attitudes, hungers and behaviors. A subjective approach to evaluating their discomfort during starvation was an automatic component of my research endeavors. Contrary to the beliefs of some people, I found obese patient-volunteers undergoing prolonged periods of fasting often ravenously hungry. Nonetheless, they were not as devastated as I would have anticipated. Most of the patient-volunteers could tolerate starvation for long periods of time. Another component of our study was to observe how starvation affected a person's cognitive abilities. Most of the volunteers showed improved scores on psychological tests as the study progressed. We thought, however, that the improvements were linked to the patients' increased familiarity with test taking rather than any changes in mentation brought on by starvation.

Recently, when I began preparing to write this chapter, I browsed through old books and articles shelved or filed in my personal library. I was surprised to find how preciously little had been published about changes in blood fuels and hormones during starvation. Detailed descriptions with reproducible data were virtually non-existent before we began collecting and publishing our data at Harvard in the mid-sixties. To me, this seems incongruous with the blight of human starvation throughout the world.[1]

Blood Fuels and Hormones

Organs of the body need energy to maintain vitality. This energy is derived from fuels. Fuels are complex compounds that, in the process of being broken down into simpler products, release energy. Cells break down fuels mostly through oxidation. This process is not unlike burning a piece of wood. But unlike burning a piece of wood in

---

[1] I read articles and books about the findings discovered after Jews were liberated from German concentration camps during World War II. The descriptions made me sick, and information helpful for understanding the results of forced inanition was either not available or of little use.

which the energy escapes into the atmosphere, some of the energy released during fuel breakdown is captured in "batteries" known as adenosine triphosphate (ATP). The energy trapped in ATP is employed to perform metabolic work. Excess caloric energy available after a meal is stored in fuel depots. These stored fuels are mobilized during periods of food deprivation or by strenuous physical activity.

The three basic fuels used by the human body are carbohydrates, proteins and fats. There is a minimum and maximum amount of each of these fuels that the body can utilize at any given time. In general, when one fuel is being maximally oxidized the others are being minimally oxidized or stored. These reciprocal patterns of utilization of storage are present in the fed and starved states. As a fuel, only a carbohydrate, glucose, is the universal fuel that can be utilized by all tissues in the human body at all times to produce the energy needed for cell survival. Stored fat at the initiation of starvation is usually available in overabundance, but it cannot be readily used as a source of fuel by all tissues. However, fat and protein can substitute for carbohydrate in providing most but not all of the metabolic needs of the body. Although a small amount of glucose must be oxidized for survival, this glucose can be synthesized mostly from amino acids derived from protein breakdown, or from glycerol derived from triglyceride breakdown.

Hormones, like fuels, play an integral role in cell survival. Hormones are molecules that regulate body processes, and scientists are discovering new ones all the time. They serve as chemical messengers that influence cellular behavior. There are many types of hormones. Most of the ones discussed in this chapter are ones that scientists and researchers identified long ago. I will concentrate on hormones produced by endocrine glands like the pituitary gland, islets of the pancreas, thyroid gland and adrenal gland. Adipose tissue as an endocrine gland is only briefly referenced because the vast majority of the research done on the production of hormones by adipose tissue has been published since I retired from the research arena. Nonetheless, it should be noted that adipose tissue may be regarded as the largest endocrine system in the body. Fat cells produce hormones that affect appetite control, obesity, insulin activity (diabetes mellitus), and blood vessel constriction (high blood pressure) and inflammation (heart attacks).

Hormones circulate through the blood to various target organs where they regulate a variety of physiologic and metabolic activities. Hormone concentrations in blood vary tremendously, but most often they exist in trace amounts. Yet hormones are crucial to regulating the uptake and release of blood fuels. They have a primary role in controlling not only glucose but also fat and protein synthesis and mobilization and conversion into fuels for oxidation. Insulin is the indispensable hormone in these actions.

Body Composition

During starvation, the body mobilizes its supply of stored fuels to meet its continuing energy requirements. Only a small quantity of glucose is present in the bloodstream. Glucose is stored in the body as glycogen; however, there is only about 0.3 kg of glycogen in the body. The majority of glycogen can be mobilized, providing a small amount of fuel. Available, stored glycogen is quickly used during exercise or periods of starvation.

The average weight of non-obese women (60 kg with 25% body fat) and non-obese men (80 kg with 20% body fat) forms a theoretical hybrid of about 70 kg. In this example, lean body mass (fat free mass) constitutes approximately 77% (58 kg) of the over-all weight. Lean body tissue is composed primarily of protein (~20%) and water (~80%). Muscle is the largest depository of protein in the body. Yet, only half of the estimated 12 kg of protein suspended in 58 kg of lean body mass can be mobilized before the muscles lose their ability to move the body, and the heart, liver and kidney lose their ability to function. On the other hand, this 70 kg, theoretical female-male hybrid would have roughly 16 kg of adipose tissue containing fat stored as triglyceride.[2] Unlike lean tissues, adipose tissue is 85% fat. This translates into 14 kg of triglyceride per 16 kg of adipose tissue. Therefore, the caloric value of triglyceride per unit mass (Kcal/gram) of fat is more than twice the caloric value of glucose or protein. At least 90% of this triglyceride can be mobilized and used without adverse effects to the body. The estimated size of the depots and caloric equivalents of the quantities of energy that are stored and can be mobilized by a theoretical female-male hybrid of 70 kg are shown in Table 1.

Depot	Calories per Gram	Total Calories	Usable Percent	Quantity Available as Calories
glycogen 300 grams	~4	1,200	66%	~800
protein 11,600 grams	~4	44,000	50%	22,000
fat 14,000 grams	~9	126,000	90%	113,400

Table 1. Estimates of fuel depots and the caloric equivalent of the quantities of a conceptualized 70 kg human that can be mobilized and consumed during starvation. Note the trivial caloric equivalents of glycogen. Only 50% of the protein mass can be mobilized and life be sustained. Virtually all of the fat depot can be mobilized and oxidized with impunity. The total fat that can be mobilized has about 5 times the caloric potential of protein.

History of Chemical Analysis and Radioimmunoassays

If a clinical investigator, or anyone, wants to study something, he or she must have access to material under study.

Blood has been recognized as long as there has been eyesight, and starvation has been present since the origin of

---

[2] Adipose tissue couples 3 long-chain fatty acids (an average of 17 carbons in length) to glycerol which is a short carbon chain (3 carbons in length) to make a single molecule of triglyceride.

life. Blood is a medium that connects the various parts of the body together. It transports oxygen, fuels and hormones and moves byproducts to organs of excretion. Blood is available for analysis through a variety of techniques. Changes can readily be measured in the blood concentrations of fuels and hormones under various nutritional conditions; however, they have only been systematically analyzed during periods of feeding and fasting for the last half of the twentieth century. This is primarily due to the fact that good analytical techniques became available after 1950. Many of the early methods used to measure blood and urine compounds, such as glucose and ketone bodies, were difficult to use, time-consuming and often inaccurate.

As early as 1500 B.C., Egyptian physicians described the illness now known as diabetes mellitus. Subsequently, the sweet taste of sugar was detected in the urine of diabetic patients. Crude blood glucose measurements became available after the 1870's. However, most methods for measuring blood glucose were not quantitatively suitable before 1915. At that time, it took large quantities of blood to determine concentrations of glucose. Because urine from diabetic patients contained excessive amounts of sugar, it could be tasted if not otherwise easily detected. Severe, dehydrating hyperglycemia (and white sugar spots from dried droplets of urine on the shoes and/or clothes of some patients) were signs or clues that helped a physician make the diagnosis of diabetes mellitus.

Only glucose has a longer history of being detected in the blood of patients with diabetes mellitus than ketone bodies.

In 1865, scientists discovered the ketone body, acetoacetate, in the urine of patients suffering from catastrophic diabetes mellitus. By 1887, researchers reported the accumulation of beta-hydroxybutyrate (another ketone body) in the urine of patients who had been fasting for two or three days. It is logical that these compounds would have been detected in the urine before the blood because the urine concentrates the excess materials that originate in the blood and need to be excreted from the body. In 1908, Magnus-

Levy discovered that beta-hydroxybutyrate, acetoacetate and, later, acetone originated from the breakdown of fatty acids. He also recognized that the breath of patients who were fasting or suffering from serious, uncontrolled diabetes mellitus exhibited a fruity smell caused by acetone in their systems.

Forty years later, the modern biochemical history of ketone body metabolism began when Kaplan and Lipmann (Nobel Prize recipient, 1953) identified an active form of acetate. These two-carbon breakdown compounds of fatty acids could be activated and reactivated with other molecules of acetate to form acetoacetate and beta-hydroxybutyrate. Acetone develops from the spontaneous degeneration of acetoacetate. During the early 1950's, researchers used analytical methods developed by Warburg (Nobel Prize recipient, 1931) to measure compounds in bodily fluids and tissue. Warburg started a revolution that put forth a specific, reproducible and sensitive method for determining concentrations of glucose, ketone bodies and other substrates (fuels/material) in blood and urine and tissue preparations. An additional new factor appeared to facilitate measurements of fuels in biological specimens: the commercial production of biochemical reagents for analysis occurred and allowed widespread application of measuring methods.

In 1962, the work of Williamson, Mellanby, and Krebs resulted in a major advance in the understanding of ketone body metabolism. Work performed in their Oxford laboratory in England laid forth a method for the rapid and accurate measurements of beta-hydroxybutyrate and acetoacetate in biological fluids. Thereafter, an accurate method for measuring acetone was described. The availability of these accurate and convenient procedures for measuring ketone bodies did much to widen the field of study.

The discovery that ketone bodies were an important fuel during periods of limited carbohydrate intake challenged conventional wisdom. For years, researchers and scientists had viewed ketone bodies as monstrous materials signaling impending death (as in the case of diabetes mellitus). It was not until good methods for measuring these compounds in urine and blood became available that the importance of these fuels was recognized.

E. Voit and his colleagues were among the first to recognize fat as a major source of energy for the body during starvation. Numerous subsequent clinical studies affirmed that the body oxidized fat during starvation. As early as 1896, F.N. Schulz recognized that if fat was oxidized in parts of the body other than fat (adipose) tissue, the fat would have to be transported by the blood to the various organs of the body. Prior to 1950, however, there were no valid indications that the blood's content of fatty acids changed during fasting. This failure to demonstrate the mobilization of fat existed because of inadequate techniques for identifying the species of lipid material mobilized and methods for measuring the lipid material. Scientists at that time identified the lipid material as long-chain fatty acids attached in very small quantities to plasma proteins. Long-chain fatty acids deriving from the breakdown of fat (adipose tissue) are oils, and oils are not water-soluble. Blood is comprised mostly of plasma. Plasma is 93% water and about 6% protein. Fatty acids, derived from adipose tissue storage sites, circulate throughout the body attached to plasma proteins. This protein/fat combination allows the oils of fat to circulate in the watery plasma. These fuels were named non-esterified or free fatty acids. In 1956, V. P. Dole and, independently, R. S. Gordon, Jr. and A. Cherkes reported that these fats could be extracted from plasma and quantified by titration techniques. Subsequently, several laboratory refinements were made, giving the clinical investigative community access to accurate, reproducible methods.

There are various organs of the body that extract fatty acids from plasma and oxidize (burn) them for energy. Some of these long-chain fatty acids are routed to the liver. There, enzymes cleave them into two-carbon fragments, which undergo several re-combinations to finally make four-carbon materials. These reconstituted, four-carbon materials are called ketone bodies, which are water-soluble and can travel in the bloodstream. Ketone bodies are synthesized specifically in the liver and require their own metabolic machinery (enzymes) to accomplish this task. Ketone bodies are not direct byproducts of fat breakdown. It wasn't until 1962 when Williams, Mellanby and Krebs designed a way to measure beta-hydroxybutyrate and acetoacetate in the blood that the scientific community recognized ketone bodies as a major source of fuel for the body.

In 1958, W. Stein and S. Moore published a pioneering technique to separate and quantitate amino acid concentrations in blood plasma. However, this method did not adequately measure the dominant plasma amino acid, glutamine. Therefore, we had to employ an enzymatic technique to measure glutamine in blood and plasma in work we conducted after 1965.

During starvation, proteins are cleaved into the twenty amino acids and released into the blood. This process is instigated by low concentrations of insulin in the bloodstream. In the face of severe caloric deprivation, the liver converts amino acids from muscle and other peripheral tissue into glucose and nitrogenous urea. Simultaneously amino acids are transported to the kidneys to undergo breakdown to produce glucose and nitrogenous ammonia. The nitrogenous compounds are excreted in the urine while the glucose is released in the blood and used by tissues for energy.

In 1959, Berson and Yalow developed a radioimmunoassay to measure insulin concentrations in the blood. This sensitive and specific assay uses a radioactive immune globulin to seek out and react with minute quantities of insulin. As time progressed, researchers used radioimmunoassay techniques to measure many other hormones in a host of biological fluids including blood, lymph, and cerebrospinal fluid. The importance of Berson and Yalow's work cannot be overstated. And many scientists believe that Berson would have surely shared the 1977 Nobel Prize with Yalow, Guillemin and Schally if it were not for his untimely death.

In our studies, we used sensitive, reproducible and specific enzymatic methods for measuring blood and urine concentrations of glucose, beta-hydroxybutyrate, acetoacetate, lactate, pyruvate, glycerol and other substrates. We employed further advances in radioimmunoassays to measure a variety of blood hormones, particularly insulin. These advances in methods made it possible for us to define fuel homeostasis in health and the lack thereof in disease states.

We slowly learned that concentrations of fuel in the blood are not determined solely by the rate at which the fuel enters and exits the bloodstream. Obviously, this is not a rule but a generalization. Further, we recognized that it can take days before the rate of fuels entering the bloodstream approximates the rate at which they exit. Again, this state of approximate equilibrium is referred to as "fuel homeostasis."

Ketosis is a condition characterized by increased concentrations of ketone bodies (acetoacetate, beta-hydroxybutyrate and acetone) in the body. Because ketone bodies were first detected in the urine of patients suffering from catastrophic diabetes mellitus, doctors thought they indicated pathological states. But like glucose, ketone bodies are beneficial fuels that play a central role in human survival when dietary carbohydrates are in short supply.

There has always been more in the lay press about blood glucose concentrations than ketone body concentrations. It wasn't until the late Dr. Robert Atkins publicized the efficacy of ketogenic diets for weight loss that the public learned about ketone bodies as a vital body fuel. Although Atkins' work revealed some important truths about ketone bodies, it is my opinion that he did not have enough data to back up his quantitative claims. Below in this chapter, I will show and describe concentrations of ketone bodies measured in patients' blood. Subsequently, in "Urine Reflects the Truth" I will display the rate at which the body excretes ketone bodies.[3]

---

[3] Although a patient's dietary intake before beginning a period of starvation can have some influence on blood fuels and hormones, it is generally trivial. That is why I have decided to limit my statements regarding dietary intake in this presentation.

Results from Studying Blood Fuels and Hormones

After an overnight fast the average blood glucose concentration of both women and men is about 80 mg/dl (4.5 mM). However, it should be noted that a woman's fasting blood glucose concentration is usually slightly lower than a man's. Even more profound is the difference between a woman and a man's blood glucose two hours after a meal. Two hours after eating, a woman's blood glucose is about 10 mg/dl lower than her fasting values while a man's blood glucose is about 10 mg/dl greater than his fasting values. However, the average value for both women and men two hours after eating is approximately equal to their average fasting blood glucose. Additionally, when fasting periods are extended, lean women may develop significantly lower blood glucose values than lean men. For many years, some physicians have misdiagnosed women with normal glucose levels as being hypoglycemic. A woman's relatively low level of glucose is a normal difference between the sexes, not a disease. Unfortunately, the majority of prolonged starvation studies measuring blood glucose concentrations in morbidly obese men and women neither recognized nor clearly demonstrated this normal difference.

The adaptive changes that occur in the concentrations of blood fuels and hormones during starvation form a time-dependent continuum that can be divided into three phases. Phase One is the post-absorptive stage which occurs after an overnight fast and extends two or three days into starvation. Blood levels of glucose, insulin and free fatty acids undergo the most acute changes during this first phase. Phase Two is called the sub-acute starvation period. It begins somewhere between the second and third day of total starvation and extends to about day 18. The most obvious change in this phase is an increase in the concentration of ketone bodies in the blood.

During the latter part of Phase Two, subtle changes can be found in the principal amino acids, glutamine and alanine. But day-to-day variations in other fuels, hormones and metabolic requirements are trivial. Phase Three of the starvation time-line is referred to as prolonged starvation and

66

spans the period between days 18-40. It leads to the premortal state in lean individuals subjected to about 60 days without food. It is during the premortal phase that lifelessness gradually develops. These changes in blood fuels and hormones are illustrated in Figures 1-3.

Because obese people have an excess of body fat, they are better able to tolerate longer periods (up to 90 days) of starvation than lean individuals. Similarly, lean young women, who have more body fat than lean men, fare better than lean men.

After an overnight fast and in the absence of food, blood (plasma/serum) glucose and insulin concentrations begin a parallel fall (Figure 1). This decrease in insulin concentration was recognized by Cahill to be the cardinal signal to the body to begin mobilizing fuels. Coupled with this drop in blood insulin is the rise of insulin counter-regulatory hormones like glucagon, cortisol, growth hormone, epinephrine and norepinephrine. This finely tuned process is central to supplying the body with fuels to meet its continuing energy requirements during starvation. After about three days of total starvation, the blood concentrations of glucose and insulin plateau (Figure 1). Nonetheless, insulin continues to circulate and has a persistent impact in regulating blood fuels. Insulin has a *braking action* on the release of all fuels into the blood. Changes in the venous concentration of other blood substrate concentrations, like lactate and pyruvate, are small. A slight increase in venous blood glycerol may reflect heightened, yet controlled fatty tissue breakdown.

In the brief postabsorptive period, the concentration of venous plasma free fatty acid (FFA) is about 0.5-0.6 mM (mmol/liter). During the first 2-3 days of starvation, plasma FFA concentration increases to about 1.2 mM and plateaus as starvation progresses (Figure 2).

Changes in ketone body concentrations are fascinating, not only during starvation but in illnesses, especially diabetic ketoacidosis. Only ketone bodies can

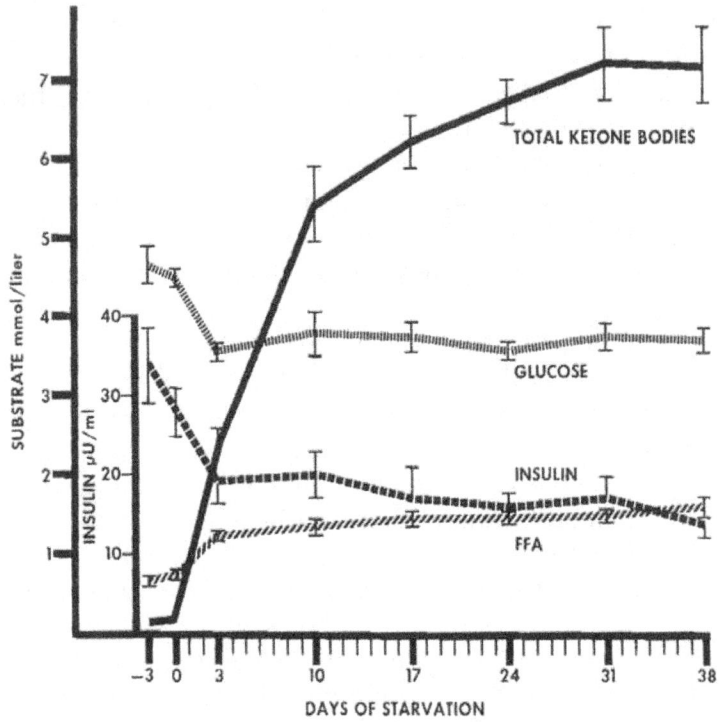

Figure 1. Concentration of fuels and insulin in the blood during starvation. The blood glucose falls from an overnight fast to its lowest value after 3 days of starvation. Thereafter it plateaus. Insulin changes parallel the blood glucose concentrations, but subsequent techniques for measuring insulin showed that all values are lower than those displayed in this figure. Free fatty acids rise and peak after a few days of starvation. Total ketone bodies, acetoacetate plus beta-hydroxybutyrate, undergo the greatest change in concentration of any mammalian fuel, peaking after 17 days of total starvation.

undergo such drastic changes in blood concentrations and still be compatible with life. After an overnight fast the concentration of the ketone body, acetoacetate, in the blood is approximately 0.05 mM. This same ketone body can drop to 0.01mM about two hours after a person consumes a high carbohydrate breakfast. The relative concentration of beta-hydroxybutyrate in the blood is comparable. The third

68

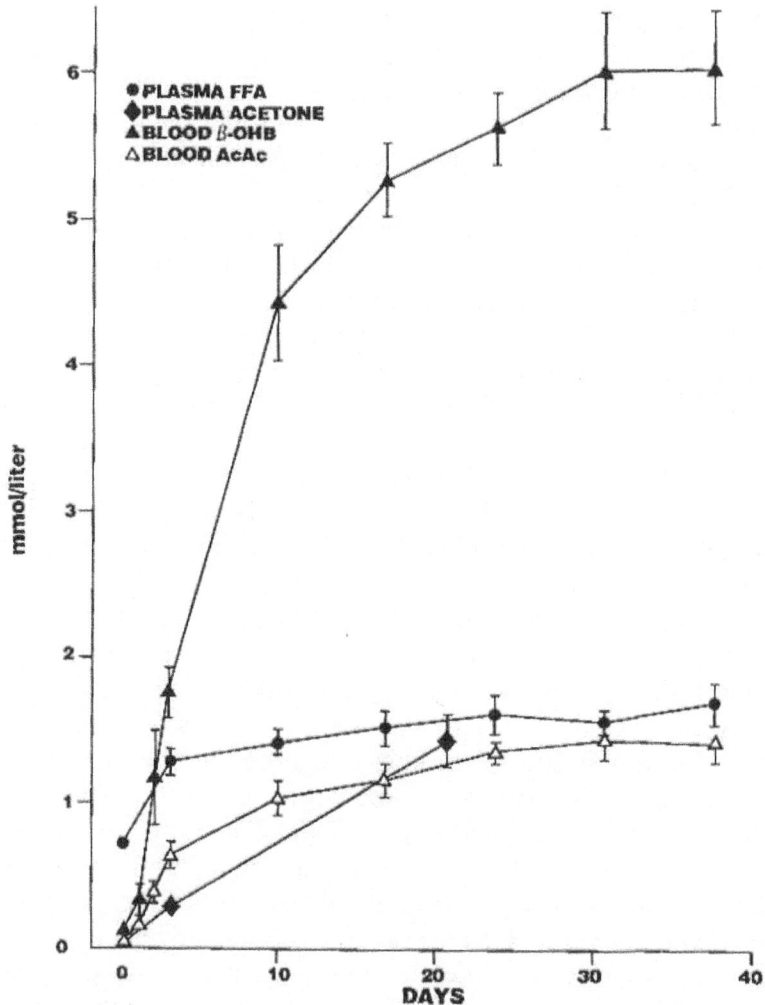

Figure 2. Displayed are ketone bodies and free fatty acids. Note that the beta-hydroxybutyrate (β-OHB) is a ketone body that undergoes the greatest change during starvation. Among the ketone bodies, acetone rises slowly. The maximum concentration of acetone is not shown in this figure. AcAc is the abbreviation for acetoacetate.

ketone body, acetone, is practically absent in the blood after meals unless individuals have put themselves on a high fat, low carbohydrate diet.

Starvation causes an exponential rise in acetoacetate and beta-hydroxybutyrate (Figure 2). These fuels plateau after about 18 days of total starvation where the rate of entry into the bloodstream equals the rate of exit either by oxidation by various tissues or elimination in the urine (and breath for acetone). At about day 18, the concentrations of beta-hydroxybutyrate (the major ketone body) plus acetoacetate (a minor ketone body) usually reach total values of about 6-8 mM. It is rare that a fasting patient's concentration of blood acetoacetate will be greater than 2mM or his/her beta-hydroxybutyrate greater than 12 mM. After two or three days of starvation, when both acetoacetate and beta-hydroxybutyrate begin to increase, the normal arterial pH of 7.40 (after an over night fast) falls to about 7.34. This change in pH is a physiological event compatible with a mild metabolic acidosis of starvation. This decline in arterial pH does not cause the respiratory center in the brain to initiate labored breathing.

Starvation also has a marked impact on acetone levels. The concentration of acetone changes from near undetectable levels to about 1-2 mM after 21 days of starvation. Chances are that acetone continues to increase as the starvation ensues. Unlike acetoacetate and beta-hydroxybutyrate, acetone escapes from the body via the lungs and can be smelled in the breath. The range of acetoacetate plus beta-hydroxybutyrate concentrations from the fed (0.02 mM) to the prolonged starvation state (6-14 mM) varies over a 700-fold range. These changes in a healthy person's blood ketone bodies are not associated with abnormal metabolism. After ketone bodies are synthesized and released into the blood, tissues oxidize them as fuels. A balance between production, utilization and kidney conservation/loss occurs by day 18 of fasting.

The human body contains 20 different types of amino acids. And like glucose and ketone bodies, amino acids undergo changes in concentrations during starvation. Overall, there is a mild but progressive decrease. However, individual amino acids respond differently to starvation. These changes form roughly three or four distinct patterns

(Figure 3). Some amino acids rise and stay elevated, noticeably glycine. Others peak and then subsequently

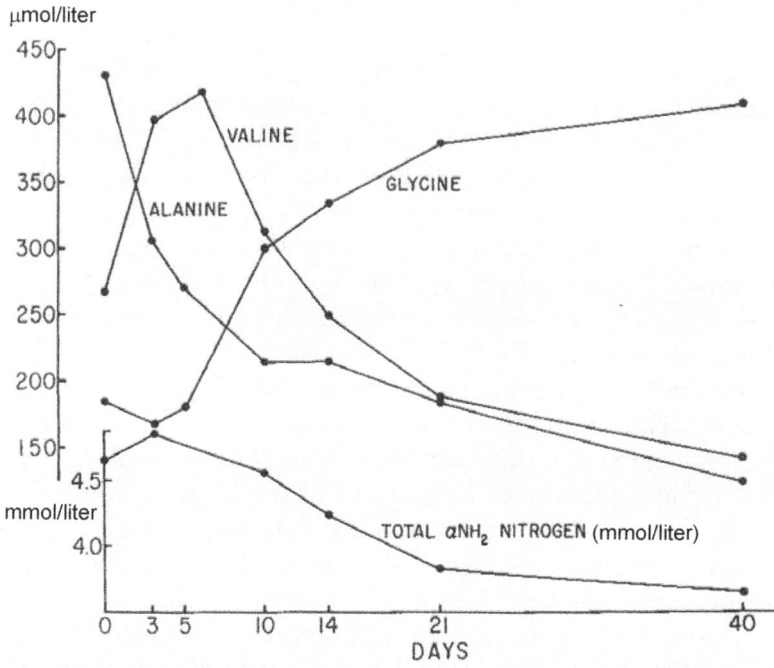

Figure 3. The bottom of the figure shows total alpha amino nitrogen which collectively reflects the changing concentration of total amino acids during starvation. However, individual amino acids show distinctive patterns. The key gluconeogenic acid undergoes a progressive decline in the first 40 days of starvation. Valine peaks at 7 days of starvation and falls thereafter. In contrast, glycine rises and plateaus only after 21 days of starvation. (Taken from Cahill, G.F., Jr., Starvation in man. *New Engl. J. Med.* **282:**668, 1970.) The major amino acid, glutamine, is not displayed. Its concentration is greater than the other amino acids, and it does not decrease during prolonged starvation.

decline. Alanine is the amino acid that has received the most attention from researchers studying starvation. In 1966, my friend and trusted colleague, Dr. Philip Felig, was the first to detect and describe the importance of this key amino acid in hepatic synthesis of new glucose.[4] Dr. Felig was a brilliant

---

[4] It was on Thanksgiving morning in 1966 that Dr. Felig discovered that alanine was the key amino acid mobilized from muscle and taken up by the liver and assumed to synthesize glucose during starvation. On this morning he was in the laboratory working because he had an amino acid

researcher with a remarkable ability to synthesize data. He was the primary person to delineate the behavior of amino acids, first in plasma (blood) and then during starvation. Dr. Felig went on to describe how amino acids responded to changes brought on by diet (consuming only protein vs. a balanced meal), exercise and mild diabetic states.

While working at Temple University, my team of researchers and I re-evaluated the area of amino acids in the blood. We paid particular attention to studying glutamine, an amino acid that had not been adequately analyzed. Glutamine comprises about 25% of amino acids in blood. Its concentration remains relatively constant during starvation. Our subsequent studies showed that, during starvation, glutamine was the principal amino acid used by the kidneys to synthesize ammonium for acid-base balance. This same study revealed that glutamine was crucial to synthesizing glucose into fuel for various tissues. However, glutamine's ability to mobilize amino acid carbon skeletons and nitrogen content from muscle to liver is diminished by its hidden partner, glutamic acid. Unlike glutamine, which is transported in plasma, glutamic acid travels inside red blood cells and behaves in an opposing manner to glutamine in the metabolism of these two amino acids. Thus, the impact of glutamine as the transport vehicle for amino acid carbon skeletons (and nitrogen) out of muscle to liver and kidney is exaggerated because its amino acid partner, glutamic acid, travels primarily inside of red blood cells and travels back to muscle from the liver. Moreover, although plasma carries glutamine from muscle to the liver and the kidneys, glutamate released from the liver carries the carbon skeleton of glutamine as glutamate inside red blood cells back to the muscle. There, glutamate picks up more nitrogen from other amino acids undergoing catabolism in muscle tissue. The reconstituted glutamine travels in plasma primarily to kidneys to form glucose and ammonium.

---

analyzing machine that needed attention. At that point alanine was shown to be the key amino acid extracted from the plasma by the liver. He continued his work and later confirmed that alanine was the principal amino acid converted into glucose by the liver during starvation.

Some people may ask how studying starving volunteers helps researchers to better understanding illnesses. How does studying the steady-state of starvation metabolism, which is beautifully orchestrated to supply fuel requirements in a finely regulated manner so that the provision of carbohydrates (glucose), amino acids and fats as fuels from various body stores exactly match the energy requirements of the organs of the body, help physicians and surgeons understand disease states? Simple answer: One needs to know normal behavior before one can identify disease state.

Doctors usually recognize severe forms of illness before they detect more subtle changes in metabolism like blood fuel and hormone fluctuations.

Summary

Our research team began studying metabolism in patients who were well fed and those who were starving at a time when methods for measuring blood fuels and hormones were accurate and available. The studies we conducted on fuel homeostasis were started at the right time and the right place. The Peter Bent Brigham Hospital and Joslin Research Laboratories at Harvard University had the resources to properly execute these clinical investigations. As time progressed, our analytical techniques improved, especially in the areas of blood (plasma/serum) free fatty acids, amino acids and insulin. Our team was able to delineate the three phases of starvation as post-absorptive (0-3 days), sub-acute (3-18 days) and prolonged (greater than 18 days). We also found that the time required to develop steady-state metabolism of fuels and hormones can vary and that it takes three days of starvation for blood glucose, plasma free fatty acids and serum insulin concentrations to become relatively constant. On average, it takes about 18 days of fasting before blood ketone body concentrations stabilize. And while individual blood amino acid concentrations can vary widely during weeks of starvation, level of one principal blood amino acid, glutamine, decreases very little. In the end, we concluded that different fuels and hormones require

73

their own time-line to develop into steady states in the blood. Nonetheless, we found that after 18 days of starvation, day-to-day changes in blood fuel and hormone concentrations are trivial and functional steady-states are achieved. It is at this point that the rate of fuels and hormones entering and exiting the blood reaches equilibrium.

Our studies on starvation metabolism demonstrated that starvation caused drastic changes in blood ketone body concentrations. These findings were the first of their kind. We found that patients tolerated metabolic adjustments during starvation very well. An explanation of how ketone bodies assured survival during food deprivation was something that the research community needed. And although it was safe to assume that the liver contributed ketone bodies to the bloodstream, we could only speculate on which organ was responsible for removing these fuels during starvation. Future studies were required to accurately identify the production rate and removal sites of ketone bodies.

Chapter IV. Nutrition, Biochemistry and Physiology

How can a physician/surgeon treat a disease if he/she doesn't know what is normal?

A simplified overview of nutrition, biochemistry and physiology may help to clarify the content of this book. Eating delicious foods is a pleasant experience. Obesity results from natural instincts to eat an excessive amount of food when it is available. Over half the people in the United States consume more nutrients than their bodies need to remain lean. The imbalance causes them to become fat. After individuals become obese and their physical activity diminishes, their weight is maintained even though the quantity of food (calories) ingested by them may not be any more than that consumed by humans who are not fat. Nonetheless, it is clear that they have eaten more than their bodies require to stay lean. The consequences of food indiscretions or functional addiction can be severe in some people who become morbidly obese with awkward body motions and physical limitations. Some have foul smelling odors because overlapping skin maintains moisture and creates fertile ground for fungal infections. In addition, complications from diabetes mellitus with excessive thirst, urgent urination and fungal infections (candida), and hypertension with strokes and heart failure may compromise their lives. Some with general low self-esteem and self-deprecation create a population that needs compassionate considerations. What a mess overindulgence can bring! Preciously little sympathy is aroused among the healthy minority, the lean. When physicians are confronted with patients suffering from the miseries of morbid obesity, hopefully they can have the knowledge and sympathy needed to help. The physician's responsibility is to comfort or eliminate the distress encountered by compromised or sick persons. Sometimes physicians fall short in this regard.

This chapter is not another compilation of good foods or recommended diets. There are enough excellent monographs on healthy nutrition. Rather, it contains a tale of a clinical investigator who was enthusiastic about solving the mysteries of human survival during adverse states.

Starvation was the first condition chosen as an instrument to understand human metabolism, and it was generally believed that morbidly obese people would benefit from prolonged periods of fasting. This chapter concentrates on survival during starvation and how the various organ systems supply, convert, conserve and select fuels for the body. It also provides information needed to grasp the intricacies of fuel utilization by the body.

When we began our studies of prolonged starvation in humans we assumed it would take about 40 days of food deprivation to develop a nutritional steady state. After years of research we learned, however, that after about 18 days of total starvation (supplemented with water), a near-steady state developed where the day-to-day change in blood fuels and hormones, urinary excretion rates, energy requirements and body compositional changes were relatively small. This steady state provided a clinical situation where if a perturbation was introduced its effect could be evaluated, e.g. giving a starving volunteer a small amount of sugar to eat.

The foods humans eat and absorb from the gut or the flesh they mobilize from the body have components that are toxic and must be cleared from the body. The body has three major routes for excreting unwanted materials, through the breath, urine and feces. During prolonged starvation defecation practically stops.

There are several ways to categorize food groups. It is important for adults to eat enough food to get the calories (energy) the body needs to function and repair itself. Meats, vegetables, fruits, dairy products, oils, eggs, nuts, etc. are eaten, digested, absorbed and converted into glucose, amino acids and triglycerides (fats). All are building-blocks or energy-yielding fuels. Vitamins are cofactors for enzymes (catalysts) essential to build or break down body parts for sources of energy. Minerals must maintain the salt content of fluids in the body. Essential nutrients must be eaten because the body cannot synthesize them. Minerals and most vitamins are essential, as well as some fats, carbohydrates and amino acids. After nutrients are eaten, digested and absorbed they are stored or slowly oxidized (burned) to provide energy for bodily functions. Carbohydrates and fats are composed mainly of carbon, hydrogen, and oxygen. The by-products of carbohydrate and fat breakdown are carbon dioxide (carbon and oxygen), water (hydrogen and oxygen), and available energy. This energy, contained in carbohydrates and fats, is released during the breakdown process. In periods that are only hours between meals, carbohydrates and fats provide 80-85% of the fuel requirements. The carbon dioxide from slowly burning these fuels is excreted from the body through the lungs (breath) and the energy eventually dissipated as heat.

Proteins usually contribute the remaining 15% of the energy needs between meals. Ingested proteins are cleaved in the gut into amino acids (there are 20 amino acids), each of which possesses nitrogen; some also possess sulfur in addition to carbon, hydrogen and oxygen. During and immediately after a meal, amino acids are used to replace those amino acids that were used by the body or mobilized during the periods between meals. At this phase of amino acid metabolism, the nitrogen components of amino acids must be converted to urea, ammonia, urate and creatinine to be excreted by the kidneys. Gaseous nitrogen is not lost via the lungs. Sulfur from amino acids, phosphorus from lipids, and other minerals are also excreted in the urine. The average nitrogen content of amino acid is about 16%. Therefore, if a person eats 100 grams of protein and digests and absorbs the amino acids, and if the quantity lost from the body is equal to the quantity absorbed (steady-state), practically 16 grams of nitrogen are excreted in the urine. In humans, two simple amino acids, alanine and glutamine, serve as primary vehicles for transporting the nitrogen content from other amino acids in the body parts (muscle proteins) to the liver for glucose and urea synthesis and to the kidneys for glucose and ammonia (ammonium) synthesis. Glucose is released into the blood, and urea and ammonium ions are excreted in the urine.

The lungs take up oxygen and put out carbon dioxide. The heart pumps blood through the body to deliver oxygen and fuels and to remove the major by-product, carbon dioxide. In adults, cardiac output is about 5 liters per minute. An approximation of where this blood flows is useful for understanding body metabolism. At rest, about 1 liter of cardiac output flows to each of the following organs: brain, liver and kidney. The remaining 2 liters of blood go to the rest of the body, primarily the muscles of the extremities. The brain is the master computer with nerves to every reach of the body. It has a large energy requirement. The liver is the chief fuel refinery of the body. It not only synthesizes needed proteins, it removes toxins. Its major metabolic function is to supply the brain with fuel for energy requirements. The brain and liver sizes and functions are tightly coupled. The kidneys are much smaller and receive a large blood supply that is grossly out of proportion to their metabolic energy needs. Their primary task is to cleanse the blood of excessive salts and by-products of metabolism - excrete protein waste products such as nitrogen, phosphorous and sulfur - and to maintain the consistency of body fluids. Muscle serves to move the body. At rest muscle energy requirements are relatively small, considering muscle is the largest organ system of the body. Exercise markedly increases blood flow and energy requirements for muscles. Adipose (fatty) tissue has a low energy requirement per unit weight. Its functions are primarily to serve as a "fuel tank," storing fuel for the rest of the body, and to cushion the body and keep it warm. During prolonged starvation the adipose tissue supplies more than 90% of the total body energy requirements. During fasting, the liver extracts large quantities of fatty acids for synthesis of ketone bodies (acetoacetate and beta-hydroxybutyrate) and releases them into the blood mainly for brain and, to a lesser degree, other tissues that need them as a source of fuel (Figure 1).

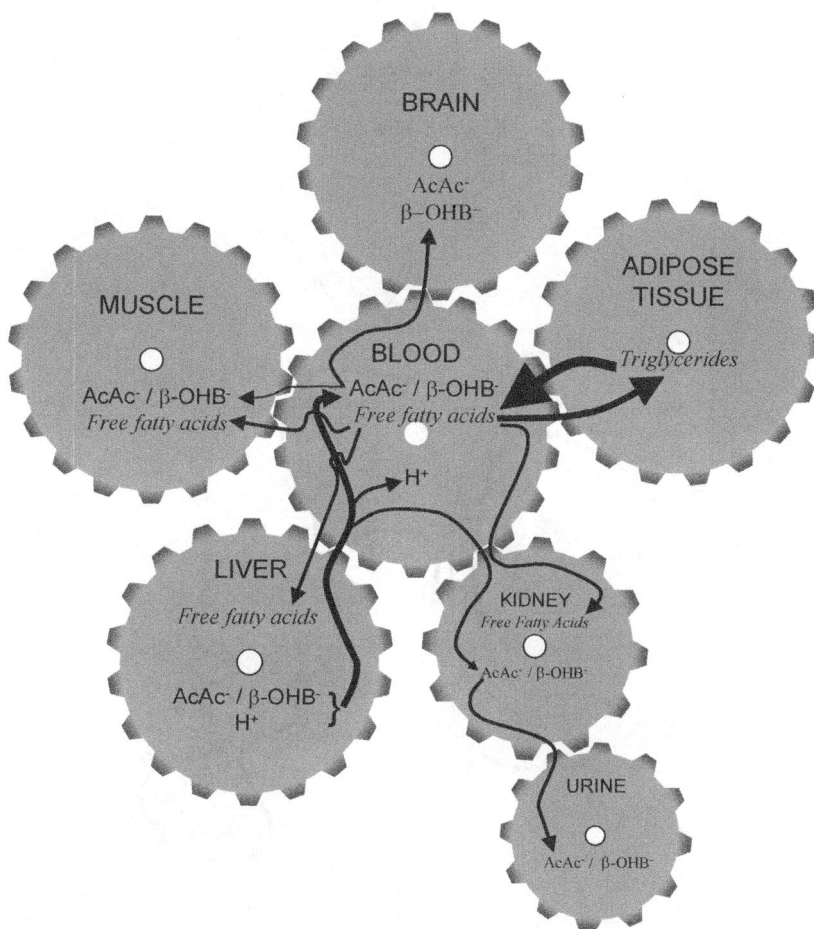

Figure 1. The organs of the body are in lock-step to provide the energy needs of the body during starvation. About 25% of the free fatty acids released into the blood and not recycled to adipose tissue is converted into ketone bodies.

Triglycerides, stored in adipose tissue, release free fatty acids, two-thirds of which are recycled. These are lipids laden with energy, providing fuel for much of the body, particularly muscle. Practically all of the fat can be mobilized for fuel before death occurs. During fasting periods, muscle breaks down its proteins and releases amino acids. Only one-half of the protein mass can be mobilized before death occurs (Figure 2). The liver, the refinery,

79

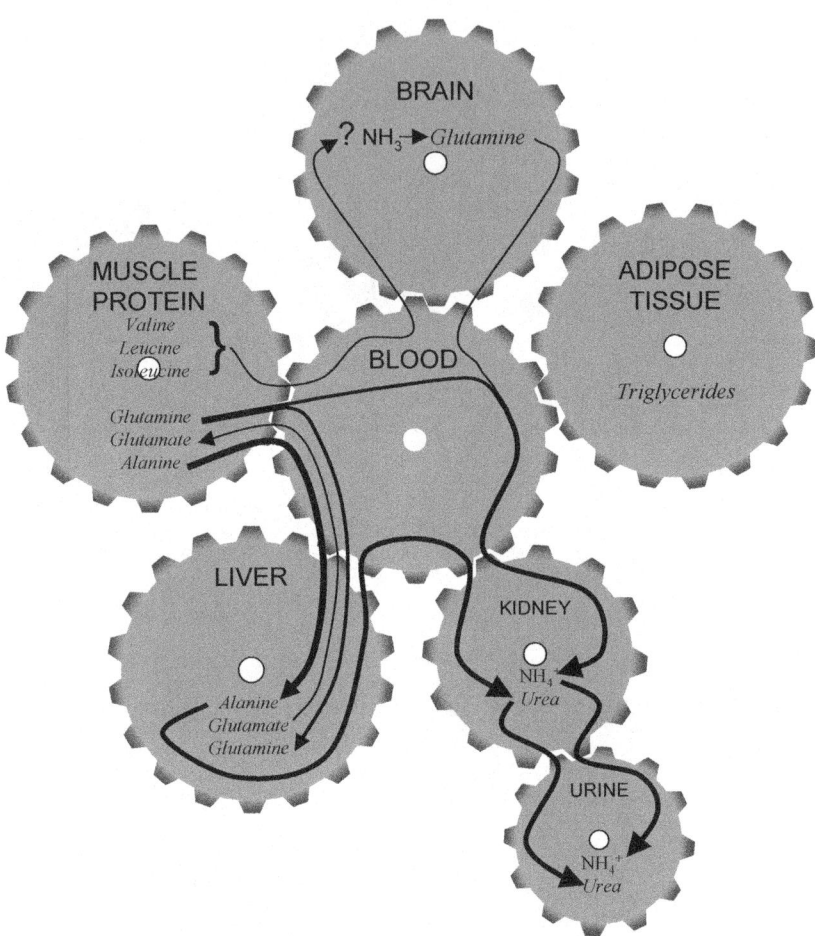

Figure 2. Muscle protein has the largest available supply of amino acids mobilized during prolonged starvation. Alanine is the principal amino acid transported to the liver for conversion into glucose and urea. Glutamine is the other major amino acid transported, but it is carried to the kidney for conversion into glucose and ammonia (ammonium). Glutamate carries the carbon skeleton of glutamine inside red blood cells back to muscle to be converted back into glutamine needed to transfer more amino acid nitrogen to the liver and kidney.

receives amino acids, glycerol and acetone [derived from fat stores (adipose tissue)], and other precursors, primarily recycled lactate and pyruvate [derived from muscle, red blood cells, and brain] , and converts them into glucose (Figure 3).

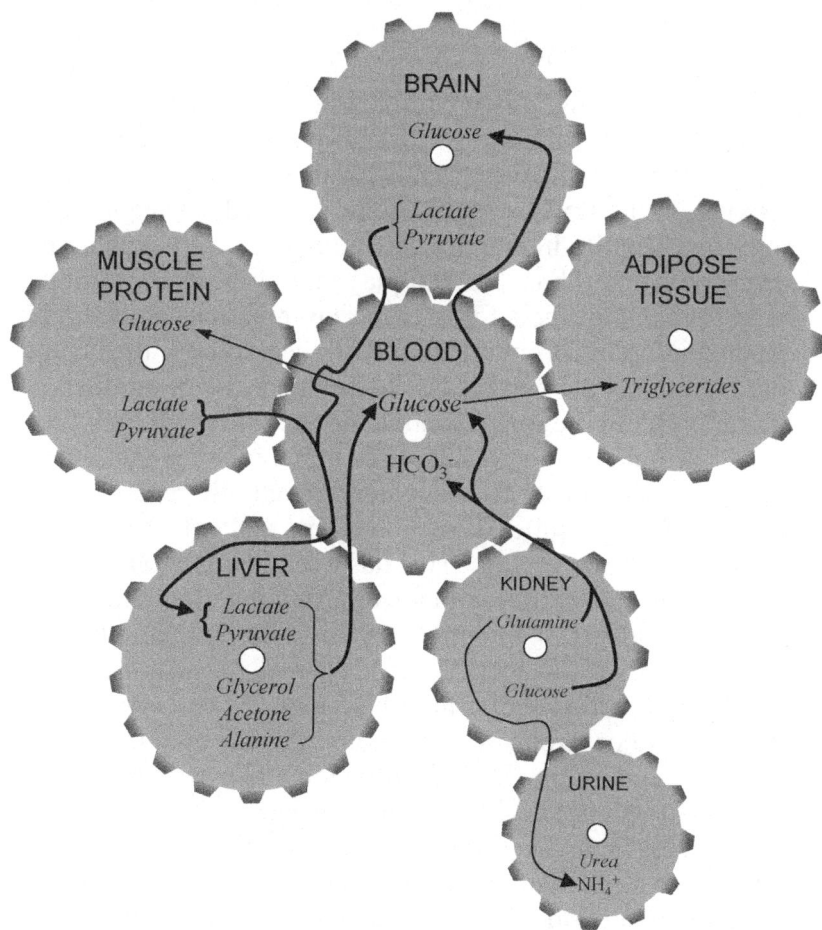

Figure 3. The liver and kidney share the role in synthesizing glucose and releasing it into the blood to support the metabolic needs of tissues during prolonged starvation.

Energy is the most crucial component of life. Cells in the body extract energy from food in the fed state and derive energy from stored fuels in the starved state. Metabolism is the sum of all biochemical processes within a living organism. Metabolic pathways that regulate energy generation or energy use in biological processes are common and simple. Those biological reactions that provide cellular energy are called catabolic reactions, or catabolism. Those

81

reactions that require energy, such as the synthesis of proteins, fats and carbohydrates (glucose) are called anabolic reactions, or anabolism. Energy (and heat) is released in the process of breaking down complex materials derived from fat, protein and carbohydrate into more simple products. The body uses energy-rich fuels for its energy-requiring activities. The flow of fuels for energy needs throughout the body may require interactions by complex systems engaging several organs. Thus, the interplay among organs within the body to maintain fuels for energy requirements can be highly dependent upon communication with each other: the cells of one organ may have to be assisted by the cells of another organ to obtain the full potential energy possessed by a fuel.

A fundamental principle of metabolism is that the number of carbon atoms that enter a metabolic reaction cycle must equal the number of carbon atoms that exit the metabolic reaction cycle. This has been likened to a traffic circle where the number of cars entering the circle must equal the number of cars that exit the circle to maintain function.

Eventually, fuels enter the metabolic [tricarboxylic (TCA) cycle or Krebs cycle (synonyms)] cycle. This cycle serves as a common pathway in which a two-carbon molecule (acetate) derived from fatty acids, glucose and amino acids is destined for oxidation. Acetate becomes attached to an activating factor (CoA) to form acetyl CoA.

Conversion of a fuel to acetate is not always accomplished in one organ. This is especially true for amino acids where some of the carbon atoms in the molecules may enter the TCA cycle but cannot all be converted to CO_2, and some of the carbon components must exit the cycle. The entry of a compound into the TCA cycle occurs by a process known as *anaplerosis* (to fill up), and exits as another compound containing part of the parent compound carbon by a process known as *cataplerosis* (to drain down). This balance is displayed in Figure 4. The metabolites that are

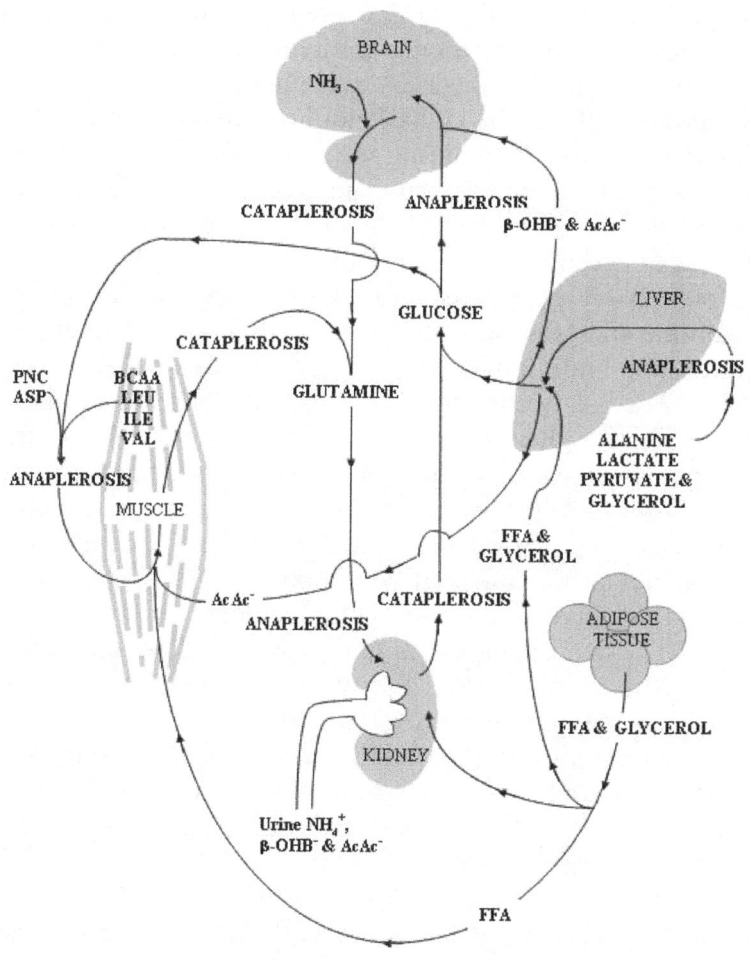

Figure 4. Anaplerotic and cataplerotic reactions in the major organ systems of the body. The inter-organ fluxes of fuels are highlighted by glucose and glutamine. AcAc⁻, acetoacetate; ASP, aspartate; ß-OHB⁻, ß-hydroxybutyrate; BCAA, branched-chain amino acid; FFA, free fatty acid; LEU, leucine; ILE, isoleucine; NH_3, ammonia; NH_4^+, ammonium; PNC, purine nucleotide cycle; VAL, valine.

routed through anaplerotic and cataplerotic reactions are highlighted by the inter-organ transport of glutamine and glucose. Glutamine drains the carbon skeleton (and nitrogen component) added to the TCA cycle by amino acids (leucine, isoleucine, valine and others). Glutamine travels through the blood and is added to the TCA cycle in the kidney. Glutamine replaces the alpha-ketoglutarate consumed (drained) in the kidney during the synthesis of glucose which is added to the blood. Thus the addition of carbon compounds added to the TCA cycle by anaplerosis equals the loss of carbon compounds from the TCA cycle by cataplerosis. Figure 4 displays the interdependence of glutamine and glucose metabolism among muscle, liver, kidney, and brain (and adipose tissue) for metabolism.

The balance of carbon atoms that enter and exit is maintained for glucose, fatty acids and amino acids. During the final stages of catabolism in the TCA cycle the carbon atoms from fuels (glucose, fatty acids and amino acids) enter the cycle as two-carbon units (acetyl CoA) and exit the cycle as two one-carbon units (carbon dioxide). The CoA remains behind to receive another acetyl molecule.

The heart pumps a large quantity of blood through the kidneys every minute. The watery component of the blood (plasma) and its various compounds are filtered through a million small membranous sieves which separate the water dissolved compounds from blood cells and particles. The fluid formed by the filtration process travels toward the small tubules and into the collecting system in the center of the kidneys and finally into the bladder; urine is formed. More than 99% of the initially filtered water, salts and other valuables is reabsorbed by the kidney before the final quantity of concentrated nitrogen waste and salt compounds are collected in the urinary bladder and discharged from the body. (See Chapter VII, Liver and Kidney Metabolism in "Normal" Adults.)

In the animal kingdom an accumulation of nitrogenous compounds in the body is incompatible with life. There are four nitrogenous compounds that animals excrete. Two are complex compounds: urate and creatinine. Two are simple compounds: urea and ammonia (ammonium ion). Birds combine urine and feces in a common excretory channel (cloaca; sewer) and expel a white chalky nitrogenous waste product that dresses automobile roofs, statues and windowsills. It is mostly <u>urate</u> (which causes gout in humans). Sharks lose a majority of their excessive nitrogen through their gills as ammonia which is pumped out of these organs and into the sea water as it flows through them. The urea and ammonia (actually, the ion, ammonium), the principal nitrogenous products in mammals, are readily smelled in animal barnyards. Fed humans discharge nitrogen from the body primarily as urea in the urine. During prolonged starvation, ammonium ion, becomes the dominant form of urinary nitrogen discharged from the body. Humans also excrete a small amount of nitrogen as urate. In addition, humans discharge part of the remnant energy of muscle housed in creatine as creatinine. These four nitrogenous compounds (urea, ammonium, urate and creatinine) make up 99% of the nitrogen excreted from the body by humans in the fed and starved states.

It is wrong to assume that meaningful discoveries in biomedical laboratories are predominantly transferred from the research bench to a patient in bed. The reverse is true. Discoveries made from studying humans can often be explored more in depth in laboratory animals to gain further insight into the clinical problems; not vice versa. In fact, the translation of basic science findings into medical practice for humans has been dismal. If society wants to cure human ailments, then people must volunteer for experimental studies. Of course, the welfare of human subjects dominates clinical investigation.

Before 1967 it was generally thought that the brain could derive its energy only from glucose. However, with time, biochemical and mathematical considerations brought this assumption into question. It was believed that, during fasting, the liver removed precursors from the blood and converted them into glucose for consumption by the brain. The by-products from glucose synthesis were nitrogenous compounds secreted in the urine. After an overnight fast, studies with humans who consumed large quantities of carbohydrates showed that the brain used an estimated 100-125 grams (3-4 ounces) of glucose daily. It was known that the liver stored about 150 grams (5 ounces) of glucose as glycogen. Muscle also stored about 75 grams (2-3 ounces) of glucose as glycogen. Muscle cannot release glucose directly from its stored glycogen; it converts glycogen to glucose and uses it for energy. Muscle can release lactate and pyruvate derived from glucose breakdown into the blood. Lactate and pyruvate circulate in the blood to the liver for conversion back to glucose, which the liver can release. This cycle has been termed the Cori cycle in honor of its discoverers. During the initial two to three days of starvation, the liver breaks down and releases glycogen as glucose into the blood. Small quantities of lactate and pyruvate may also be released from muscle and circulate to the liver for synthesis and release of glucose.

The recycling of lactate and pyruvate to the liver from the muscle produces no glucose oxidation to carbon dioxide (one carbon and two oxygens, CO_2) and water (two hydrogens and one oxygen, H_2O). During the Cori cycle there is no net loss or gain of carbon or water.

The quantity of glycogen stored in the body (liver and muscle) is only enough to supply glucose for the energy requirements of the brain for two to three days. Yet, it was well known that if humans only drank water they could fast for weeks, if not for months. The question became, how was this possible if the brain continued to use glucose as the only fuel?

Studies using rodents suggested that the liver synthesized glucose not only from lactate and pyruvate but also from glycerol derived from the breakdown of fat and amino acids from protein breakdown. The brain could then oxidize the glucose to CO_2 and H_2O. Biochemical pathways for glucose synthesis by the liver were clearly established and enzymatic machinery for doing this was augmented during fasting. In contrast to the Cori cycle, the brain breaks glucose down completely to the end products, CO_2 and H_2O. This results in a net loss of carbon dioxide and water (glucose) from the body. Where do the precursors come from that allowed glucose to be terminally burned (oxidized) to CO_2 and H_2O if the brain is obliged to use only glucose?

Ammonia (NH_3) is a gas that freely penetrates cell membranes whereas ammonium (NH_4^+) is a charged molecule. Ammonia is formed by the kidney cells surrounding the tubules containing fluid destined to become urine. Once ammonia enters the tubular space where urine is being formed, it is trapped as ammonium in the urine and is bound for excretion. It cannot readily diffuse back into the blood. Some of our studies done in the 1980's employing catheterization techniques for measuring renal exchange rates of ammonia (gas of ammonium) coupled with urinary excretion rates of ammonium reveal that about 1/3 of the ammonia produced in the kidneys escapes renal excretion. Ammonia is released into the blood for subsequent extraction by the liver (and other organs) where it is converted into urea, and thereafter excreted in the urine. Recent estimates of renal ammonia production and hepatic urea synthesis suggest that renal ammonia release could account for about one-half of the total urea excreted after 3 weeks of total starvation. It took a long time and a lot of work before we gained the knowledge related to total nitrogen excretion and the various components that comprised nitrogen excretion.

The interplay between the concentrations of thyroid hormones in the blood and urinary urea nitrogen and ammonium nitrogen excretion during starvation in humans is fascinating. The most potent thyroid hormone, T_3, is known to fall in concentration during starvation. This fall is associated with a decrease in urinary urea excretion and a subsequent increase in ammonium excretion. After about 18 days of total starvation urinary ammonium excretion exceeds urinary urea excretion. Thus, a fall in blood T_3 during starvation is followed by a shift of nitrogen excretion from urea to ammonium. This reversion is exactly the opposite pattern seen when the ammonia-excreting (ammoniotelic) tadpole is given T_3 to induce metamorphosis and convert the tadpole into a frog with urea-excreting (ureotelic) nitrogen.

Multiple processes have evolved to maintain a supply of fuels for the body during starvation. Ammoniagenesis and ureagenesis are closely related processes and both are coupled to amino acid breakdown (catabolism) following proteolysis, mostly from structural proteins, and specifically muscle. The carbon skeletons of amino acids are converted into glucose. As glucose release from the liver decreases, alternate fuels are needed. Fat stores are mobilized and ketone bodies are synthesized in liver. These valuable fuels replace glucose as the predominant source of energy for the brain. Ketone bodies are negatively charged compounds lost in the urine. They must be accompanied by positively charged compounds, principally ammonium (NH_4^+). All body fluids have restrictions on the concentrations of hydrogen (acid) allowed in them.

The loss of ketone bodies in the urine generates a complex, yet simple solution to providing part of the essential glucose needed by the body during starvation. There was a time that medical scientists thought that ketone bodies were filtered from the blood by the kidney and only a limited amount of these fuels could be reabsorbed by the kidney. This is not true. However, the body has an essential requirement for a small amount of glucose. Part of the glucose requirement is synthesized from the carbon skeleton of amino acids that surrenders its nitrogen to make ammonia.

Ketone bodies are negatively charged compounds in biological fluids. The urine, like all biological fluids, requires a high degree of electrical neutrality where negatively charged compounds are nearly matched by positively charged compounds. Ammonium is positively charged. Thus, the quantity of ammonium (NH_4^+) lost in the urine during starvation needs to be closely matched by the amount of ketone bodies (beta-hydroxybutyrate$^-$ plus acetoacetate$^-$) lost in the urine to maintain near electrical neutrality. The caloric content of ketone bodies lost in the urine during starvation (or a high protein-low carbohydrate diet) is trivial. However, the kidney's generation of glucose as a consequence of excreting ammonium is essential for survival during starvation. A reciprocal relationship between renal ammonium and glucose synthesis versus liver ketone bodies, glucose and urea synthesis exists.

NASA contacted Dr. George F Cahill, Jr. approximately 37-40 years ago seeking advice on survival of humans during periods of food deprivation with "space travels." He recommended sending up fat people with no food. He also suggested feeding astronauts tablets of sodium bicarbonate ($NaHCO_3$). I was working with him at that time (1967), and we did not understand that ketonuria was essential to generate ammonia and renal glucose. Because of my lack of understanding, I never interpreted and published the data we collected, and still have, on patients undergoing weeks of starvation and given oral $NaHCO_3$ or $NaCl$. Now, I realize that ketonuria is essential for renal gluconeogenesis (and ammoniagenesis). Ketone bodies are 47% oxygen derived from atmospheric oxygen. The loss of ammonium nitrogen in the urine is the most cost-effective way the body has of discharging a nitrogenous by-product. Thus, the loss of ammonium and ketone bodies in the urine is an extraordinarily efficient system for producing the small quantity of glucose that is essential for survival during starvation.

During a period of about 24 years, colleagues and I studied well over 1,000 volunteers and patients. Roughly 100 of these individuals were volunteers who underwent prolonged starvation studies. About half of the starving volunteers could not tolerate the prolonged hospitalization and/or the protocols. Nonetheless, those volunteer-patients were noble in their effort to promote the understanding of body metabolism: food intake, energy expenditure and organ behavior to store or mobilize fuels so the body maintains a near-steady state of metabolism during the resting, fed and starved states.

The most important task the body has during the fed and starvation states is to maintain a flux of fuels that perfectly matches the energy requirement of the various organs. In this process the body must conserve as much energy as is possible. Physical activity during starvation is usually limited, and most of the energy consumed is done in the resting state. Multiple processes have evolved to maintain a supply of fuels for the body organs during starvation.

Starvation studies showed that the organs of the body have more than one choice of fuel for survival. The body calls upon all of its organs to provide, select and conserve fuels.

Urinary excretion of nitrogenous compounds, predominantly urea and ammonium, suggested that the body's (brain's) consumption of glucose was curtailed during starvation. Alternative fuels were searched for and found.

Subsequent chapters provide detailed information regarding brain, liver, kidney, and muscle metabolism. Comparisons between the fed and fasted states are delineated.

Chapter V. Urine Reflects the Truth

In the book, *The Idiot*, Dostoyevsky used Marie (who was consumed by starvation and tuberculosis) to illustrate that if you understood poor health and suffering you could clearly and simply recognize the discomfort experienced by others. Although I believe I understand some of the causes of obesity and why starvation was studied to comprehend how the body supplied fuels needed by the various organs during food deprivation, I find it difficult to explain how the excretion of nitrogenous compounds in the urine were instrumental in our research to delineate brain metabolism in humans.

In this chapter emphasis is placed on urine because the first, but poorly defined, clues that biochemists and physicians had misconceptions regarding survival mechanisms in starvation, and perhaps other states, arose from urinary excretion rates of nitrogen.

The fundamental job before me is to state how the analyses of urine led to insightful thoughts regarding the need to reevaluate energy sources for organs, especially the brain, during starvation.

How on earth can any author make a tale about excreting urine interesting? Maybe it is not so difficult when it is recalled that urine was among the first specimens available to biomedical scientists for studying the human body. Urine is used to detect poisons, anemia, pregnancy, infections, kidney diseases, diabetes mellitus and other endocrine diseases, narcotic use, heart failure, malnutrition and numerous other disorders. Therefore, it is reasonable to expect that adults would be able to grasp the clues provided from analyzing urine to develop new perspectives on whole body and individual organ metabolism.

Urine is normally light amber in color and has a characteristic, peculiar and pungent odor. The quantity excreted from the body usually reflects the body's hydration status. The daily excretion rate is one to two liters (1-2 quarts). Urine is the primary way the body excretes the breakdown products from ingested proteins and body proteins and excess ingested body salts and toxins. Drinking urine provides no useful benefit when dying from dehydration because it usually has a higher content of excretory products than body fluids, particularly during dehydration. Urine reflects healthy and diseased states and contains many clues to understand these states. The daily urinary nitrogenous excretion rates not only reflect the moment-to-moment fluctuations which occur in metabolic processes across one organ, but also integrate the metabolism across all organ beds (liver, kidney, brain, extremities, etc.). Collecting all the urine a patient eliminates at 24-hour time intervals is not as easy as it may seem. A patient half asleep gets up in the middle of the night and urinates in the toilet and flushes it before he/she remembers that the entire amount of urine needs to be collected for analysis. It costs at least $1,000 per day to study a patient or volunteer in the hospital. Lost specimens are lost time, money and results. One of the differences between an excellent clinical research center (hospital) and a poor research center is the ability to accurately collect specimens (urine, blood, sputum, etc.) and retrieve laboratory data that are needed to define the problem under investigation.

Urinary excretion of nitrogen during prolonged starvation provided the first inkling that some of the concepts from biomedical sciences regarding survival during fasting were wrong. In the mid 1960's millions of dollars were spent on research to determine how the liver was able to synthesize enough sugar (glucose) to meet the body's requirements for energy from this fuel. The body absolutely has an essential need for glucose to survive. However, the quantity needed for survival is far less than that hypothesized in the 1960's. This mistake was largely due to the misconception that the brain had to have a quantity of glucose for normal function that was grossly overestimated. The liver was thought to be the primary if not the sole organ that contributed glucose to the blood for brain energy requirements. Most of the work on glucose synthesis was done on the liver from animal models, usually the mouse, rat, and guinea pig. The pathways for forming glucose from compounds that can be converted to glucose were demonstrated in these animal models. However, the quantity of glucose released from the liver could not be measured from slices or homogenates of liver (or kidney). Further, the brains of these animals did not need much glucose because of their small sizes or ratios of brain to body mass. Humans have the largest brain-to-body ratio in the animal kingdom. The brain requires a constant delivery of fuel to supply its energy requirements to permit function. The brain is encased in the skull which prevents it from expanding to store fuels. Energy for the nervous system must be mobilized from other organs and delivered by the blood in the fed and starved states. It took human studies to delineate the fuel requirements for human beings.

During starvation the stores of fuels in tissues are mobilized and consumed. Waste products are eliminated almost entirely through urine (nitrogen) and breath (carbon dioxide). During starvation, defecation usually stops and the gut has a trivial energy requirement. As noted in Chapter III, Fuels and Hormones, glycogen availability is limited, but fat stores and protein supplies are available for many weeks. Only a small quantity of glucose can be derived from fat stores. The major source of new glucose is from amino acids derived from protein breakdown (largely muscle). A cardinal characteristic of amino acids is presence of nitrogen in each of the 20 amino acids that make up protein. *The conversion of an amino acid to glucose, a compound with no nitrogen, results in the formation and release of nitrogenous waste by-products that must be excreted in the urine.* The accumulation of nitrogenous waste compounds can be lethal; they must be excreted in the urine. Thus, if amino acids are converted to glucose to provide fuel for the brain, nitrogen has to be excreted in the urine. The approximate ratio of urinary nitrogen excreted to glucose formation was established. Therefore, if the quantity of urinary nitrogen excreted is measured, the quantity of glucose synthesized from the remaining carbon skeletons of amino acids could be estimated.

A large quantity of blood flows through the kidney every minute. The kidneys maintain fluid, electrolyte (salts) and acid-base balance (near neutral) and rid the body of waste products. The body has two kidneys, each about the size of a human fist. Each kidney receives its blood supply from a large artery. These arteries divide repeatedly until they form small arteries (arterioles) which split into a cascade of minute, web-like structures that ultimately function as sieves or filters which are part of the functional unit of the kidney, the "nephron" (Figure 1). Each kidney

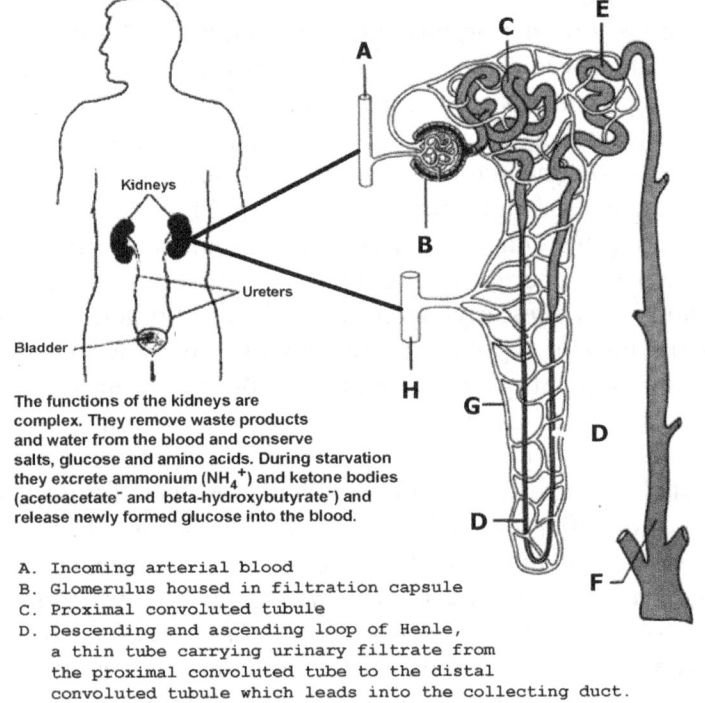

The functions of the kidneys are complex. They remove waste products and water from the blood and conserve salts, glucose and amino acids. During starvation they excrete ammonium (NH_4^+) and ketone bodies (acetoacetate⁻ and beta-hydroxybutyrate⁻) and release newly formed glucose into the blood.

A. Incoming arterial blood
B. Glomerulus housed in filtration capsule
C. Proximal convoluted tubule
D. Descending and ascending loop of Henle, a thin tube carrying urinary filtrate from the proximal convoluted tube to the distal convoluted tubule which leads into the collecting duct.
E. Distal convoluted tubule
F. Cortical collecting duct leading to renal pelvis which is connected to the bladder
G. Capillaries leading to outgoing venous blood
H. Venous blood leading to the major vein flowing toward the heart

Figure 1. Nephron – the functional unit of the kidney: a tiny coiled tube with a "bulb" at the end.

has about one million nephrons. Each nephron consists of a filter, a cluster of tortuous vessels (glomerulus) permeable to small molecules derived from the arterial blood supply. The filtrate is collected in a surrounding space and funneled to a tiny tube (tubule). Downstream from where the small arteries became capillaries in the glomerulus they rejoin to form another set of arterioles that divide into the second group of capillaries that run along adjacent to the tubules and serve to reabsorb most of the filtrate produced through the glomerular sieves, leaving the molecules to be excreted remaining in the tubule. The capillaries rejoin to form venules that coalesce with numerous other venules to form the renal vein which returns the reconstituted blood to the body's large venous system. About 180 liters/day of fluid are filtered through the kidney's sieves. Approximately 99% of this fluid is reabsorbed during the passage down/along the tubules. The remaining fluid in the tubule is a concentration of nitrogen compounds, salts and other waste products. Practically all of the glucose present in blood entering the kidney is reabsorbed by the kidney of healthy humans. The remaining concentrate in the tubule is sent to the center of the kidney and then into the urinary bladder for storage before being expelled as urine.

Twenty-four hour urinary excretion rates are among the most accurate measurements made in a research laboratory. As noted above, it was the daily urinary nitrogen excretion rate that provided useful insight into the production rate of glucose from amino acids during starvation.

For each gram of nitrogen excreted in the urine, the liver and kidney synthesize about 3.6 grams of glucose. After two to three days of starvation the liver is functionally depleted of glycogen and the urinary excretion of nitrogen is only 8-9 grams/day. Multiplying the grams of urinary nitrogen by the grams of glucose equivalent (8-9 x 3.6) gives an estimate of glucose production from amino acids, which is somewhere between 29-32 grams per day. There are another 20 or so grams/day of glucose that can be derived from other materials which can be burned to CO_2 and H_2O. Nonetheless, the quantity of glucose that can be totally oxidized to CO_2 and water is less than the100-125 grams/day previously believed to be needed by the nervous system.

95

Brain function is normal after weeks to months of starvation. Urinary nitrogen excretion continues to decline as starvation progresses. Therefore, some fuel other than glucose must provide the energy for the brain during starvation.

When we began studying metabolic adaptations during starvation in humans we did not know how long a person should fast and what fuels would be used by specific tissues. Further, once new insight began to accumulate, the energy requirements of all organs and the body as a whole had to be reevaluated.

Only one or two clinical investigators thought that during fasting there was not enough nitrogen in the urine to account for the alleged amount of glucose the brain was thought to need for normal function. However, accurate, reproducible urinary excretion rates of nitrogenous compounds were not widely known. Therefore, clinical investigators had to develop protocols for studying people to gather data about urinary nitrogen excretion and couple the data with oxygen consumption and carbon dioxide excretion.

By the middle of the 1960's obesity was noticeably on the rise in the USA. People whose weights were twice that predicted by the Metropolitan Life Insurance Tables had a two-fold risk of dying compared to age- and sex-matched individuals with the average weights for heights. Providing adequate water for drinking was given, starvation was the classic method for reducing body weight. Some insurance companies would pay for brief hospitalization of patients to undergo periods of starvation to initiate a weight reduction process thought to be most worthy of the expense. Dr. George F. Cahill, Jr. and I thought that if patients were going to be subjected to starvation they should be thoroughly studied.

The purpose of starving people was two-fold. First, doctors wanted to help patients lose weight, especially if they suffered from morbid obesity (200% of ideal body weight) and were subjected to premature death; and second, a few doctors wanted to study the processes of starvation so they could learn what was safe for patients: How did people maintain the appropriate supply of energy to meet the needs

96

of the brain, liver, muscle, kidney and other organs during starvation, and what were the warning signs, if any, of impending danger from starvation? When our pioneering studies of starvation were initiated in the mid-1960's, clinical scientists knew very little about how the body maintained its energy requirements so people could safely tolerate food deprivation.

When I arrived at Harvard, Dr. Cahill was "on the speakers' circuit." He frequently traveled to various cities to address medical audiences regarding metabolism. Dr. V.K. Vance of Buffalo, New York, was aware of Dr. Cahill's interest in starvation. He referred an obese nurse with chest pain to Dr. Cahill for evaluation and for prolonged and radical fasting. The patient, Ms. B., was motivated from fear of having a heart attack. Her father had died from a heart attack and her mother had suffered several heart attacks (myocardial infarctions). Ms. B. worked as an assistant director of nursing service in Buffalo. She was large at birth and during childhood, and her weight during nursing training varied from 180 to 200 pounds. Her weight continued to increase. At 39 years of age she weighed 260 pounds. Her resting metabolic rate and thyroid functions were normal. As she grew larger, her physical activities had decreased. She recognized she had a lifetime history of excessive eating. Intermittently, she experienced several episodes of feeling suffocated. In addition, she had infrequent feelings of substernal, oppressive pain radiating to her left shoulder blade and down the left arm to the elbow. She had used nitroglycerine for angina with questionable benefit. Her weight continued to increase before being admitted to the hospital for diagnostic and research studies.

Physical examination revealed a large framed woman with generalized plethora (redness) and gross obesity. Her body weight was 280 lbs., her height was 5 feet 8 inches, and her blood pressure was borderline elevated at 140/90. She was a bright, pleasant, and mature person. Her plasma total cholesterol had been elevated to 360 mg/100 ml (definition for "normal" is changing, but probably <165 mg/100 ml), and her fasting blood glucose was 112 mg/dl (normal <110 mg/dl). Other routine laboratory tests were normal. Her resting electrocardiograms did not suggest she had inadequate circulation of blood to the heart. More sophisticated noninvasive tests had either not been developed or evaluated in 1965. From her history, however, it was thought that she had insufficient blood flow through her heart. The most definitive test for determining blood flow through the heart was coronary angiography with left ventriculography. These tests required placing catheters into a peripheral artery in the thigh or forearm and threading the catheter into the coronary arteries and into the major chambers of the heart and filling these sites with contrast dye that could be seen on x-rays. [At that time in the medical history of evaluating heart blood flow, the major vein of the heart (coronary sinus) was also catheterized to measure arteriovenous lactate concentration differences to reflect the lack of oxygen availability for the heart muscle.]

In 1965, a service/research catheterization laboratory with imaging (x-ray) equipment could usually only do about 5 studies a week. After 1998, a proficient diagnostic catheterization laboratory could do about 14 studies in an eight-hour period. It is now a different medical world!

At the time Ms. B. was hospitalized on The Clinical Center of Peter Bent Brigham Hospital, none of us knew that she was godsend. She understood the research starvation protocol and the catheterization studies that were planned in addition to her diagnostic heart studies. She admired Dr. Cahill, and Ms. B. and I developed a mutual trust. I never wavered in my commitment to protect her or any other patient-volunteer's welfare. Ms. B. knew how 24-hour urinary collections were supposed to be done, and she was compulsive in voiding urine and collecting her specimens accurately. The other patient-volunteers followed the pattern she and the researchers developed.

Dr. Cahill and I had another blessing on The Clinical Center of Peter Bent Brigham Hospital. There was a tremendously motivated hospital orderly who wanted to go to medical school but did not have the financial means to do so. While helping us oversee the health of the obese volunteers and collecting the specimens for analysis, he received notice that he had been granted a 6-year scholarship to a medical school in Great Britain, effective the following year. He was a key figure in executing the early obesity and starvation experiments. We learned a great deal from the studies with this first obese patient who underwent prolonged starvation, and subsequent studies were largely based on the information gathered from the data obtained from Ms. B.

During a noontime teaching session at the Peter Bent Brigham Hospital in Boston where the starving patients were studied, someone asked me why we chose the six-week period. I replied that "Jesus fasted forty days and forty nights; he was afterward an hungered" (St. Matthew 4:2, King James version).

After Ms. B. fasted 41 days and lost 54 pounds she underwent diagnostic cardiac and research catheterization studies.[5]

After the brain and liver research catheterization studies were completed, selective right and left coronary artery cine-angiography was performed. During right coronary artery injection, the patient developed ventricular

---

[5] In writing this book I rummaged through some of my medical souvenirs. I found a letter dictated by Dr. Cahill on October 8, 1965, to the personnel of The Clinical Center. It stated that, "It has been shown by many laboratories that during a prolonged fast, the amount of nitrogen in the urine falls to extremely low levels, such as a gram per 24 hours." (This turned out not to be true.) "Only a small quantity of glucose can be synthesized from this small amount of protein and one is then faced with the question as to what supplies the necessary fuel for the central nervous system during a prolonged fast … We will monitor her urinary nitrogen … and repeat the glucose turnover. If the turnover indeed should be markedly diminished, this will be proof that her central nervous system is capable of utilizing some other fuels such as ketone bodies." (The glucose turnover studies were never completed.) "It is then our hope (if patient-volunteer agrees) to perform cardiac catheterization at which time fuel balance (utilization) across the myocardium (heart muscle) can be ascertained and possibly the catheter can be turned up into the jugular bulb in order to do a cerebral blood flow and A.V. (arteriovenous) differences across the brain." The authors were Drs. G.F. Cahill, Jr., M.G. Herrera, O.E. Owen and N. Ruderman.

fibrillation which lasted approximately 20 seconds. She was reverted to a normal rhythm with an electrical shock. Although her abnormal heartbeat was rapidly corrected, it created considerable physician anxiety. Before this serious and potentially fatal ventricular arrhythmia developed, multiple simultaneous blood samples had been taken from the major artery, the aorta, and major vein, internal jugular vein, to measure brain extraction of glucose, oxygen and ketone bodies (beta-hydroxybutyrate and acetoacetate) and production of CO_2, lactate and pyruvate. In addition, a hepatic vein was catheterized to measure liver production of glucose, ketone bodies and other exchangeable materials.

On the day of the vascular catheterization study we had not analyzed all of Ms. B.'s 24-hour urinary specimens. However, we knew that her urinary excretion of nitrogen was low. Therefore, we expected that the brain was deriving its energy from a fuel or fuels other than glucose. We expected that ketone bodies, beta-hydroxybutyrate and its redox couple, acetoacetate, were the likely fuels that the brain was using after prolonged starvation. Further, we expected that the liver's production of glucose was low. However, it was extraordinarily low, less than the diminished quantity of glucose extracted by the brain. Thus, our accounting of glucose consumption and utilization showed a deficit. Hepatic production of glucose was inadequate to account for the brain's low extraction of glucose. What was happening in the body to allow life to continue with normal brain function during starvation? Clues to where the glucose was being produced during starvation only came forth later when the urine was analyzed not only for total nitrogen, but for the various components that made up the total nitrogen (urea, ammonium, urate and creatinine nitrogen). The clues from analyzing urine of many starving volunteers to overall body metabolism were evaluated and re-evaluated several times.

The findings displayed in Figure 2 took years to accumulate, analyze and display. They are inconspicuous but display the crux of this chapter on urinary excretion. They show the average daily total urinary nitrogen excretion

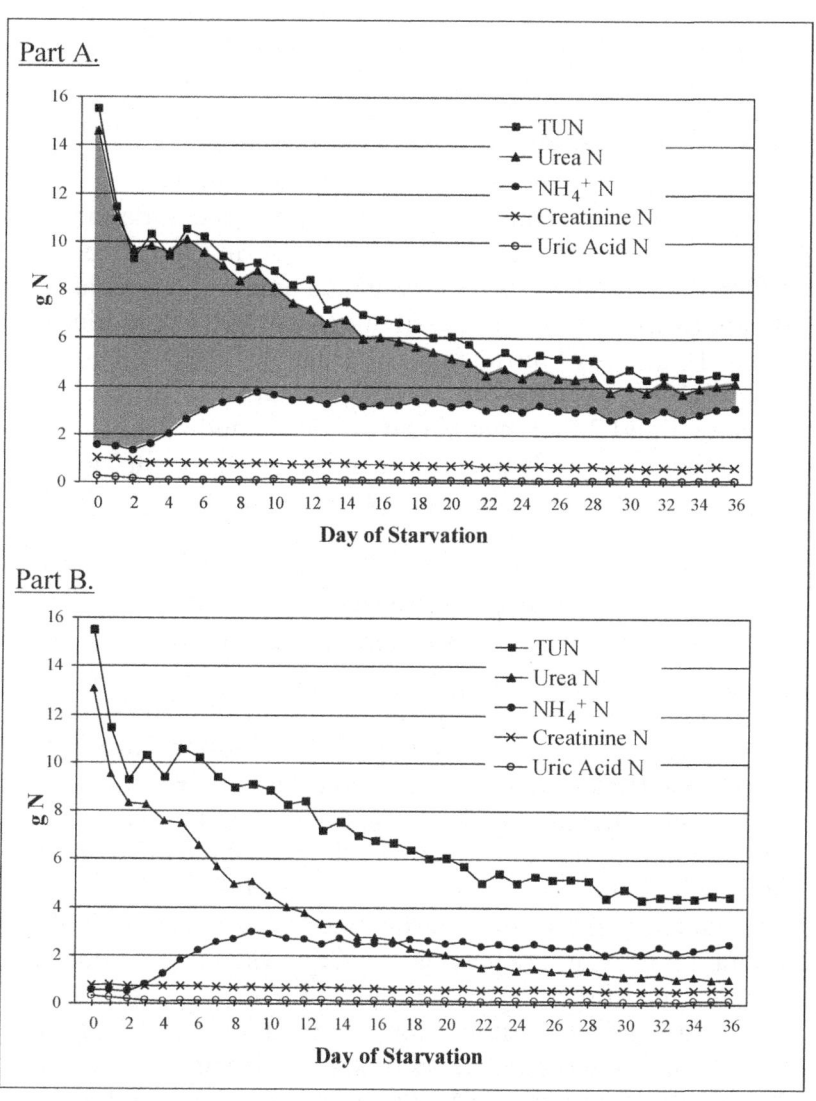

Figure 2. Total quantities of urinary nitrogen (TUN), urea nitrogen (Urea N), ammonium nitrogen (NH₄⁺N), creatinine nitrogen (Creatinine N) and uric acid nitrogen (Uric Acid N) excreted daily by five obese women and five obese men who starved for a minimum of 36 days. Quantities of nitrogenous components excreted have been "stacked" so their sum can be compared to total urinary nitrogen excretion. Shaded area represents urea nitrogen. Clear area between urea and total urinary nitrogen represents unmeasured urinary nitrogenous compounds. Part A is stacked, and Part B is unstacked.

101

rates in 10 obese women and men who starved for a minimum of 36 days. All of the urinary nitrogenous compounds have individual or unique, time-dependent excretion rates during total, prolonged starvation.

Part A displays "stacked" urinary total, urea, ammonium, urate and creatinine nitrogenous compound excretion rates for the 10 obese people during starvation. When the volunteers were eating a balanced and weight-maintenance diet containing about 100 grams of protein with about 16 grams of nitrogen, total urinary nitrogen excretion was 15.5 ± 3.7 g/day. Starvation induced a sudden decline on days 1 and 2, a transient rise on days 3 and 4, and subsequently a gradual decrease in total urinary nitrogen excretion approaching an asymptotic value of 4.6 ± 1.6 g/day near the end of the 36 day starvation study. After about day 5 of total starvation, total urinary nitrogen loss from the body follows an exponential decay curve.

After the first day of starvation, urea nitrogen excretion acutely diminishes as the total urinary nitrogen excretion decreases, but the rate of exponential decay for urea nitrogen is greater than that for total urinary nitrogen during the first 14 days of starvation. In contrast, ammonium (the positively charged ion of ammonia) excretion does not change during the first three days of starvation but rises 5 to 6-fold between days 3-9. Subsequently there is a slow decline to a plateau value of about 2.2 ± 0.2 g/day between 26-36 days of starvation. Ammonium directly excreted by the kidneys becomes the major urinary nitrogenous compound after about 18 days of starvation. After many years of study it became widely known that renal (kidney) ammonium formation and glucose synthesis are coupled. However, the cardinal point to be taken from this figure is that urinary nitrogen excretion during starvation is too low to allow the brain to extract from the blood 100-125 grams of glucose per day.

In essence, it was analyses of urine that provided the initial clues that biomedical concepts of metabolism during starvation had to be realigned.

Chapter VI. Brain Metabolism

"In 1967, Owen and colleagues (8) at Harvard Medical School catheterized cerebral vessels in 3 obese patients and demonstrated that under conditions of prolonged (5-6 weeks) starvation, when carbohydrates stores are reduced to just such a low level, the brain could turn to the metabolism of the fat-derived ketones β-hydroxybutyrate and acetoacetate to replace glucose as its primary fuel (by the process of ketosis). Historically, ketosis was considered to be a pathological condition associated with diabetes, which resulted in the view that ketone bodies were toxic waste products. This finding triggered a reversal in our way of thinking, and we now know that these two ketone bodies are the only free soluble fats that the body can use." Paul A. Marks, Editor-in-chief 1967-1971, *The Journal of Clinical Investigation.* (*J. Clin. Invest.* 114:1019, 2004.)

When a system works, most people don't care *how* it works. But the intellectual curiosity of a few clinical investigators led us to seek answers about the sources of energy for the brain.

In 1965, I was awarded a fellowship position in metabolism under the tutelage of Dr. George F. Cahill, Jr., Associate Professor of Medicine, Harvard Medical School. Dr. Cahill served on the professional staff of the Peter Bent Brigham Hospital and was Director of the Joslin Research Laboratories in Boston, Massachusetts.

After studying the literature, I began helping Dr. Cahill and his colleagues develop protocols to study whole body and organ metabolism.

We were initially interested in determining how the body responded to starvation and how the brain functioned during prolonged fasting. At the time, scientists believed that glucose was the only fuel furnishing the brain with energy. Our research team at Harvard, however, found this theory perplexing. Why? Because during starvation for two to three months, the body is unable to generate enough glucose from body protein to satisfy the brain's energy needs. So we set out to investigate the possibility that the brain utilized alternate sources of fuels during starvation.

It is important that the reader understand that the brain is the master organ of the body. Its energy requirements take precedence over all other organ systems. This is particularly true during starvation when the body mobilizes adipose tissue (fat), muscle, the gastrointestinal tract, liver, and finally the heart, to keep the brain functioning.

Although the brain's relative size and energy requirements, compared with the rest of the body, diminish from infancy to adulthood, its metabolic demands remain enormous compared to other bodily tissue. An infant's brain requires an inordinate amount of energy compared to the rest of the body. Although the brain's energy requirements relative to the rest of the body diminish in adulthood, it still needs more fuel based on organ size than most other bodily tissue. The brain, which accounts for about 2% of body weight, requires about 20% of the body's resting energy requirements. Because the brain is encased so closely in the skull, there is little room to store a large supply of fuel. The brain, therefore, must rely on the fuel-rich blood circulating through the head for energy.

After arterial blood passes through the lungs its composition is the same throughout the body. Thus, the arterial blood supplying brain, liver, kidney and muscle is practically identical in its concentrations of oxygen and fuels. Since different organs have varying energy needs, venous blood draining the organs varies in composition, depending upon the function of the organ. For example, organs, like the brain, extract large quantities of oxygen and fuel, like glucose, from the arterial blood. In contrast, subcutaneous fatty tissue uses only small quantities of oxygen and fuel per unit weight.

The pathway to gaining knowledge on how fuel was supplied (via the bloodstream) to the brain for normal function was a long and circuitous route. It is easy to understand how physician-scientists initially formulated erroneous concepts regarding brain requirements for glucose.

Studying a pathologic condition in order to gain knowledge about brain metabolism complicated, rather than clarified, the understanding of normal function.

Early research regarding brain metabolism was hindered by the widespread, yet erroneous, hypothesis that developed as a consequence of treating diabetic patients with insulin. The most severe form of diabetes mellitus is manifested during diabetic ketoacidosis: It is a fulminant state of catastrophic tissue breakdown where all the fuels used by the body for energy production are simultaneously dumped into the bloodstream. This diseased state floods the blood with an overabundance of most usable fuel. Thirst develops and profuse urination occurs even as the body becomes progressively more dehydrated. The flesh of the body melts away and is drained out of the body in the urine as glucose and ketone bodies. Excessive skin drapes the remaining skeleton of a severely emaciated body. The acidosis of ketoacidosis stimulates breathing. Respiration becomes forced. The acidosis and dehydration cause the cardiovascular system to fail, and shock followed by death occurs. Severe insulin deficiency induces a horrible death. However, extracts of pancreatic islets containing insulin reverse this devastating tissue breakdown.

The treatment for diabetes, a catastrophic disease in metabolism, became available with the discovery of insulin at the University of Toronto in 1921-1922. This scientific breakthrough was one of the most dramatic events for the management of any disease. By lowering the blood glucose, insulin's impact on a diabetic patient was sensational and miraculous.[6]

---

[6] "Late in 1923 the Nobel Prize was awarded for the discovery of insulin. It was awarded to Banting and J.J.R. Macleod. This raises what seems to be the single really controversial point about the discovery: why should Macleod have shared a Nobel Prize for work done in his lab while he was on holiday? It is fairly well known that Banting was dissatisfied with the Nobel Committee's decision. He immediately announced that he was sharing his half of the award with Best. Macleod announced that he would share his half with J.B. Collip, a biochemist who had joined the team late in 1921 and worked on the development of the extract." (Taken

But early insulin therapy was not perfect. Although insulin saved lives of experimental animals, and subsequently humans, initially, researchers had no way of knowing how much or how to best administer it to diabetic animals or humans. They recognized that in the absence of insulin the blood sugar (glucose) rose to high levels and death occurred. They also realized that injecting too much insulin lowered the blood sugar to a point where "peculiar" behavior occurred before animals and humans began frothing at the mouth, became unconsciousness, developed convulsions and died. Naturally, researchers concluded that a severely low level of blood glucose (insulin-induced hypoglycemia) was responsible for the suffering. This theory was further substantiated by the fact that drinking or eating carbohydrate-rich foods (i.e. orange juice or candy), or receiving intravenous glucose reversed these adverse signs.

Ketone bodies in the blood and urine of insulin-deficient diabetic patients were recognized in the 1880's. These compounds were associated with severe disease states and viewed as culprits. In the 1920's, when it became evident that insulin lowered the content of blood and urine glucose, it was also learned that insulin removed detectable quantities of ketone bodies from the blood and urine of diabetic animals and humans. Nonetheless, the idea that insulin affected only glucose and that too little glucose in the blood led to brain dysfunction (and sometimes death), was incomplete and detrimental to a true understanding of brain metabolism.

It wasn't until the 1950's-1960's that researchers learned insulin lowered not only glucose in the blood and urine, but a host of other fuels including free fatty acids, ketone bodies and amino acids. Unfortunately, this discovery was not enough to correct the misconception that ketone bodies were unhealthy and glucose was the brain's only source of fuel. In 1965, we demonstrated that the brain

---

from The Discovery of Insulin by Michael Bliss, The University of Chicago Press, 1982.)

106

utilized alternative forms of fuel in the bloodstream and that ketone bodies were essential to healthy brain metabolism during starvation.

In 1960, I was in a medical school classroom when one of our classmates lost consciousness and began salivating and having convulsive twitching. He was covered with sweat. He was an insulin-dependent diabetic and was exhibiting the classic signs of insulin-induced hypoglycemia. Even we medical students knew that brain cells die when the nervous system has inadequate supplies of fuel or oxygen. We rushed him down the hall into the emergency room and gave him intravenous glucose. He quickly and completely recovered.

Prior to 1965, numerous studies conducted after an overnight fast showed that the only fuel the brain consistently extracted from blood to meet its energy requirements was glucose. Patients suffering from insulin-induced hypoglycemia experienced mental dysfunction, and this fact supported the erroneous concept that glucose was the only fuel that could supply the brain with its energy requirements. However, during these early studies it was not recognized that insulin not only decreased the availability of glucose, but it limited the availability of all fuels in the blood to every organ in the body: insulin lowers the blood concentrations of glucose, free fatty acids, ketone bodies and amino acids, to name a few. Although glucose is the preferred fuel for the brain after an overnight fast, it was erroneous to assume that glucose was the only fuel the brain could use for energy. Nonetheless, this misconception persisted for three decades before new findings showed that the brain could use alternative fuels when they were supplied to the brain through the blood.

Studies by numerous other investigators revealed an interesting connection between the brain and liver metabolism. The central nervous system (including the brain) is approximately the same size as the liver, and both have similar blood flow rates. However, these studies revealed that the brain and liver meet their energy requirements in distinctly different ways. The liver can use

107

glucose (a carbohydrate), amino acids (from protein) and/or free fatty acids (from fat). But the brain requires glucose or other specific water-soluble fuels like the ketone bodies, beta-hydroxybutyrate and acetoacetate. Both glucose and ketone bodies have access to the central nervous system after crossing the blood/brain barrier. Another marked difference is that the brain can only extract fuels from the blood while the liver both extracts and/or adds fuels to the blood. This happens when the liver (and kidney) removes substrates (lactate, pyruvate, glycerol, free fatty acids, amino acids, etc.) from the blood and converts and releases them into the blood as fuels for brain energy. [The kidneys share the role of extracting an amino acid (glutamine) and adding glucose to the blood with the liver. See Chapter VII.]

For years researchers believed that the brain survived solely on glucose produced by the liver. Our studies of obese patients proved otherwise. In an attempt to lose weight, obese volunteers subjected themselves to long periods of starvation. After starving for 5-6 weeks the patient-volunteers underwent catheterization studies to determine the metabolic requirements of their brain and liver. (We subsequently studied their kidneys as well.) We were very interested in how the body both produced and used various fuels during long periods of starvation.

But gleaning information from patient-volunteers was not easy. I still remember our first patient-volunteer, Ms. B. She was obese and had checked herself into the Clinical Research Center at the Peter Bent Brigham Hospital to participate in a prolonged starvation study. Her hope was to lose weight and have heart evaluation studies done. She also agreed to have her brain and liver studied after fasting.

We began by putting Ms. B. on a balanced diet of proteins, fat and carbohydrates. After a few days, we initiated the approved starvation protocol. Ms. B. received water, salt tablets and vitamins. Our research team made daily recordings of her weight, blood pressure, body temperature and pulse. We also measured Ms. B.'s total body energy requirements and drew periodic blood samples for analyses. Each day we collected the urine to measure her excretion rates of nitrogenous waste compounds.

As mentioned in Chapter V, after Ms. B. had fasted for approximately 41 days, we inserted multiple catheters into her blood vessels to measure the exchange rate of metabolic materials between the brain and liver. Although our team at the cardiac catheterization laboratory had provided for every safety precaution, there was a palpable tension in the air. We were concerned about the inherent risks of obtaining multiple artery and venous blood samples from a patient who had not eaten for 41 days. (Today, such a procedure would not cause such concern since it has been proven relatively safe.)

Our team drew simultaneous arterial and venous blood samples over a 10-second timed period from around Ms. B's brain and liver. Her blood volume was replaced with normal saline. We waited fifteen minutes before proceeding to make sure that the patient had suffered no ill effects. Once we assessed that Ms. B. was stable, we repeated the process with fresh syringes to withdraw arterial and venous blood for a second and third time.

It took a couple of hours to do the diagnostic studies and to collect the experimental blood specimens. After obtaining the needed blood samples from the brain and liver, we sent them off to be analyzed. When our research team received the initial results, we were thrilled to learn Ms. B.'s brain had survived by extracting blood ketone bodies (beta-hydroxybutyrate and acetoacetate) and a very small quantity of blood glucose (Figure 1). The fact that the brain could derive energy from substrates other than glucose was of monumental importance for understanding human survival during starvation. Our findings resolved the inexplicable reality that humans can survive 60-90 or more days without

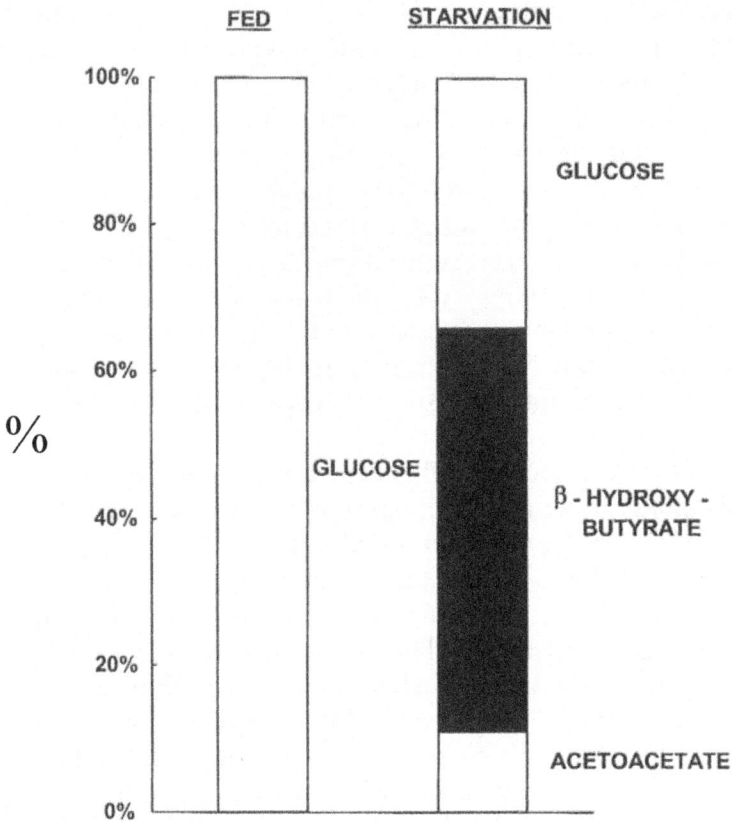

Figure 1. This figure displays the percent energy provided by glucose, beta-hydroxybutyrate and/or acetoacetate for brain metabolism in the fed and prolonged starvation states. Glucose is the predominant, if not the sole, fuel extracted by the brain after an overnight fast. During prolonged starvation, beta-hydroxybutyrate plus acetoacetate provide about 66% of the energy requirements for the brain. Glucose consumption is curtailed to about 34% of the energy requirements. Not shown are extraction and release of amino acids.

food because the brain obtained most of its energy requirements from fuels other than glucose.[7]

---

[7] For another example, consider a larger man of 75 kg (165 pounds) who has roughly 15 kg (33 pounds) of fat stored in 16 kg adipose tissue, and about 12 kg (26 pounds) of protein suspended in 60 kg of lean body mass, mostly muscle. Practically all of the body fat is expendable without serious adverse effects. In contrast, only one-half of the body's protein can be mobilized and used as fuel before death occurs. The

Hepatic vein samples revealed another shocking discovery. According to our findings, Ms. B.'s liver produced less glucose than what her brain had extracted from the blood. Before we did the catheterization studies, we knew that after about 3 days of starvation the blood glucose concentration stabilizes. This means that the body's organs are extracting the same amount of glucose from the blood that other organs are adding to it. There is a balance between utilization and production of glucose. Although Ms. B.'s brain was extracting only a small amount of glucose, it was more than the liver was producing and her blood glucose remained constant. We set out to figure out how there could be an imbalance between brain utilization and liver production of glucose while the arterial blood glucose remained stable. There must be another source adding glucose to the blood.

As is often the case in medical research, our preliminary data raised more questions than it answered.

A few days later, we received the results of Ms. B.'s urine samples (collected over each of the 24-hour periods). From these results, we began to suspect that both the kidney and the liver were synthesizing glucose during prolonged starvation. Before examining Ms. B.'s urine samples, we were under the impression that urea produced by the liver constituted the body's principal source of excreted nitrogen. How much glucose is produced by the liver is in part dependent upon the liver's production of urea, and shortly thereafter urea is excreted in the urine. Thus, the liver's production of glucose is coupled to liver production of urea and renal excretion of urea. Turns out that during prolonged starvation, the body relies more on ammonium production and excretion by the kidneys than it does on urea excretion to

---

conversion of 6 kg of protein to glucose results in the formation of only 3.4 kg of glucose. If the brain oxidizes 100-125 grams of glucose daily, this human could starve for only 27-34 days. The fact that the brain can derive two-thirds of its energy from ketone bodies, synthesized mostly from fat, allows humans to survive total starvation for 60-90 days. This period is compatible with the time known to induce death in humans from starvation.

111

rid the body of nitrogen waste. Further, kidney production of ammonium is coupled to kidney production of glucose.

At the Joslin Research Laboratory at Harvard University, Drs. Robert Fuisz, David Goodman and Donald Kamm had noticed a link between the output of ammonium and the production of glucose in rat kidney slices. Our combined findings led me to predict that part of the glucose used by Ms. B.'s brain during prolonged starvation had been generated by her kidneys. Hearing my prediction, Dr. Cahill leapt out of his chair and shouted, "You're right!"

As confident and excited as we were by our initial findings, we knew that the brain and liver results had to be confirmed, and our research had to include the kidney's role in producing glucose.

Mr. N. was our second patient-volunteer for the starvation study. He was 49 years old and had attended both Yale and Harvard. He attributed his weight problem to overeating when depressed. Over the years, his 5'11" frame increased to 300 pounds, with most of the fat concentrated in the regions of his chest and abdomen. According to our laboratory results, Mr. N.'s thyroid, blood cell counts and liver functions were all normal. Resting energy requirements for his weight were also within the normal range. Laboratory tests revealed impaired glucose tolerance (a risk factor for type 2 diabetes mellitus), and we suspected problems with his kidneys after detecting traces of protein in his urine. Mr. N. also suffered from high blood pressure (180/110 mmHg) and small bouts of exercise left him fatigued and short of breath. An EKG (electrocardiogram) revealed left ventricular hypertrophy, an enlargement and thickening of the heart. He required a lot of psychological support during a 38 day fast. Nonetheless, he managed to get through without complications other than he was demanding during the fast. He lost 55 pounds and was most satisfied with this accomplishment. His blood glucose concentration and blood pressure became normal. He underwent brain, liver and kidney catheterization studies before a re-feeding period with a low caloric diet.

The third patient-volunteer, Ms. L., was a 26 year old woman. She had been heavy as a baby, child, adolescent and adult. By the time Ms. L. signed up for the study, she weighed 324 pounds. She had chaotic menstrual irregularities (known to occur with morbid obesity) and at times heavy vaginal bleeding every 3-4 months requiring surgical treatments (dilatation and curettage) and hormonal therapy. Her weight reduction program was done to reestablish normal menstrual periods. When she entered the starvation study, she weighed 317 pounds at 5 feet 9 inches. Her subcutaneous tissue was flabby and skin was pale. Laboratory screening tests revealed no diabetes mellitus or thyroid, liver or kidney disease. She fasted for 39 days, tolerated the food deprivation surprisingly well, and lost 51 pounds. She underwent brain, liver and kidney catheterization studies. She tolerated these procedures easily. Thereafter, she returned to the care of her regular physician.

Retesting our theory on Mr. N. and Ms. L. confirmed our initial results: During starvation, the brain survives by extracting significant quantities of acetoacetate and beta-hydroxybutyrate from the blood. The utilization of these ketone bodies as the predominant source of energy, rather than glucose, allows humans with fat in their body to survive during severe caloric deprivation (Figure 1).

In 1967, our results were published in the *Journal of Clinical Investigation* (Owen, O.E., A.P. Morgan, H.G. Kemp, *et al*. Brain metabolism during fasting. *J. Clin. Invest.* 46:1589-95, 1967). The article went on to become a Citation Classic.

A human being's ability to survive extreme variations in caloric intake depends, at least in part, on their body's ability to economically store fuel. This means that the storage depot, like subcutaneous and abdominal fat, should have a high calorie:weight ratio. It should be capable of meeting the energy requirements for most, if not all, tissues and should be usable without adverse effects. Survival during prolonged starvation also depends upon the body's ability to spare vital proteins in the liver, muscle, heart, kidney, blood, etc. that allow the body to function.

Fat has the greatest caloric value per weight, and fat is readily expendable. Adipose tissue mobilizes fat, and fat circulates through the liver, surrendering about one-half of its caloric value as it is broken into fragments which provide materials that can be used to synthesize ketone bodies (beta-hydroxybutyrate and acetoacetate). These ketone bodies contain the remaining one-half of the caloric value of lipids originating from the fat stores. During starvation, these energy-rich ketone bodies circulate through the central nervous system, and provide the brain with its primary source of energy. This process minimizes the liver's need to convert amino acids derived from proteins into glucose for the brain. This means that during prolonged starvation, humans can continue to accomplish physical tasks like protecting themselves and foraging for food.

Three patient-volunteers and two clinical investigators made a contribution to biomedical science when they demonstrated that ketone bodies could serve as valuable fuels for brain metabolism during starvation.

Cerebrospinal Fluid Analysis

People have long used fasting to lose weight, and fasting is a widespread method of weight reduction. In the late 1950's, some physicians hospitalized patients to undergo a few days of starvation. Other individuals fasted over the weekend to lose weight. While fasting, some of the individuals complained of headaches. Others experienced precipitous drops in blood pressure when getting up out of bed. Some physicians suspected that these symptoms and signs arose from an infection in the central nervous system. The brain is suspended and bathed in the cerebrospinal fluid. As a diagnostic test for an infection in the central nervous system, physicians compared the concentration of glucose in the patients' blood to that in their cerebrospinal fluid. In healthy individuals, the glucose concentration in the cerebrospinal fluid is two-thirds of that found in the blood (e.g. 60 mg/dl cerebrospinal fluid compared to 90 mg/dl blood). An infectious process is suspected when the difference between the cerebrospinal fluid glucose and the blood glucose increases (e.g. 30 mg/dl cerebrospinal fluid compared to 90 mg/dl blood).

Because we had found and reported in 1967 that the brain derived most of its energy from ketone bodies rather than glucose, we wondered if the usual ratio of glucose in cerebrospinal fluid to blood remained 2:3 (60:90 mg/dl) in starving patients. Our finding at Harvard showing the brain's use of ketone bodies during starvation brought up another intriguing question. Did the 2:3 glucose ratio detected in people undergoing an overnight fast (or during the postprandial period between meals) persist in patients who did not eat food for long periods of time? We suspected the answer was "no," but this suspicion had to be confirmed. We also thought that if the brain was extracting ketone bodies, these fuels had to pass through the blood/brain barrier to be accessible to the nervous tissue and should be present in the cerebrospinal fluid during starvation. In 1973, while working at Temple University Hospital, we tested this hypothesis by measuring the glucose and ketone bodies in the blood and cerebrospinal fluid in volunteers who had fasted overnight. Next, we compared these results with samples taken from the same starving volunteers 21 days later. After fasting for 21 days, glucose in the cerebrospinal fluid was closer to 50 mg/dl compared to 60 mg/dl in the bloodstream. Our findings challenged the standard use of cerebrospinal fluid:blood glucose ratios to indicate an infection of the nervous system. Thus, in the absence of a greater difference between cerebrospinal fluid and blood glucose, an infection is unlikely. This same study also demonstrated that during starvation, cerebrospinal fluid contained high concentrations of the ketone bodies, beta-hydroxybutyrate and acetoacetate, and some insulin.

Brain Enzymes for Ketone Body Utilization

It was fortunate that Mulchand S. Patel, Ph.D. joined the faculty at the Temple General Clinical Research Center and Department of Biochemistry. Dr. Patel was trained in nutrition and biochemistry and had a high energy level and a perceptive mind. He recognized avenues of fruitful research before other investigators did in biochemistry. He bridged the gap between basic science and clinical medicine with extraordinary insight. Of equal importance was his ability to use basic science to advance knowledge first described in human volunteers. Thus, he demonstrated that basic science expanded clinical investigation. It was Dr. Patel's research effort in a basic science laboratory that further substantiated that ketone bodies were metabolized in the nervous system of fetal, newborn and adult tissue samples (taken from rats and humans).

From the first clinical studies we did at Harvard in 1965-1968, we were under the impression that during starvation, the brain needed time to adapt the enzymes needed to process the oxidation of ketone bodies for fuel. Dr. Patel and colleagues, and other groups, subsequently learned that these enzymes were always present and abundant in the brain's nervous tissue. Therefore, no adaptation time for the brain is required for animals or humans to be able to use ketone bodies.

Brain Synthesis of Lipids from Ketone Bodies

In follow-up studies in developing animal brains, Dr. Patel and colleagues showed that ketone bodies could be incorporated into lipids (fats) and proteins located in the brain. This makes sense because we know that breast milk is high in fat content, and lipid (nutrient) serves as a source for generating ketone bodies in the babies' livers. These ketone bodies in the babies' blood subsequently furnish the brain energy and building blocks. The brain cells are insulated by sheaths of fatty material, much like electrical wires are wrapped with a protective material. During normal pregnancy a transient mild ketosis may occur during the intervals between meals; therefore, the metabolism of circulating ketone bodies may contribute to cerebral energy metabolism and the synthesis of brain lipids. Thus, ketone bodies are readily utilized for the biosynthesis of fatty substances (fatty acids and sterols) in human fetal brains. It is likely that ketone bodies contribute to cerebral lipid synthesis even greater when the infant is nursing. Dr. Patel and his colleagues must be credited with demonstrating that the carbon elements in both acetoacetate and beta-hydroxybutyrate could be incorporated into brain lipids and proteins (Patel, M.S., C.A. Johnson, R. Rajan, and O.E. Owen. The metabolism of ketone bodies in developing human brain: development of ketone-body-utilizing enzymes and ketone bodies as precursors for lipid synthesis. *J. Neurochem.* 25: 905-8, 1975).

Summary
For many years the majority of the scientific community regarded ketone bodies as deleterious. Our initial work at Harvard, however, demonstrated that they are crucial for survival. Ketone bodies supply the brain and other tissues with essential water-soluble fuels when glucose is in short supply (i.e. during starvation or when consuming a high fat/low carbohydrate diet). Our later work at Temple showed that ketone bodies also serve as building blocks for brain lipids and proteins in fetal, newborn and adult nervous tissues. Our brain metabolism studies opened up a whole new avenue of scientific inquiry. When the master organ of the body shifts from oxidizing glucose to ketone bodies, it has a global effect on the body. To better understand metabolism in health and disease states, we were motivated to expand our research to the whole body and liver, kidney, brain, muscle, and adipose tissue to gain the knowledge needed to understand the availability of and use of fuels.

117

Chapter VII. Liver and Kidney Metabolism in "Normal" Adults

What makes sense depends on what is known at a given time. Facts don't change, but the interpretation of facts may change as more knowledge is gained.

Liver

The subtle but dominant function of the liver is production of glucose and ketone bodies that can be used by organs lacking the ability to use alternative fuels as sources of energy.

The liver is located in the center of the body, just under the right ribcage. It is the largest organ concentrated in one location, unlike muscle. At birth the liver accounts for 1/15 of body weight. It is easily felt in infants through the abdominal wall because it extends well below the rib cage. With aging, its relative size to the body diminishes, being 1/40 of the adult body weight. Nonetheless, it maintains its many vital responsibilities.

Gross manifestations of liver disease are readily detected. Hallmarks are jaundice, wasting of the muscles of the extremities, fluid accumulation with voluminous swelling (ascites) of the belly (spider-like appearance), massive gastrointestinal hemorrhage, and swollen ankles and legs accompanying emaciation. In addition, loss of appetite, fever and abdominal pain are early signs and symptoms of hepatic (liver) diseases. The stools may become yellow in color, and fatigue and lassitude usually occur. These signs and symptoms are visible or noted by the patient.

The liver is a hotbed of enzymes (catalysts). It assumes more diverse tasks than any other organ. It has a dual blood supply: blood from both arteries and veins enters the liver and several large veins drain the liver. The liver is the basic organ responsible for integrating fuel homeostasis: extracting some fuels from blood and releasing others. It adds one-half of the fuels needed to meet the energy requirements for the rest of the body. The liver also excretes toxins and by-products into the intestine (and urine) and secretes vitamins into the bloodstream.

The liver is subjected to the influences of available substrates (precursors, fuels), and it is modulated by hormones. Thus, both the availability of substrate and hormonal concentrations dictate hepatic behavior. For example, after eating a meal and when glucose (substrate) and insulin (hormone) concentrations are high in the blood, the liver extracts glucose, spares amino acid uptake and releases fats. In contrast, during the non-fed state when glucose and insulin concentrations are low, the liver extracts amino acids and fat and releases glucose and ketone bodies. Thus, the liver can make diagonally opposed flux rates of fuels. It is the key organ of the body for modulating and maintaining a constant availability of fuels in the bloodstream. Insulin, glucagon and other hormones modulate the various processes involved in fuel homeostasis. In the starved state, the liver is central in removing compounds funneled into it from muscle and adipose tissue and releasing glucose and ketone bodies as a source of fuels for peripheral tissues. This responsibility is the largest task the liver has to do.

The adult liver stores about 150 grams of glucose as glycogen. This stored source of fuel can be quickly mobilized to meet energy demands. Liver glycogen is replaced after meals but nearly depleted after physical activity or during starvation.

Glycogen is stored inside of liver cells. It is a large molecule that must be suspended in a salty water environment. For each gram of glucose stored as glycogen inside the cell, about 3 grams of salty (potassium phosphate) water are required to suspend the gigantic glycogen molecule. (Stored glycogen is analogous to seaweed flotating in the ocean.) At least another 75-150 grams of glycogen can be stored in muscle. Other tissues contain a small amount of glycogen. However, the total content of glycogen in most human bodies is not very much fuel compared to other potential body fuels stored as fats and contained in proteins.

At birth the relative quantities of fat and muscle are small. Babies must be fed frequently or they die. However, the healthy 60 kg (132 lb) woman with 25% body fat and the average 80 kg (176 lb) man with 20% body fat have approximately 15 kg (33 lb) of body fat. Fat is stored inside of fat cells (adipocytes) as oil droplets. Other than the ring of active protoplasm surrounding the droplet, no water is required. Therefore, the caloric content of fat cells (adipose tissue) is very high. Protein is mostly housed inside lean body tissue. Muscle, the largest mass of lean tissue, is approximately 80% water and 20% protein. Only one-half of the lean body mass can be lost before death occurs. Since the protein content of lean tissue is low and the quantity of lean tissue that can be used for energy is limited before death occurs, the total available store of calories as protein is usually much less than that present in adipose tissue. (See Chapter III, Fuels and Hormones.)

Adults can starve for days, weeks or months if water is available because they can mobilize practically all of their fat mass and one-half of their protein (muscle) mass before they die. Survival during starvation depends primarily upon the body's ability to derive over 90% of its energy requirements from fat utilization. Some of the body's fat mass is converted into water-soluble ketone bodies, and part of the protein mass is converted into water-soluble glucose to supply tissues with specific fuels to meet their energy requirements.

Before showing data derived from our patient-volunteers reflecting hepatic (liver) metabolism under different clinical circumstances, notes of caution should be provided. It is important to state that the accuracy from any research study must be guardedly accepted. All data should be confirmed before assumed to be accurate. Measurements made in biological systems have many limitations. For example, reporting the results derived from measuring small concentration differences between an artery and a vein that are not meaningfully significant and then multiplying these insignificant differences by large blood flow rates may produce values that are mathematically significant but not physiologically significant. The reader has to realize that measurements of concentrations of fuels made from arterial and venous bloods have technical limitations. Further, the accuracy in determining blood flow rates is not precise. Nonetheless, combining the arteriovenous concentration differences with blood flow rates may provide the best information available at a given time. In the past, it reflected the state of the medical art employed.

Another difficulty with clinical investigation is that the subjects under study do not always behave exactly as the researcher expects them to behave. Maybe the hypothesis under which the research proposal was developed predicted finding one thing, but something else appears during the research efforts. This occurence always surprises everyone, and practically no one will accept the findings as real unless the research team has unequivocal data to support the strange finding. Most humans, including researchers and review personnel, sometimes fail to remember that each person is an individual, and individuals have unique DNA and, thus, unique profiles. Thus, everyone does not fit the average. Further, the average is not necessarily right and the misfit necessarily wrong. The merit of each may be equal, but different.

After the first three patient-volunteers (Ms. B., Mr. N. and Ms. M.) were studied following periods of prolonged starvation (See Chapter VI, Brain Metabolism), more patients were studied under similar circumstances. Mr. B., the fourth patient-volunteer to undergo liver and kidney studies after prolonged starvation, was a 19 year-old college student from Dallas, Texas. He was a large framed man with central obesity. He was 5 feet 11 inches tall, and his weight before the first of two prolonged starvation studies was 339 pounds[8]. After a starvation study of 35 days he was discharged on a diet over the Christmas holidays. He was subsequently readmitted, with a weight of 275 pounds, for a second study and weight reduction. At the end of the second starvation period his weight was 224 pounds. Thus, during

---

[8] One pound equals 0.45 kilograms

the two fasting periods, each lasting 35 days and interrupted by a vacation and feeding period, he lost 115 pounds or an average of 1.6 pounds per day. A unique characteristic about this young patient-volunteer was his activity during starvation. He wanted to continue his college education so he walked from the Peter Bent Brigham Hospital to Boston College (approximately 8 miles round trip) five days a week to attend classes. He tolerated this walking activity very well and had the greatest weight loss per day starved among all patient-volunteers over the periods of studies.

My memory is more vague, and I have no personal records outside those published, regarding the fifth patient-volunteer, Mr. F. He was a 32 year-old man of 5 feet 11 inches tall who weighed 279 pounds. After 35 days of starvation at the time of catheterization studies, his weight was 233 pounds. As I recall, other than obesity, he was healthy before and after starvation. The 46-pound weight loss benefited his employment circumstances.

The initial three patients studied at Harvard's Peter Bent Brigham Hospital in Boston showed that the brain could use ketone bodies as well as glucose for a source of energy during starvation. However, in the first patient-volunteer the production of glucose by the liver was less than the quantity of glucose extracted by the brain.[9] We had a deficit in "explainable" glucose production. Therefore, we directed our attention not only to the liver but also to the kidney as an additional source of glucose.

The results from the first five patient-volunteers demonstrated that the liver and kidney shared the role in producing glucose after prolonged starvation. However, the grand picture of the role of the liver and kidney in maintaining fuel homeostasis in health and disease was far from complete.

With colleagues at Temple and other academic institutions, I continued to evaluate liver and kidney metabolism for the next two decades. We studied patient-

---

[9] We employed the Indocyanine green dye technique developed by S. Sherlock and coworkers to estimate hepatic (liver) blood flow rates.

volunteers after an overnight fast, a 3-day fast, and periodically during prolonged starvation periods. In addition, we studied these organs in patients with scarred livers from alcoholic cirrhosis and liver metabolism in patients suffering from diabetic ketoacidosis. The results from studying alcoholic and diabetic patients are covered in other chapters.

Some of our results outlined in this chapter were combined with the peer reviewed data published when Dr. Philip Felig, *et al* were at Yale University School of Medicine and Dr. John Wahren, *et al* were at the Karolinska Institute in Sweden. It took many years of study to integrate organ metabolism under various nutritional circumstances. Eventually, we demonstrated that there was an orchestrated harmony among organ systems that store nutrients after eating or mobilize fuels during caloric deprivation in a way that maintains a near steady-state of fuel availability in the blood to meet the body's energy requirements. Specifically, after meals the body removes glucose, fats and amino acids from the blood. During fasting the fuels are released into the blood. Some of the amino acids and fats are converted into glucose and/or ketone bodies, respectively, by the liver and less so by the kidney. We ultimately were able to state with reasonable certainty the roles of liver and kidney in producing fuels, specifically glucose and ketone bodies, in health and disease states. It was a long journey that required a lot of work with great cooperation from patient-volunteers.

We standardized the production rates of glucose and ketone bodies to the average human weighing 70 kg or having 1.73 meters body surface area. Standardization has many limitations; nonetheless, it is an accepted method of reporting data. We also converted production rates of glucose and ketone bodies into caloric equivalents so the reader would have a better grasp of the contributions liver (and/or kidney) made to total body energy requirements in the resting state. The data presented in the following figures are not always in the sequence that the data were accumulated. Rather, the complex data are displayed in a manner that is more understandable.

Although the figures in this chapter are somewhat pedantic presentations designed for the deeply committed intellectual who must have details, some of the information provided in these figures is essential for understanding how the liver is able to supply glucose and ketone bodies to the blood for use by other organs during various states of fasting. In the figures, the production rates of glucose and ketone bodies are converted to the caloric equivalents of these fuels because the purpose of synthesizing and releasing these materials into the blood is to provide energy for organs that lack other sources of fuels. Expressing data as caloric equivalents eliminates the need for the reading audience to convert mmole values into energy equivalents.

During fasting, numerous materials are funneled into the liver from its periphery (extrahepatic tissues). The amino acids, glycerol, lactate, pyruvate and propanediol (precursors) are extracted and converted (gluconeogenesis) into glucose (product). Stored glycogen in the liver also breaks down (glycogenolysis). The combination of newly synthesized glucose and glycogen breakdown delivers about 0.86 mmol/min/70 kg or 1.73 m^2 of glucose to the blood.[10] The majority ($\sim$60%) of hepatic glucose released after an overnight fast comes from the breakdown of glycogen. The remainder ($\sim$40%) of glucose is derived from newly synthesized glucose. Data from catheterization studies may exaggerate hepatic glycogenolysis and underestimate gluconeogenesis. However, these possible inaccuracies in glycogenolysis and gluconeogenesis do not affect estimates of total hepatic glucose output. The expression of the data as caloric equivalents eliminates the possible errors made in estimating what amount of glucose released is attributable to glycogenolysis or gluconeogenesis.

---

[10] The data derived from patient-volunteers of different body sizes are standardized by correcting their body weights to 70 kg or their body surface areas to 1.73 m^2. This is not an ideal correction because brain and liver sizes do not fluctuate in adult humans as much as other body changes with different weights. Nonetheless, it was a standard method used to correct for body size during the 20th century.

About one-half of the synthesized glucose comes from recycled lactate and pyruvate. Some glycerol is also recycled as glucose. Recycled glucose is not available for terminal oxidation to carbon dioxide and water; however, some of the glucose derived from glycerol after fat breakdown is not recycled and is available for oxidation. The rest of the newly synthesized glucose is derived from amino acids from protein breakdown (proteolysis). Thus, the amount of glucose that can be derived from amino acids and some of the glucose derived from glycerol can be completely consumed by extrahepatic tissues. The quantity of glucose not recycled was used to calculate caloric equivalents that could be derived from glucose oxidation.

Figure 1 shows the glucose and ketone body production after an overnight fast and after 3 days of starvation. After an overnight fast, a small amount of ketone bodies is synthesized from free fatty acids flowing to the liver. The combined energy equivalents of these fuels when oxidized to CO_2 and H_2O are also displayed. After an overnight fast the liver is the only significant, net source of glucose added to the blood. The kidneys extract and add small quantities of glucose simultaneously. The kidney's net contribution of glucose to the blood becomes significant after more prolonged periods of starvation or under special circumstances.

After 1-2 days of starvation the hepatic glycogen stores are practically depleted, and most of the glucose released from the liver is derived from newly synthesized glucose. However, the total release of glucose from the liver after 2-3 days of starvation is depressed to less than 50% of what it was after an overnight fast. Analysis of tracer techniques using radioactive lactate and/or glucose have shown that approximately one-half of this glucose is derived from recycled lactate and pyruvate and does not contribute to oxidation to carbon dioxide and water (terminal oxidation). By contrast, both catheterization and radioactive tracer techniques show that ketone body release from the liver is

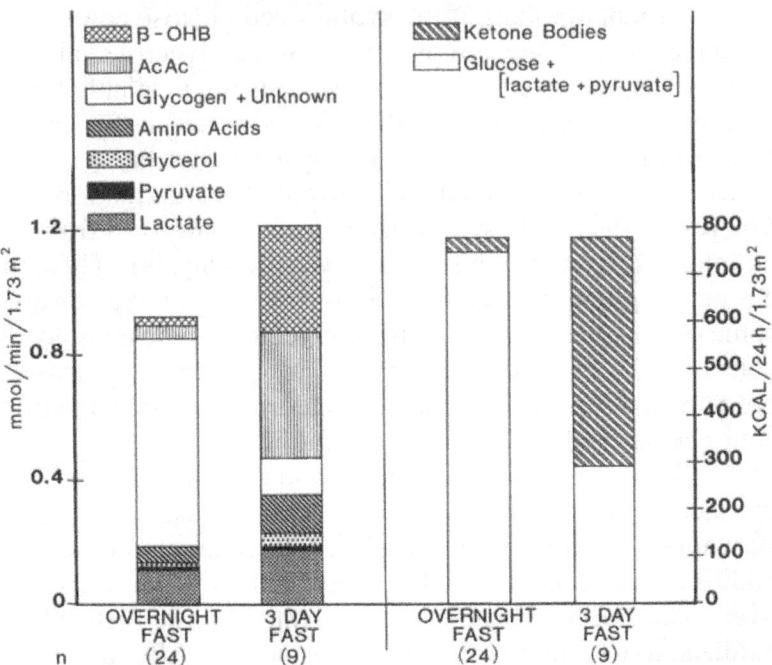

Figure 1. Liver or hepatic (splanchnic) glucose and ketone body production rates and energy equivalents in overnight and 3 day fasted humans. The left side of the figure shows the relative contributions of glycogenolysis and gluconeogenesis to total glucose production as well as ketone body production. The right side of the figure shows the energy equivalents of glucose and ketone body production. Liver glucose and ketone body production rates account for approximately 50% of the body's total energy requirements. These values should be considered as estimates because of the limitations in the measuring techniques and the methods used to calculate energy equivalents.

increased about 10-fold after about 3 days of fasting and remains elevated for many weeks during starvation. The vast majority of the ketone bodies can be oxidized to carbon dioxide and water, releasing their chemical energy. Thus, the nature and quantity of hepatic fuels are different. Ketone bodies produced by the liver become a quasi and persistent fuel substitute for glucose. Therefore, the caloric equivalent of the fuels released from the liver after overnight and 3 or more days of fasting are approximately equal.[11] The combination of hepatic release of glucose and ketone bodies provides the caloric equivalent of about 800 Kcal/day /1.73 m^2 or 70 kg (Figure 2). This is about one-half of the body's total daily resting energy or caloric requirements of a theoretical 70 kg (1.73 m^2) person needed to maintain resting body functions.

As starvation progresses to many weeks, the body size diminishes. Accompanying the loss of body weight (and body surface area) is an appropriate but small decrease in hepatic production and release of glucose and ketone bodies (Figure 2).

Two major accomplishments regarding liver metabolism came out of the work initiated at Harvard's Joslin Research Laboratories and the Clinical Research Center of Peter Bent Brigham Hospital and continued at Temple University's General Clinical Research Center and other research facilities.

First, the liver maintains its role of providing one-half of the body's energy requirements by delivering both glucose and ketone bodies to the blood after an overnight and more prolonged fasts. Further, there is a reciprocal relationship between hepatic production of glucose and hepatic production of ketone bodies. When glucose release from the liver is high, ketone body release is low. Conversely, when glucose release is low, ketone body release is high. This reciprocal relationship allows the liver to exchange the production of one water-soluble fuel (glucose) for other water-soluble fuels (ketone bodies) so the

---

[11] The caloric values of a gram of glucose, beta-hydroxybutyrate and acetoacetate are nearly equal. However, glucose weighs 1.8 times more than either ketone body. Therefore, on the molar basis (a term frequently used in scientific literature), glucose has about 1.8 times the caloric value of either ketone body. But there is another catch. All of the glucose released from the liver is not oxidized to carbon dioxide and water. Therefore, the total caloric potential of glucose released by the liver is not used by the body for energy production. An additional complication is related to the small loss of ketone bodies in the urine during ketotic states.

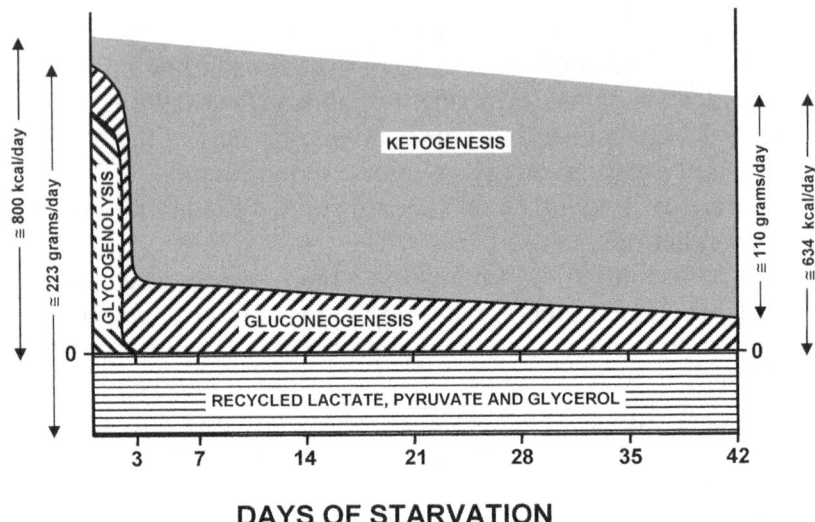

DAYS OF STARVATION

Figure 2. Hepatic (Liver) Metabolism. A theoretical human weighing 70 kg with a body surface area of 1.73 m² should require about 1600 Kcal/day while lying down to rest. The liver provides fuels to meet about one-half of the caloric requirements. After an overnight fast, glycogen breakdown (glycogenolysis) provides the largest (~60%) component of hepatic caloric delivery. Hepatic gluconeogenesis (newly synthesized glucose from amino acids and some of the recycled glycerol) contributes about 20% of the glucose which can be terminally oxidized to carbon dioxide and water. Recycled glucose from lactate, pyruvate and glycerol adds an additional 20% to glucose release. Obviously the glucose from recycled lactate, pyruvate and glycerol is not oxidized to CO_2 and H_2O. However, in the process of breaking glucose down to lactate and pyruvate (glycolysis), about 7% of the innate energy of glucose is released for use. Some of the glucose derived from glycerol is recycled to esterify fatty acids in adipose tissue.

brain can have access to a constant supply of fuels during fasting. Hepatic ketone body synthesis and release into the blood spares the lean body mass (primarily skeletal muscle) from mobilizing its protein content (amino acids) to synthesize glucose.

Second, after 2-3 days of starvation the liver synthesizes and releases approximately 110 grams (0.74 mmol/min/1.73 m²) of ketone bodies (acetoacetate plus beta-hydroxybutyrate) day after day during prolonged starvation. There is no other metabolic function of liver that equals this relatively huge synthetic process. As long as the body has

128

fat stores and can mobilize free fatty acids during starvation, the liver synthesizes and releases ketone bodies (Figure 2). Thus, the liver maintains a constant supply of water-soluble fuels during starvation by substituting ketone bodies for glucose. The magnitude and duration of this task for the liver may not be fully recognized or appreciated by either the scientific or lay groups. *It should be noted that the constant supply of fuels by the liver, with its persistent synthesis of ketone bodies for energy requirements of extrahepatic organs, is the largest task the liver has to accomplish so life can continue during starvation. This does not negate the fact that the amount of glucose produced by the liver after 3 or more days of starvation is insufficient to meet brain and total body requirements for water-soluble fuels.*

Kidney

The body has many organ systems operating simultaneously. Each organ system must sense the behavior of the other organs to function in a coordinated manner. Similar to the fuel interplay between the brain and liver, the kidney and liver have a close collaboration on excreting nitrogenous waste products and synthesizing glucose. *There is cross-talk between the liver and kidney.*

The body has two kidneys, one located on each side of the backbone, behind the abdomen and below the lowest rib. Each kidney weighs about one-quarter of a pound and is about the size of a fist. They have a huge blood supply considering their small energy or oxygen requirements.

Like the liver, the kidneys have a multitude of tasks to accomplish. However, the primary role of the kidney is to maintain the water volume, salt content and acid-base balance in the body. They are the "master chemists of the body, constantly assisting the body's internal environment." Included among the essential roles of the kidneys is to provide glucose during total, prolonged starvation to body organs that have a constitutional need to use the energy content present in glucose (e.g. brain). In this section of the chapter, emphasis is placed on the kidneys' fine regulatory role of blood glucose, ketone bodies and ammonium excretion. However, previously and throughout this book, I describe in detail how we discovered that the various metabolic mechanisms during healthy states are all in lockstep. Figures 1-3 in Chapter IV demonstrate this concept. Figure 4 in Chapter IV puts forth the concept of anaplerosis (fill up) and cataplerosis (drain out). In essence, the number of carbon and nitrogen atoms entering an organ must equal the number of carbon and nitrogen atoms exiting an organ. More than one organ may be required to accomplish this balance.

After studying our first patient-volunteer, Ms. B., in 1965, we observed that during prolonged starvation, the quantity of glucose released from the liver that could be terminally oxidized to carbon dioxide and water was less than the quantity extracted and oxidized by the brain. There had to be another source for adding glucose to the blood during long term fasting. Our attention was turned toward the kidneys because urinary excretion of nitrogen showed that the most abundant excretory product during prolonged starvation was ammonium. We began to believe that there may be a relationship between renal (kidney) ammonium excretion and renal glucose production and release into the blood.

Different methods were needed to study glucose production by the kidney. In order to use the Fick principle (blood flow rates multiplied by the differences in arterial and venous blood concentrations) we had to use credible techniques to measure blood (plasma) flow rates. We employed the legendary techniques of sodium *para*-aminohyppurate developed by Dr. Homer W. Smith to measure renal blood flow.

Before I left Boston in 1968, we confirmed the hypothesis that the kidney shared with the liver the role of producing glucose during prolonged starvation.

The results from our first five patient-volunteers who underwent liver and kidney catheterization studies after 35-41 days of starvation were reported (Owen O.E., P. Felig, A.P. Morgan, *et al.* Liver and Kidney Metabolism During

130

Prolonged Starvation. *J. Clin. Invest.* 48:574-83, 1969).[12]
This manuscript has since been quoted well over 1,000 times
in highly regarded scientific journals. We showed that the
liver and kidney together produced enough glucose to meet
the small glucose requirements by the brain and the rest of
the body tissues. The fact that they shared the role for
glucose production was firmly grasped.

Before we began studying the kidney function in
1965, we thought that the work of others supported the
teachings that there was a "renal threshold" for ketone bodies
and glucose. It was well known that patients with
uncontrolled diabetes mellitus, with high blood levels of
ketone bodies and glucose, excreted large quantities of
ketone bodies and glucose in their urine. In essence, when
blood ketone bodies and glucose concentrations were
elevated and the kidneys were presented with more of these
materials than they could reabsorb, ketone bodies and
glucose were excreted in the urine.

For many years, ketone bodies (acetoacetate, beta-
hydroxybutyrate and acetone) were found in the urine not
only of diabetic patients but also in the urine of starving
people. Blood passes through the kidney and some of the
blood (plasma) undergoes filtration through the renal
glomeruli (see Chapter V, Urine Reflects the Truth). The
filtrate of plasma contains ketone bodies and glucose. The
majority of these fuels is reabsorbed into the blood and exits
the kidneys. Nonetheless, reabsorption is rarely 100%
effective, and ketone bodies and glucose are present in trace
amounts in the urine practically at all times. However, when
these fuels are elevated in the blood, they are excreted in the
urine in large amounts. These findings formed the erroneous
concept that ketone bodies and glucose had renal thresholds
for excretion. Specifically, the misconceptions promoted the
thinking that when ketone bodies or glucose were elevated to
high concentrations in the blood, they were "spilled over in
the urine." These misconceptions were propagated by

---

[12] There is a long time between gathering research data and having the
data published in a reputable medical journal.

several reputable groups of investigators. Early studies performed in dogs and humans suggested there was a maximum rate that filtered acetoacetate and beta-hydroxybutyrate (and acetone and glucose) could be reabsorbed from the renal tubules before being discharged down the renal tract into the urinary bladder. This *idea* was wrong. There were, in addition, other concepts that needed to be modified regarding the loss of ketone bodies (anions) in the urine and kidney generation of ammonium (cation) for excretion in the urine.

Studying metabolism of the kidney after an overnight fast and periodically during prolonged starvation required collaboration. We had to expand and employ different techniques to measure renal function. We had to use methods to measure glomerular filtration rates using the inulin (not insulin) clearance techniques. This, coupled with urinary excretion rates, allowed us to determine the quantity of ketone bodies (and glucose) filtered and reabsorbed or excreted in the urine.

There seems to be no question that near-electroneutrality (compounds with positive charges $\cong$ compounds with negative charges) in urine and other biological fluids is essential in living forms. Acetoacetate and beta-hydroxybutyrate exist as negatively charged compounds (anions) in body fluids, including the glomerular filtrate. The loss of these negatively charged compounds in the urine obligates the near-equal excretion of positively charged elements or compounds (cations) to maintain a close balance of negatively charged and positively charged compounds. However, if the loss of negatively charged ketone bodies in the urine required the body to excrete nearly equal quantities of positively charged compounds, specifically sodium and/or potassium, from the body fluids, death induced by diminished fluid volume would occur in less than one or two weeks.

We were in the process of studying urinary excretory compounds during starvation when we noticed that shortly after the blood ketone body concentration rapidly increased, urinary ketone body excretion (ketonuria) developed.

132

Initially, urinary electroneutrality was maintained primarily by sodium (Na^+) excretion. Shortly thereafter, ammonium (NH_4^+) excretion rose and replaced sodium excretion to cover the negatively charged ketone bodies. Ammonium excretion progressively increased in parallel with the loss of ketone bodies in the urine (ketonuria), peaking after about 14 days of starvation. Ammonium excretion slightly exceeded the loss of acetoacetate⁻ and beta-hydroxybutyrate⁻ because NH_4^+ is also needed to balance the other anions (negatively charged compounds) excreted mainly as phosphate and sulfate (Figure 3). Thus, the total equivalents of ammonium slightly exceeded the total equivalents of acetoacetate plus beta-hydroxybutyrate lost in the urine. (Another ketone body, acetone, has no electrical charge and, therefore, does not require neutralization.) We found a positive relationship between the urinary excretion rates of ammonium and acetoacetate plus beta-hydroxybutyrate ($r = 0.95$).

Upon leaving my fellowship training position at Harvard to become a full time faculty member at Temple University Hospital in 1968, my responsibilities changed. I became a member of the Division of Endocrinology and Metabolism and the day-to-day Director of the General Clinical Research Center (GCRC). I took care of inpatients and outpatients, taught medical students, made teaching rounds with the residents, and provided consultation rounds and taught residents and fellows. The time for research shrunk. Obviously, there was less time than needed to devote to research activities. No one has the freedom to devote time to research like a fellow in training does. Nonetheless, my clinical research activities were not stopped, just dampened.

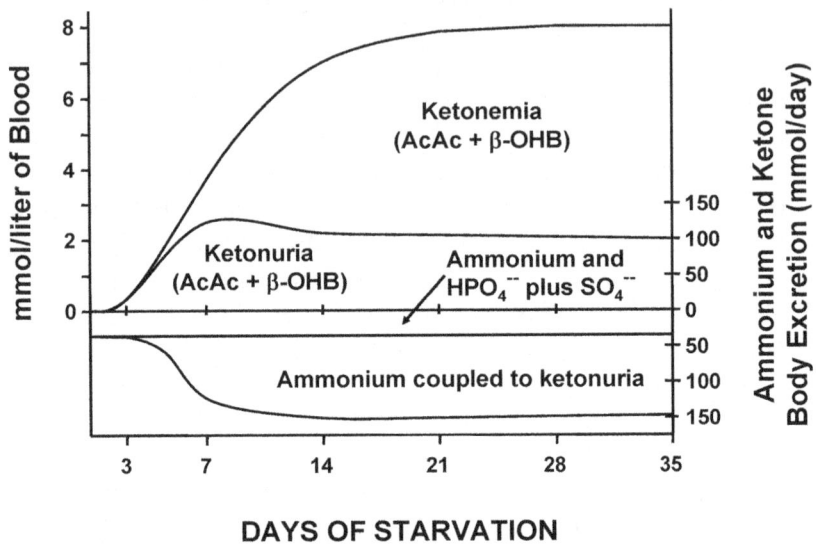

Figure 3. There is a dissociation between blood ketone body concentrations (ketonemia) and ketone body excretion (ketonuria). On the other hand, ketone body loss plus phosphate (HPO_4^{--}) plus sulfate (SO_4^{--}) losses in the urine (ketonuria) and ammonium losses are closely related.

In the early 1970's, while at Temple's GCRC, I began collaborative studies with a physician-educator, the late Dr. Daniel G. Sapir, a kidney specialist at Johns Hopkins University School of Medicine and Hospital. Dr. Sapir was a physician of the highest caliber whose enthusiasm for clinical research and ability to analyze renal function were superb. He was a practical realist who cast light on disease states and elucidated a better understanding of renal function in health and disease. His research focused around diseases collectively related to the excretion of nitrogenous waste products: diseases where there was an inability to excrete in the urine the by-products of protein breakdown due to kidney failure. One approach to correcting these disorders was to prevent the breakdown and the loss of body protein, primarily muscle or lean body mass, as reflected in the urinary excretion of nitrogen. Dr. Sapir made many pertinent discoveries regarding the preservation of lean body mass. Studying renal function during starvation provided an ideal opportunity for him to gain knowledge related to the loss of urinary nitrogen and the loss of body proteins. In collaboration with Dr. Sapir and his colleagues at the GCRC at Johns Hopkins, we began to tease apart complex interactions on how the kidney spared body protein and what was excreted in the urine as a consequence of trying to conserve lean body mass. In addition, we investigated the loss of body fluids, salts and ketone bodies during starvation. We were able to accomplish these joint research efforts because support staff on both GCRCs frequently traveled between Johns Hopkins in Baltimore and Temple in Philadelphia to transport blood and urine specimens.

Dr. Sapir, other colleagues, and I collaborated on studies of 9 obese volunteers admitted to the Johns Hopkins Hospital's GCRC to undergo therapeutic starvation for weight reduction. We showed that ingestion of 2-4 teaspoons of sugar per day could reduce urinary nitrogen excretion from protein breakdown by 50% in humans undergoing prolonged starvation (Figure 4). These results were published (D.G. Sapir, O.E. Owen, J.T. Cheng, *et al.* The effect of carbohydrates on ammonium and ketoacid excretion during starvation. *J. Clin. Invest.* 51:2093-102, 1972). Prior to these studies, no one knew that the human body was so exquisitely sensitive to small quantities of ingested carbohydrates. This was the beginning of more new light being shed on metabolic mechanisms essential for survival during starvation. Just eating a small quantity of sugar (e.g. as in rice, honey or berries) daily had the potential to salvage life during starvation.

Subsequently, in another collaborative study on the conservation of lean body mass, Dr. Sapir and colleagues hospitalized 11 obese volunteers on the GCRC at Johns Hopkins Hospital. We gave these obese volunteers the sodium salts of alpha-ketoanalogues (the amino acid carbon skeletons without the nitrogen component) and inhibited the body from breaking down its protein mass. The primary purpose of this study was to demonstrate that protein wasting

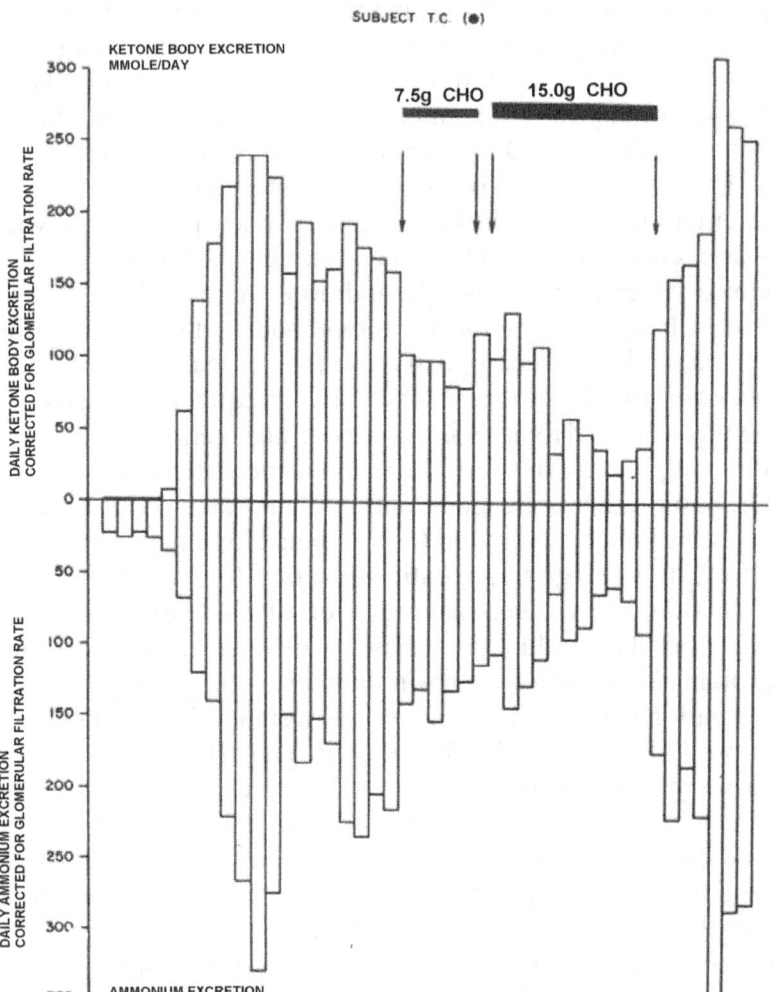

Figure 4. Changes in daily acetoacetate plus beta-hydroxybutyrate (ketone bodies) and ammonium excretion corrected for glomerular filtration rates during starvation of an obese patient-volunteer who received 7.5 grams and 15.0 grams of supplemental sugar during a prolonged starvation study.

could be curtailed by giving starving people these amino acid analogues. Specifically, urea nitrogen excretion derived from protein breakdown was decreased in these starving volunteers. Thus, these amino acid analogues could be used to treat patients with protein wasting disease and dying from kidney failure who could not properly conserve lean body mass or excrete nitrogenous by-products in the urine. The analogues could substitute for amino acids, and there was less of a need to excrete waste nitrogenous urea. The results of these studies were published (Sapir, D.G., O.E. Owen, T. Pozefsky, and M. Walser. Nitrogen sparing induced by a mixture of essential amino acids given chiefly as their keto-analogues during prolonged starvation in obese subjects. *J. Clin. Invest.* 54:974-80, 1974). We also recorded, but did not properly emphasize, an incidental finding that the sodium salts increased ketone body excretion. In retrospect, it seems obvious that ketone bodies were used as expendable anions to balance the excretion of sodium cations given as the salts of alpha-ketoanalogues of amino acids. Thus, we unintentionally showed that ketone bodies were excreted to maintain electroneutrality. This was a very subtle but key finding. It should have, but did not, raise the question: Is ammonium cation loss in the urine during starvation there to cover ketone body anion loss in the urine or is ketone body anion loss to cover ammonium cation loss? Because the intravenous infusion of the sodium salts of ketoanalogues during starvation causes an increase in ketone body anion excretion to cover not ammonium but the sodium cation excretion suggests that maintenance of electrical neutrality is one driving force. In hindsight I suspect that the essentiality of renal synthesis of glucose coupled to the excretion of ammonium during starvation was another and independent driving force. During total, prolonged starvation, ketonuria was probably a secondary event promoting renal gluconeogenesis. However, the fact that both urinary electroneutrality and renal gluconeogenesis have persisted through the millennia suggests that there may be more than one reason for ketonuria.

In another collaborative study, Dr. Sapir hospitalized 12 obese individuals on the GCRC at Johns Hopkins Hospital. These volunteers were given only water during 24 days of total starvation. The results of our collaborative efforts were reported and showed that both acetoacetate and beta-hydroxybutyrate reabsorption rates in the kidney increased linearly when plotted against their filtered loads (Figure 5).

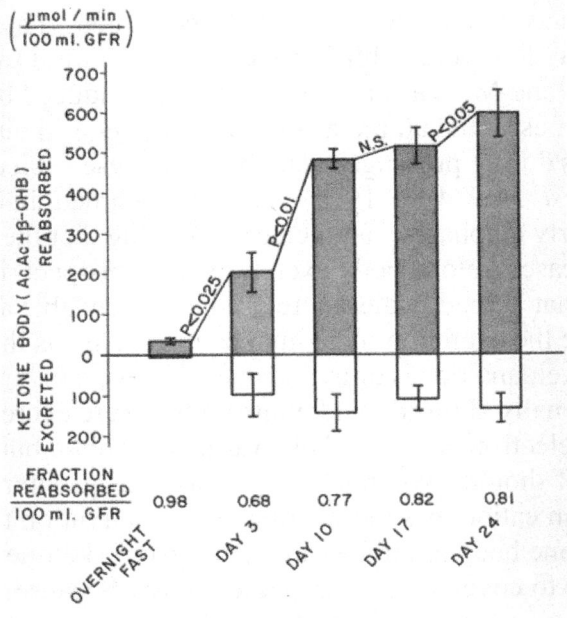

Figure 5. The renal conservation of ketone bodies (acetoacetate plus beta-hydroxybutyrate) during starvation ketosis. The rates of ketone body reabsorption and excretion were plotted against data obtained on successive days of study. GFR = glomerular filtration rate

Thus, no tubular maximal transport rate existed for either ketone body during physiologic ketonemia and starvation. Further, the conservation of a huge quantity of filtered ketone bodies by the kidneys prevented a large loss of these valuable fuels during prolonged starvation. Dr. Sapir and I showed that the conservation of ketone bodies minimized the body's loss of sodium and protein during starvation and aided in maintaining a high concentration of acetoacetate and beta-hydroxybutyrate in the blood. Such circumstances probably aided the brain in consuming ketone bodies during starvation (Sapir, D.G. and O.E. Owen. Renal conservation of ketone bodies during starvation. *Metabolism* 24:23-33, 1975).

Although our first published manuscript on renal gluconeogenesis in the *Journal of Clinical Investigation* in 1969 was factual, we did not have enough information to synthesize the grand scheme of renal metabolism made from our early observations.

First, the quantitative aspect of low liver and kidney glucose production was not fully recognized. Second, we subsequently learned that several days of starvation were required before loss of ketone bodies in the urine was accompanied by ammonium loss in the urine. We established that in humans, renal ammoniagenesis and gluconeogenesis were coupled. Third, I believe the time frame for ammoniagenesis and low quantity of renal gluconeogenesis were not properly grasped by everyone. Fourth, I recognized that one-half of a small quantity of glucose is not very much glucose. Fifth, I initially failed to recognize the difference between the small quantity of glucose produced by the kidney and the physiological and/or biochemical significance of the glucose produced. It was many years later when we revisited the issues and began to fully recognize that the small quantity of glucose added to the blood by the kidney was absolutely essential for survival during starvation. Before reevaluating renal glucose production, the question was raised of whether or not there was a minimum quantity of glucose that had to be synthesized from amino acids (causing protein to be broken down) to maintain survival during starvation. Was there a built-in turnover of proteins during starvation in which the rate of protein breakdown exceeded the rate of protein synthesis and nitrogenous by-products from amino acid catabolism were simply excreted in the urine? Was it possible that urinary nitrogenous excretion during starvation was a mechanism of removing waste from the body, and the generation of glucose, a universal fuel, was simply a by-product? Could gluconeogenesis merely be an economical process for conserving the carbon skeletons of amino acids?

If there is a minimum need for glucose, it should be demonstrated. Later, we did just that, but in the interim, administrative work, teaching and patient care consumed me while I was Professor and Chair of Medicine at Southern Illinois University. The results of the research studies done in 1986-1989 were not published until 1998.

With the lack of financial support from the state government for education, the intellectual environment at Temple University Hospital (and across the nation) began to slowly but progressively decay in the early 1980's. By 1985, most of the clinical faculty were heavily engaged in taking care of patients. Administrators thought educators who were medical doctors could earn their salaries by taking care of patients. Accepting teaching responsibilities was understood as a requirement to work at a university hospital. The fact that there was little time left to pursue research was their hard luck. In addition, there was practically no time set aside to sit quietly and to think. Nonetheless, a few of my colleagues were trying to advance health care by collaborating in an attempt to understand overall body metabolism. *Some of us realized that clinical research is not a luxury; it is a necessity!*

We knew that humans had a considerable amount of metabolic versatility during the fed state for fuel utilization to maintain energy requirements. However, were there lower limits of flexibility for the catabolism of one or another of the major fuel classes during starvation? In 1986, we began this reassessment of protein, fat and carbohydrate requirements during starvation. I designed a research protocol to answer the question of whether or not there was a minimum requirement for glucose during starvation. It was the most complex study that my colleagues and I had ever formulated. We used all the simple old and modern techniques we had mastered over the previous two decades to answer this question. We selected patients who could benefit from weight reduction. We studied their rate of weight loss, body composition before and after weight loss, energy requirements before and throughout weight reduction, urinary excretion rates of nitrogenous compounds and ketone

140

bodies, blood concentrations of fuels (glucose, free fatty acids, ketone bodies, alanine, glutamine and glutamate), and finally, the impact of administering sodium phenylacetate intravenously and measuring the effect of this compound on body metabolism. The final component of this research protocol involved catheterizing an artery that supplied blood to the liver and kidneys and the veins that drained the liver and kidneys so that the quantity of glucose produced by these organs could be measured and related to blood fuels and hormones, and to urinary excretion rates of nitrogenous compounds (specifically ammonia and urea) and ketone bodies. The consent form is included in an appendix of this chapter. However, there are sentences in this consent form to which I want to draw the reader's attention:

"I understand that this is a research study, and that other than weight reduction, it may not benefit me directly. However, it might benefit others in the future from what we learn from these investigations. *I also understand that I may withdraw from this study at any time. Such action will not jeopardize my medical needs. .... Neither failure to join in the study nor my stopping before it ends will in any way affect my medical care at Temple University Hospital.*"

The foregoing information provided in the consent form is emphasized here because patients often agree to undergo a study and then decide that it may not be in their best interest to continue their research efforts.

The National Institutes of Health require that any human who is going to be subjected to a medical experimentation be well informed on the proposed research and sign a consent form that is clearly and simply written in language that defines the risk associated with the research effort as well as the possible benefit or lack thereof to the subject, relatives or society. The consent forms are modified with experience, knowledge and medical-legal considerations. I am sure that the consent form in the appendix of this chapter would probably be modified to conform with the current societal demands and Institutional

Review Board's requests. Modifications are necessary to stay abreast with current state of knowledge used to protect the welfare of patients/volunteers.

In 1986-1988, again we turned to starvation as a circumstance employed to determine whether or not there was a minimum requirement for glucose synthesis (production) during starvation. In essence, did the body have to mobilize amino acids from proteins to synthesize glucose for the brain and other organs during starvation or could the body derive more of its energy from stored fat? This question could not be answered by starving obese volunteers until they reached a steady state of metabolism where the day-to-day changes were trivial. During this state of steady-state metabolism we could administer a compound, phenylacetate, which is known to combine with one of the principal amino acids (glutamine) for synthesizing glucose. Phenylacetate traps and causes glutamine to be lost intact in the urine without contributing its carbon skeleton to glucose production or its nitrogen component to ammonium (or urea) production (See Chapter IV, Figures 2-4). Thus, could we decrease the production of glucose and waste nitrogenous compounds (ammonium by the kidney and urea by the liver) during starvation by administering phenylacetate? We knew that phenylacetate caused no harm to humans. (Phenylacetate was routinely given to sick children who could not adequately form urea in the liver and excrete urea in the urine. The children tolerated phenylacetate treatment and their health improved.) We decided to give phenylacetate to obese starving adults to rob glutamine from their bloodstreams and determine if such perturbation decreased their liver and kidney production of glucose and ammonium and urea excretion in their urine. However, phenylacetate is the smelly ingredient sprayed on adversaries by stink-pot skunks. Preparation of phenylacetate to administer to patient-volunteers "drove the pharmacist up the wall." To protect our patient-volunteers from the offensive smell, we added phenylacetate to bottles of saline and gave the mixture to them intravenously.

There were a number of patient-volunteers who wanted to try starvation, while under close clinical supervision in the hospital, as a mechanism to lose weight. We selected five obese patients who we thought would benefit from undergoing research studies designed to determine whether or not a given quantity of glucose had to be synthesized by the liver and kidneys from amino acids, especially glutamine, during prolonged starvation. The research protocol was approved for scientific merit by the Advisory Committee and for safety by the Institutional Review Board of Temple University Health Sciences Center. Thereafter, informed, written consent was obtained from each of the patient-volunteers

The patient-volunteers were admitted to the GCRC of Temple for a 23-day study, 21 days of which were for starvation. They consumed a balanced weight-maintaining diet before hospitalization. Most of the patient-volunteers had diseases in addition to obesity, but they had compensated kidney functions and completely normal liver functions. Their body compositions (fat and fat-free body masses) were determined by underwater weighing techniques before and after weight loss. This allowed us to determine how much of the weight loss was due to fat mass and how much was due to lean body mass losses. Resting energy requirements were measured before and periodically during the starvation periods. This provided a check on the caloric value of masses lost. Blood specimens were periodically collected and analyzed. This permitted us to estimate the benefit of weight loss on their diabetic status. Twenty-four hour daily urine excretion rates were measured, and urinary ketone bodies and nitrogenous compounds (total nitrogen, urea, ammonium, creatinine and urate) were measured. This gave insight on the crux of the matter under investigation. It was the last time I oversaw human research studies on patient-volunteers hospitalized for study.

These last five patients were of special interest to me. They were only starved the length of time required to assure steady-state conditions plus the days needed to do the experimental studies. This starvation period was long

143

enough to show clear signs of weight reduction with improvements in blood glucose, blood lipids, and blood pressure. Individual weight management programs were planned after their starvation periods were completed.

Mr. R. was a 25 year old man. He had previously lost weight by consuming a liquid protein diet and the Atkins diet. However, after weight loss he would regain his fat mass. He was particularly concerned about his weight because his obese mother had diabetes mellitus. He was 5 feet 7 inches tall and weighed 375 pounds. His blood pressure was slightly elevated at 145/85, and his resting pulse rate was clearly elevated at 98/min. His blood glucose before starvation was elevated (226 mg/dl two hours after breakfast). His fasting blood glucose of 188 mg/dl on day 1 of the fast fell to 107 mg/dl on day 21 of the fast. He met the criteria for the diagnosis of type 2 diabetes mellitus. Early in the course of starvation he developed worrisome headaches which subsided spontaneously as fasting was extended. Otherwise, he tolerated the starvation period, phenylacetate infusion and renal and liver catheterization without difficulties. During the fast he lost 29 pounds.

Ms. S., 51 years old, also had type 2 diabetes mellitus and hypertension accompanying her obesity. She volunteered to undergo the starvation-phenylacetate study because her increased weight had caused her diabetic state to deteriorate. She had undergone a right nephrectomy (surgical excision of kidney), had a left staghorn kidney stone, and had pus in her urine, but urinary cultures for bacteria failed to show growth of infectious organisms. She needed to be in a controlled environment with medical help to lose weight. Ms. S. had an unusually pleasing personality. She always displayed a positive attitude and a helpful demeanor. Her fasting blood glucose fell from a high value (238 mg/dl) to a tolerable value (132 mg/dl) after 21 days of starvation. Her weight during 21 days of starvation fell from 306 pounds to a low of 277 pounds, a loss of 29 pounds. She tolerated the intravenous phenylacetate administration and catheterization studies very well. The entire research team enjoyed working with this cooperative patient-volunteer and wished her special success in combating her diseases.

Mr. R. was a 27 year old divorced man who had gained weight to 300 pounds. He was 6 feet tall. He requested help to reduce his body mass. He initially seemed to be in good physical health. He had no complaints during the first few days of starvation; however, he began spitting frequently. He had to be encouraged continuously to drink water. After day 7 of the starvation study he developed nausea and would vomit small amounts of gastric content. Dehydration developed and intravenous salt and water were repeatedly administered. This patient-volunteer's starvation was characterized by excessive time in bed and swings in mood with intermittent depression. He also developed a low body potassium content. During the 21 day fast he lost from 295 pounds to a low of 263 1/2 pounds, a loss of 31 1/2 pounds. He tolerated kidney and liver catheterization without a problem. His refeeding period was handled conservatively, and he was discharged and followed in the outpatient clinical facilities. Although he made a significant contribution by allowing us to confirm the essentiality of renal gluconeogenesis during starvation, he also demonstrated the importance of close clinical monitoring of some patient-volunteers during starvation.

The last patient-volunteer that underwent liver and kidney catheterization studies after weight reduction by starvation in the GCRC was Ms. M. She was 41 years old and suffered with asthma and questionable inadequate blood circulation to the heart (angina). During early fasting, diuresis caused large weight loss. She was cheerful over this phenomenon. Headaches developed. She slept long periods of time and smoked cigarettes incessantly when awake. She complained of chest pain, but there was no evidence that it was related to her heart. Later during the starvation period she developed a generalized itch. Maybe the itch was caused by the detergents used to clean the sheets and pillow cases. Liver function studies were normal. She maintained good spirits throughout the fast and was sociable with other patients and staff. Her weight on admission to the hospital was 309 pounds. Her height was 5 feet 7 1/2 inches. Her lowest weight, 276 pounds, occurred after 18 days of starvation and before the phenylacetate was given intravenously. Her weight loss after 18 days of starvation was 33 pounds. The catheterization study was easily accomplished and well tolerated. During the refeeding she felt bloated and full. However, after a day or two following the catheterization study she began eating more food than recommended to her for continuous weight loss. Her behavior suggested she may have thought the weight loss was not worth the effort.

The fifth patient-volunteer was a 27 year old female who weighed 315 pounds at the time of admission. Height was 5 feet 7 inches. She had a history of migraine headaches. Her maximum body weight was 357 pounds. She admitted to overeating and tried intermittently to lose weight. During hospitalization she was sociable and requested walks outside the hospital with a nurse escort. She had an itchy rash. The question of possible allergy to the detergents used to clean gowns and bed coverings was again raised. However, her spirits remained high. Unfortunately and unintentionally she lost some of her urine down the toilet. The rest of her urine was collected and saved in an ice chest in a manner similar to that used for all specimens from patient-volunteers until measured and divided for analysis. She tolerated the sodium phenylacetate infusion without complaints. However, she was bored during the prolonged hospitalization. At the end of the phenylacetate infusion she was concerned about being allergic to the dye that would be used during the study. She stated just before the catheterization study was to be done that she was allergic to iodine. (Contrast materials used in catheterization studies contain iodine.) Therefore, no liver or kidney vessels were catheterized. The other components of the research protocol were completed. Analyses of her urine specimens provided data that were not in keeping with our expectations. Like all of the patient-volunteers, she underwent underwater weighing to determine her fat and lean body masses before and after fasting. She was prescribed a diet and refeeding was initiated. Similar to all the other patient-volunteers who had undergone starvation studies for weight reduction, she was taught the caloric content of foods and given written dietary instructions. Follow-up visits as an outpatient were arranged.

We were in the process of revisiting the question of whether or not there was a minimal requirement for glucose during total and prolonged starvation when I accepted the position of Professor and Chair of Medicine at Southern Illinois University School of Medicine. As the data from Johns Hopkins and Temple were being gathered and synthesized at Temple's GCRC, I left Pennsylvania for Illinois. It was seven years later that I took a study leave from Southern Illinois University School of Medicine and began evaluating the data, so skillfully collected and stored by Ms. Maria Mozzoli at Temple, regarding whether or not there was a minimal requirement of glucose during prolonged starvation.

I thought it would take me about 3 months to analyze and submit the data for publication. Instead, it took me 18 months of uninterrupted study time to complete and submit the manuscript for publication. Our results were published as a special article (O.E. Owen, K.J. Smalley, D.A. D'Alessio, *et al.* Protein, fat and carbohydrate requirements during starvation: anaplerosis and cataplerosis. *Am. J. Clin. Nutr.* 68:12-34, 1998).

Sure enough, there was a minimal requirement for glucose synthesis during starvation, and renal gluconeogenesis was essential for the body to synthesize a small but constitutive amount of glucose for survival. During starvation the body must mobilize enough amino acids, predominantly alanine to the liver and glutamine to the kidney to synthesize this minimal, but absolutely required, amount of glucose to maintain body functions. In fact, when phenylacetate was administered to starving patients in the steady state of metabolism, phenylacetate latched onto glutamine in the body, and induced the loss of phenylacetylglutamine in the urine. Compensatory protein breakdown occurred, and total nitrogen excretion as urea and

147

ammonium reflecting liver and kidney gluconeogenesis did not diminish; specifically, the nitrogen in urea and ammonium remained constant but was accompanied by an augmented amount of nitrogen loss due to the excretion of phenylacetylglutamine nitrogen (Figure 6).

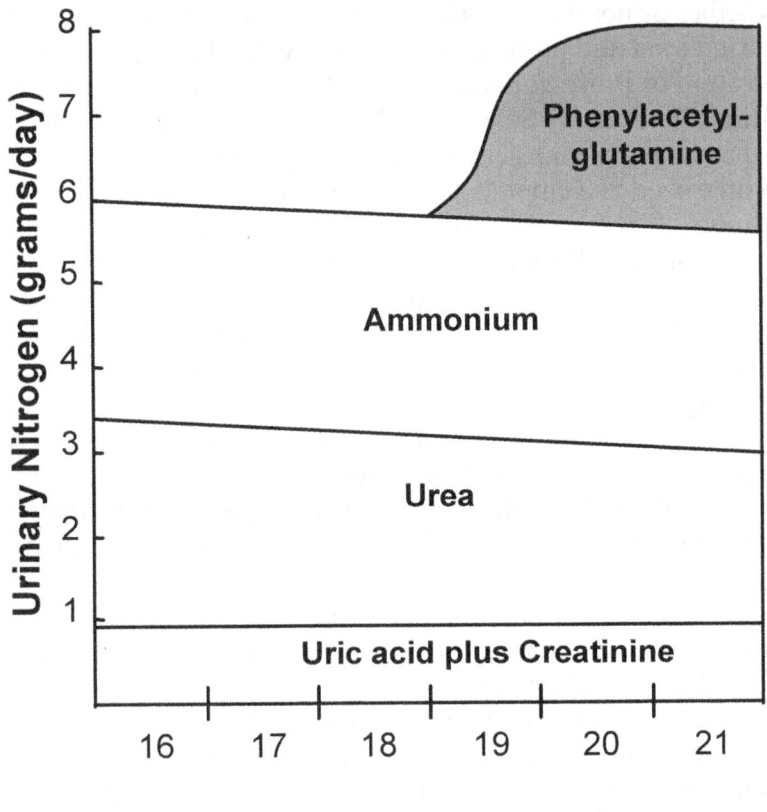

DAY OF STARVATION

Figure 6. A schematic illustration of the data presented in the 1998 *American Journal of Clinical Nutrition* article. It shows increased urinary nitrogen excretion in 5 patient-volunteers because of the urinary nitrogen loss in phenylacetylglutamine. Ammonium, urea, uric acid and creatinine urinary excretion remained relatively constant between days 16 and 21 of starvation.

Catheterization studies for measuring renal arteriovenous blood concentration differences multiplied by blood flow rates showed glucose production persisted during phenylacetate administration and phenylacetylglutamine urinary excretion. These studies clearly demonstrated that there is a minimum requirement for glucose during starvation, and the kidneys contributed their allotment. Thus, glucose production was not depressed by robbing the body of one of the primary amino acids, glutamine, that normally contributes to gluconeogenesis. Instead, more protein was broken-down to supply more glutamine.

There is a minimal amount of glucose that must be synthesized for metabolic activities during starvation; the kidney has to make its contribution to glucose synthesis. It does this in the most economical way imaginable. The kidney produces glucose from the carbon skeleton of glutamine and excretes the nitrogenous waste compound, ammonium, into the urine. The synthesis of glucose is essential and excretion of ammonium is cheap in energy cost. The excretion of ketone bodies to maintain electroneutrality is a trivial loss of energy from the body. Therefore, the use of the carbon skeleton of glutamine to make glucose and the excretion of the nitrogen waste from amino acid degradation as ammonium is an extraordinarily resourceful way to use the body's stored fuels.

Collectively, we showed that 1) administering alpha-ketoanalogues of amino acids, 2) giving small amounts of carbohydrates, and 3) the more ketone bodies filtered from the plasma, the more ketone bodies were reabsorbed by the kidneys, all suggesting that renal ammoniagenesis and gluconeogenesis cause the loss of ketone bodies in the urine and not vice versa. It appears that the synthesis of acetoacetate and beta-hydroxybutyrate provides both the anions and cations needed in the renal intra-tubular spaces to trap the non-charged gas, ammonia (NH_3), and convert it to charged cations, ammonium (NH_4^+), and induces the loss of by-product nitrogen from glutamine. Thus, the loss of ammonium in the urine induces acetoacetate and beta-hydroxybutyrate loss in the urine. After all, in most humans undergoing starvation, a little more fat can be mobilized to produce and excrete ketone bodies with impunity. Ketone

149

bodies are produced primarily in the liver from mobilized fat and from atmospheric oxygen. The caloric content of urinary ketone bodies is trivial when the amount of fat present in most humans is considered.

The kidney is the master chemist for maintaining body water, electrolytes and acid-base balance. It also complements the liver as a fine integrator of fuel homeostasis by maintaining glucose production.

In retrospect, it seems reasonable to draw the conclusions that there are at least two driving forces pushing ketone body excretion in the urine. First, the positively charged materials in the urine must be balanced by the negatively charged materials in the urine. Electroneutrality has to exist. Second, ammonium excretion in the urine has to occur so the kidneys can synthesize a small but essential quantity of glucose.

The coupling of ammonium and ketone body excretion with glucose synthesis by the kidneys is ingenious. This fortunate stroke of evolution also links ammonium production to the generation of bicarbonate (HCO_3^-) which allows the kidneys to produce bicarbonate and reabsorb chloride with renal conservation of sodium and potassium and thus maintain the fluid (water) volume needed for the body and to maintain acid-base balance.

Glucose synthesis is essential during starvation. More energy from newly synthesized glucose is needed than can be derived from glycerol stored in body fat and acetone derived from the spontaneous breakdown of acetoacetate. Body protein is the only large source of amino acids that can be mobilized and used to synthesize glucose.

The conservation of energy is also essential for survival during starvation. The body is faced with synthesizing a required amount of glucose in the most economical way possible and conserving body protein. Ketone bodies not only substitute for glucose as a source of energy for the brain, they also promote renal glucose synthesis in the most economical manner possible. First, the availability of fat that can be used with impunity is greater than the amount of protein that can be used without serious consequences. Second, about one-half the weight of ketone bodies is oxygen. Oxygen is available from the atmosphere; it does not have to be stored in the body. The loss of energy from the body as ketone bodies in the urine is trivial, about 3% of the daily energy requirements. Ketone bodies, formed in the liver, release hydrogen, the element responsible for the mild metabolic acidosis of starvation. Acidosis augments the kidney enzymes that synthesize both glucose and ammonium. Glutamine is the predominant amino acid that contributes its carbon skeleton to glucose synthesis in the kidney and nitrogen for urinary ammonium excretion. The caloric value of protein is greater when amino acid nitrogen is excreted in the urine as ammonium because only one molecule of ATP is needed to form ammonium. The synthesis of urea requires two molecules of ATP for each nitrogen atom used to form one molecule of urea. In addition, even more energy from ATP is required for the synthesis of creatine and uric acid, the other two major nitrogenous waste compounds used for excretion. Thus, the energy cost of excreting nitrogen as ammonium is the most economical way possible for the body to excrete nitrogenous waste from amino acid breakdown during starvation. Further, the carbon skeleton of glutamine is used to synthesize glucose, a constitutive compound for energy metabolism during starvation.

If I were a theorist, I would make the following speculation: The kidney absorbs practically all of the beta-hydroxybutyrate and acetoacetate that undergoes glomerular filtration. The amount of these ketone bodies lost in the urine is secondary to tubular secretion of beta-hydroxybutyrate and acetoacetate. The driving force behind ketonuria is the constitutive (essential) need for the kidney to synthesize glucose. This is done by eliminating ammonium in the urine and using the residential amino acid carbon skeleton to synthesize glucose. Ketone bodies excreted neutralize the ammonium lost in the urine. In essence, it is the energy requirement of the body from newly synthesized glucose that drives the excretion of ammonium, and ketone bodies are lost in the urine to maintain electroneutrality.

Acetone passes freely across all membranes and is not considered physiologically important in this process of electroneutrality. Nonetheless, the biochemistry and physiology of acetone metabolism is incomplete.

Liver and Kidney Interactions
    Understanding the multiple roles of the liver and kidney in maintaining a constant state of fuel content in the blood is extremely difficult because so many systems are involved in this process (Chapter IV, Figures 1-4). For example, starvation is characterized by low concentrations of blood glucose and insulin. Free fatty acids are mobilized, primarily from adipose tissue. Some of these lipids pass through the liver and are broken down into two-carbon fragments, acetate, and used for synthesizing four-carbon fuels, ketone bodies. In the process of synthesizing acetoacetate and beta-hydroxybutyrate (ketone bodies), hydrogen (H^+) is released into the bloodstream. H^+ is the element responsible for inducing the metabolic acidosis of starvation. The H^+ combines with blood bicarbonate (HCO_3^-) to generate carbonic acid (H_2CO_3). This compound is quickly converted in the lungs to carbon dioxide (CO_2) and water (H_2O). The CO_2 is excreted from the body as it continues to pass through the lungs. This leaves a deficit in the blood content of HCO_3^-, the dominant chemical compound for buffering the acid, H^+, from ketone body synthesis in the liver. However, the acidosis associated with hepatic production of ketone bodies also augments kidney ammonium formation which regenerates HCO_3^- for release into the blood for reacting with H^+ continuously produced by the liver as it synthesizes more ketone bodies. However, most of the H^+ generated during hepatic ketogenesis is consumed from the body when ketone bodies are utilized as fuels: The oxidation of ketone body anions (AcAc⁻ and ß–OHB⁻) drags H^+ into the process and clears hydrogen from the body.
    The two nitrogen groups that form ammonia are derived from glutamine mobilized from body protein. The residual carbon skeletons of glutamine are converted into

glucose. The kidney releases the glucose into the blood for utilization by brain and other tissues requiring glucose for energy. In addition, the renal ammonia (NH_3) generated passes into the intra-tubular space of the nephron and reacts with H^+ to form ammonium (NH_4^+). Adding H^+ to NH_3 traps the nitrogen as NH_4^+ because the charged compound has difficulty in diffusing back across the tubular epithelium. The NH_4^+ cation neutralizes the $AcAc^-$ and β–OHB^- anions derived from liver ketogenesis and, thus, maintains electroneutrality. Thus, ketogenesis and its related acidosis augment ammoniagenesis and ketonuria. Ammoniagenesis serves to synthesize glucose and, in the process, generates ammonia which aids to maintain acid-base balance.

Summary

The most important task the body has during starvation is to maintain a flux of fuels that perfectly matches the energy requirements. The liver is the principal organ that controls the availability of water-soluble fuels for the brain and other organs. Amino acids, lactate, pyruvate, glycerol and other precursors are funneled into the liver to synthesize glucose. Adipose tissue, however, is the predominant source of fuel furnishing free fatty acids as a source of energy to organs that can use them. In addition, the adipose tissue supplies the free fatty acids used to synthesize ketone bodies for brain fuel and releases hydrogen to promote renal ammoniagenesis and gluconeogenesis. The kidney supplements the liver's role in synthesizing small but essential quantities of glucose. The kidney also reabsorbs and conserves fuels. However, renal delivery of fuels into the bloodstream is small compared to the total quantity of fuels needed to meet the energy requirements.

The kidneys extract glutamine from the blood. Glutamine provides the nitrogen for forming ammonia (NH_3). The carbon skeleton is converted into glucose which is added to the blood. Ammonia becomes trapped inside the intra-tubular space of nephrons by accepting the hydrogen (H^+) responsible for inducing acidosis. NH_3 plus H^+ becomes ammonium (NH_4^+). The latter neutralizes $AcAc^-$

and ß-OHB⁻. Thus, ammoniagenesis, gluconeogenesis, acid-base balance and ketonuria are interrelated.

ADDENDUM
CONSENT FORM TO BE SIGNED BY PATIENTS
PARTICIPATING IN THE PHENYLACETATE
(BENZOATE) AND AMMONIUM METABOLIC STUDY
DURING STARVATION

I understand that I will be admitted to the General
Clinical Research Center at Temple University Hospital to
undergo total starvation for weight reduction and to take ...
phenylacetate ... during the fasting period. The use of
phenylacetate ... during starvation is for research purposes.
It combines with amino acids (early breakdown products of
protein). Amino acids are composed of carbon, hydrogen,
oxygen and nitrogen. The body excretes nitrogen during
starvation. Nitrogen is lost from the body during starvation
in the urine primarily as urea and ammonium, both being
derived from amino acids. However, the nitrogen present in
amino acids can be excreted from the body in another way.
Amino acids can join with phenylacetate ... and be lost from
the body in the urine. Thus, combining the amino acid with
its nitrogen element to phenylacetate ... is another way of
losing nitrogen from the body. The purpose of this study is
to determine whether the body has to lose nitrogen (waste)
from the body as ammonium and urea during starvation or
whether the body can lose nitrogen from the body as amino
acids conjugated with phenylacetate ... The quantity of
phenylacetate ... given during starvation will be enough to
neutralize ammonium excretion. This will involve infusing
intravenous sodium phenylacetate.

I agree to participate in a research study to determine
the effects of ... sodium phenylacetate ... on ammonium
excretion and amino acid metabolism during prolonged
starvation.

Three peripheral arterial punctures will be done, once
after an overnight fast and once on days 15 and 18 of the
fast. The artery located at the wrist (radial) or if necessary,
at the elbow (brachial) will be the vessel punctured. About
an ounce of blood will be withdrawn from me each time an
arterial puncture is performed. A local anesthetic will be
used to numb the site where the artery is punctured. I

recognize that an arterial puncture can be painful and that I may bleed from the site or form a blood clot at the site of the puncture wound. However, a serious complication from the repeated arterial punctures is unlikely.

The administration of phenylacetate ... may influence the behavior of the liver and kidney. These are the organs that synthesize the nitrogen containing compounds, urea and ammonium. If so, this can best be determined by inserting small, flexible tubes (catheters) into the veins of the arm and groin and advancing the tubes into the veins of the liver and kidney by using x-ray machines to localize the catheters so that blood can be drawn from these organs, and thus, to measure the effects of phenylacetate ... In addition, arterial blood will also be needed to evaluate the influences of phenylacetate ... on the liver and kidney. Therefore, an additional arterial puncture wound will be made with a needle or similar device so that arterial blood can be drawn from my body.

Anytime an artery or vein is catheterized a risk of injury is possible. However, arterial and hepatic and renal vein catheterization studies are routinely done at Temple University Hospital to investigate the causes of diseases. Although my (your) catheterization procedure will be done for research purposes, I (you) have been told that there is very little chance that any form of permanent injury will occur as a result of being catheterized. The quantity of radiation (x-ray) received by the skin and internal organs is within the guidelines set by the Food and Drug Administration for annual exposure. The total dose of radiation received should not exceed 15 rads. It should be noted that this is a significant quantity of radiation.

After 21 days of starvation I will be taken to a vascular catheterization lab where an artery and a hepatic and renal vein will be catheterized so that blood samples can be drawn from these vessels. About 6-8 ounces of blood will be drawn from me at that time. Equal volumes of fluid will be infused during the catheterization study, and after the study is completed nourishment will be initiated.

The study has other potentially harmful components:

A 21 day study of total starvation will be done. Blood, urine and breath specimens will be closely monitored. We have not observed any detrimental effects from starvation for weight reduction.

... Sodium phenylacetate is thought to be a non-toxic compound when used in humans with various diseases. The effects of phenylacetate ... during starvation are unknown. However, there is no reason to expect adverse reactions from the dosages given in this study while a human is being closely observed for undesirable reactions.

Catheterization of peripheral arteries and hepatic and renal veins is associated with pain, bleeding, blood clots and infection. In addition, scars over the site used to stick the catheters into the vessels can develop. Lastly, cardiac irregularities may be induced by catheters placed near the heart.

I understand that this is a research study, and that other than weight reduction, it may not benefit me directly. However, it might benefit others in the future from what is learned from these investigations. *I also understand that I may withdraw from the study at any time. Such action will not jeopardize my medical needs.* The doctor may also terminate the study if he/she believes it is to my benefit. Furthermore, I understand that I should not undergo this study if I am pregnant.

Dr. Owen, or his delegate, will be in constant attendance throughout the study and will answer any questions that I have. *Neither failure to join in the study, nor my stopping before its end will in any way affect my medical care at the Temple University Hospital.*

I understand that if I sustain injury as a result of my participation in this research project, only physician fees and medical expenses in excess of my medical and hospital coverage or other third party coverage will be paid. I understand that financial compensation is not available. The following is the name, address and telephone number of the person to contact in the event of any research related injury and for information regarding available medical treatment.

Oliver E. Owen, M.D.
Temple University Hospital
3401 N. Broad Street
Philadelphia, PA 19140
Telephone: 215-221-3088

I have received a copy of this consent form.

Signature of Patient _____ Date _____

Signature of PI/Investigator _____ Date _____

Signature of Witness _____ Date _____

Chapter VIII. Muscle Metabolism

Muscles comprise the largest and most diversified organ system of the body. In normal adults, they account for about 40% of body weight and have the greatest changes in metabolism and energy requirements. In the resting state, the metabolic rate for this huge organ mass is relatively low, consuming only 25-30% of total energy requirements. During extreme exercise, the metabolic rate can briefly increase 20-fold, with 80-90% of energy requirements being consumed by muscle: a physically active human needs to ingest more food to maintain body weight and strength than does a physically inactive human.

After measuring brain consumption and liver production, and kidney excretion and exchange of ketone bodies, colleagues and I thought that very little acetoacetate (AcAc) and beta-hydroxybutyrate (ß-OHB) would be available to support energy requirements for muscles after prolonged starvation. Therefore, we directed our attention to muscle, measuring the fuel use of this organ during starvation when high blood ketone body concentrations were present.

There are two distinctive types of muscles: striated muscles, which can be voluntarily contracted, and non-striated muscles, which are involuntarily contracted. The heart is unique in that it is a striated muscle with its own control system but also has some characteristics of non-striated muscles.

This chapter is by no means a comprehensive review of muscle metabolism. It deals with the striated or voluntary muscles which are under the control of the conscious brain signals. The activities of these muscles are vast and varied. They are responsible for speech as well as for non-verbal body language; they are the motors required for powerful clashes of football players; they convey the body language of lovers; they perform violent acts of warriors.

The voluntary muscles are the most beautiful structures of the body with their fusiform shape extending

159

along bones and crossing joints. Italian sculptors chiseled silhouettes of men athletes out of marble. The profiles of these muscular men with very little fat were fascinating. And among women with subcutaneous fat covering muscles, the curves of the body provide attractiveness; some of these statues were gorgeous. Thus, muscles bestow beauty upon the bodies of men and women.

Muscular machinery converts chemical energy into mechanical energy. This process is well developed in the muscles.

Without muscles human beings could not move and could not survive food deprivation. Individual components of the muscular organ can display extraordinary strength. For example, the biceps of a man can readily curl or lift 50-fold its own weight. On the other hand, we often take for granted muscles' more subtle role in providing amino acids to synthesize a small quantity of glucose essential for survival during starvation.

During starvation, muscles are broken down faster than they are rebuilt. As a consequence, the muscle mass decreases. This loss of muscle mass during starvation is visually evident, especially in the lower extremities. The loss of thigh and calf muscles is easily seen after prolonged starvation. The knees look enlarged (pseudohypertrophy) because loss of adjacent soft tissue, including muscle tissue, occurs.

Muscles have the largest quantities of protein in the body. Proteins are composed of 20 amino acids. During starvation, amino acids are released by the muscle into the venous blood, but most of them are converted into alanine and glutamine inside the muscle before being released into the venous blood. About 80% of the amino acids' nitrogen components and carbon skeletons are transported to liver and kidney using alanine and glutamine as vehicles. However, the intramuscular breakdown of protein, and the release of alanine and glutamine to liver and kidney, respectively, is a highly regulated complex.

Muscles are richly supplied with blood, and the flow of blood to an exercising muscle can increase many-fold so the energy consumption by muscles during forced physical activity can increase 20-fold. There is no other healthy organ system in the body that can adapt to its environment in a manner comparable to muscles. On the other hand, voluntary muscles also herald one of the first signs of mental deterioration by showing the loss of the ability to perform fine, coordinated muscular movements, like writing or buttoning down the collar of a shirt or blouse.

The upper extremities extend from the body, and the muscles in the forearm are practically isolated in this appendage. The forearm extends from the elbow to the hand. This part of the body contains striated muscles. The brachial artery supplies blood to the deep muscles of the forearm, and the deep vein drains the forearm muscles. These vessels can be readily identified (Figure 1).

A near perfect setup for measuring the exchange rates (uptake and/or release) of respiratory gases (oxygen and carbon dioxide) and fuels (ketone bodies, free fatty acids, glycerol, glucose, lactate, pyruvate, amino acids etc.) by striated, forearm muscle was developed by Andres, Zierler, Anderson, *et al* as early as 1954. Both the artery supplying blood and the vein draining blood from the deep muscles of the forearm can be catheterized: small flexible tubes can be inserted into the artery supplying the forearm muscle with blood and the vein draining the blood from deep muscles. By knowing the concentration differences between the gases and fuels entering and leaving the forearm muscle, and knowing the blood flow rate, the extraction or release of gases and fuels can be measured: multiplying the arterio-venous concentration differences by the blood flow rate allows an investigator to calculate the exchange rates of respiratory gases and fuels. Further, placing a small (pediatric) blood pressure cuff around the wrist and inflating it will eliminate blood flow through the hand. This action will decrease blood flow through the forearm by about 50% and double the arterio-venous concentration differences of gases and fuels, thereby significantly increasing the accuracy in determining small arterio-venous concentration differences. The volume of the forearm between the wrist

161

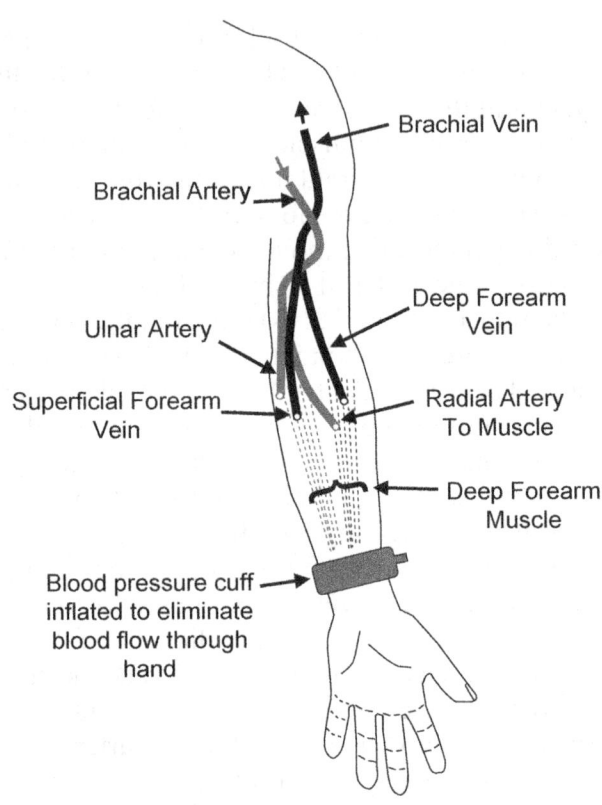

Brachial Vein

Brachial Artery

Deep Forearm Vein

Ulnar Artery

Superficial Forearm Vein

Radial Artery To Muscle

Deep Forearm Muscle

Blood pressure cuff inflated to eliminate blood flow through hand

Figure 1. This is a schematic drawing of the arm and forearm used to measure striated muscle metabolism during progressive starvation.

and the elbow can be measured by displacement of water in a glass cylinder. Thus, the uptake or release of respiratory gases and fuels can be calculated per 100 ml of forearm tissue.

We used the basic technique of measuring the exchange rates of respiratory gases and fuels to characterize metabolism of muscle after overnight, 3- and 24-day fasting periods. These stages of starvation represent times when the availability of arterial fuels and hormones initially change drastically and then stabilize. Blood glucose and insulin concentrations fall to low levels and plateau by 3 days of starvation. Free fatty acids rise quickly with fasting, and ketone bodies undergo marked increases in arterial blood concentrations. All the blood fuels are constant after 2-3 weeks of total starvation. Chapter III, Fuels and Hormones, describes these changes in detail.

We began our initial studies of muscle metabolism during starvation on the General Clinical Research Center shortly after I arrived at Temple University Hospital in 1968. Eight obese patient-volunteers were selected for treatment and research. Most of these individuals had illnesses in addition to obesity. However, their diseases were mild and probably did not affect the study results in a significant manner. Informed consent was obtained. Then baseline laboratory evaluations for heart, lung, blood, liver, kidney and endocrine states were done before a starvation protocol was initiated. I have arbitrarily selected one of the patient-volunteers to illustrate that both patients' needs and our research interests were served.

Mr. C. was a 54 year old white male jitney driver with longstanding obesity complicated by polycythemia (an abnormal increase in number of red blood cells in the body). His huge belly (Figure 2) may have contributed to his breathing difficulties while lying on his back. He had mild heart failure and diabetes mellitus. A low caloric diet had been recommended, but he had not lost weight. His height was 5 feet 11 inches and he weighed 307 pounds. His electrocardiogram was abnormal (complete right bundle block). After his initial historical and physical evaluation was done, his blood was drawn to measure liver and kidney functions and fuel and hormone concentrations. Thereafter, he began a 24 day starvation study during which time he consumed water, salt tablets and vitamins. Daily urines were collected and analyzed. He underwent forearm catheterization studies after overnight, 3- and 24-day starvation periods. He tolerated the starvation and catheterization studies without complications. He lost 34

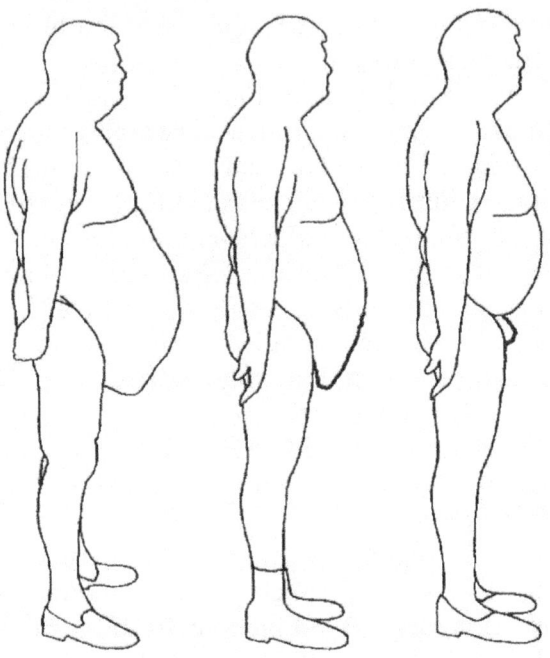

Figure 2. This graphic outline of Mr. C. reflects his abdominal obesity before a prolonged starvation study and his silhouette after weight reduction and surgical excision of his redundant abdominal apron of skin and fat.

pounds. His diabetic state resolved[13], and his shortness of breath (heart failure) decreased. The weight loss resulted in a long apron of skin-fold that covered his genitalia when

---

[13] A point aside from muscle metabolism is the concentration of blood glucose in obese humans subjected to starvation. About one-half of the obese patient-volunteers we hospitalized to study brain, liver, kidney, muscle and whole body metabolism had some degree of glucose intolerance. It has been known for 3-4 decades that obese individuals who are able to reduce body fat mass have improvement in their blood glucose concentrations. Furthermore, reducing body weight improves not only diabetes mellitus, but often decreases blood pressure and diminishes coronary artery disease, kidney disease and the possibility of suffering from a stroke. Spending less money on high caloric foods and medicines to treat the disorders induced by obesity should cut healthcare cost.

standing. He was taken to the surgical operating suite where the large skin-fold was excised; it weighed about 10 pounds. His final weight after starvation and surgery was about 253 pounds. The profiles of his body are shown in Figure 2 before and after starvation and a mockup subsequent to excision of his long, redundant skin-fold and fat mass that hung down from his abdominal wall.

Mr. C. returned to work and was followed as an outpatient. He transiently regained some weight which is typical after total, prolonged starvation. (Swelling of the body transiently occurs with salt and water retention during the early re-feeding period. Thereafter, a reduction in body weight resumes after excreting the excess in body fluids if a weight reduction diet is eaten.) He was maintained on a low caloric diet and continued to lose weight while being monitored in the outpatient clinic. Eventually, his follow-up visits ceased.

In addition to Mr. C., seven other patient-volunteers underwent forearm catheterization after overnight, 3- and 24-day fasts. Arterio-deep-venous differences of respiratory gases (oxygen and carbon dioxide), and the various fuels (glucose, glycerol, lactate, pyruvate, free fatty acids, AcAc and ß-OHB) along with simultaneous forearm blood flow rates were measured. Thus, both rates of respiratory gas utilization (oxygen) or release (carbon dioxide) were measured and combined with arterio-venous concentration differences of fuels. The nature and quantity of fuels extracted by muscle changed as starvation progressed. These patterns of fuel consumption by forearm muscle during progressive starvation are graphically displayed in Figure 3.

By measuring the arterio-venous concentration differences for oxygen, ketone bodies and other fuels, and multiplying the measured differences by blood flow rates, we could calculate the consumption of oxygen and fuels and release of carbon dioxide, lactate and pyruvate and amino acids (alanine and glutamine) by muscle in the resting and fasting state. We found that during the resting state, oxygen consumption (and carbon dioxide production) and lactate and

165

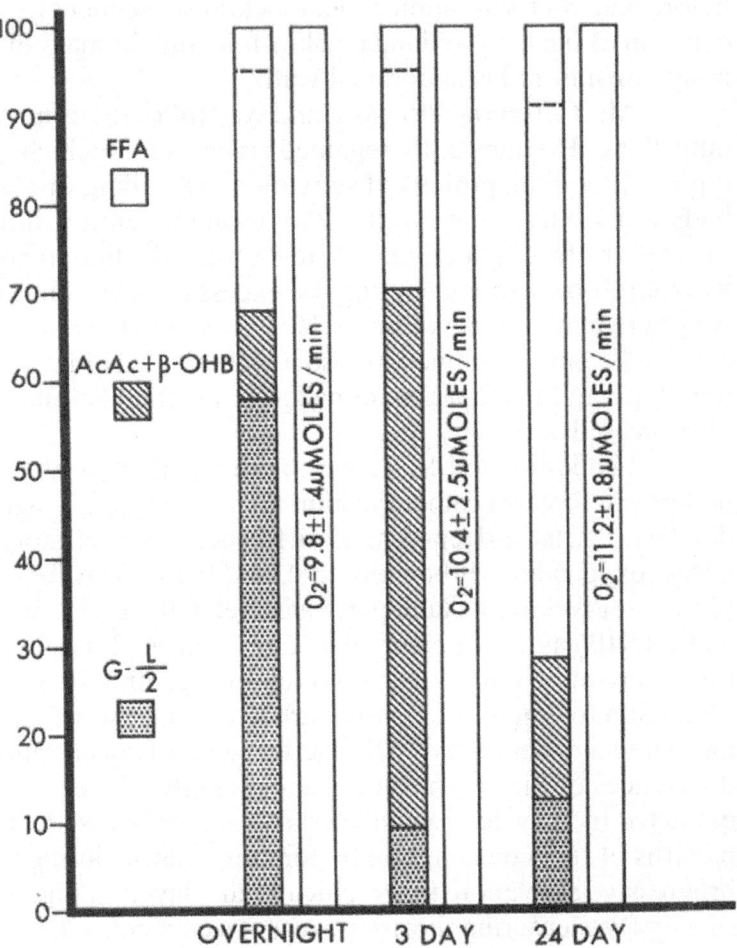

Figure 3. The clear bars to the right show the total uptake of oxygen per 100 ml of forearm tissue (mostly muscle). The bars on the left show the percent of oxygen used to breakdown (oxidize) glucose (after correcting for the release of lactate and pyruvate), AcAc plus ß-OHB (ketone bodies) and free fatty acids. Amino acid exchange rates were subsequently measured by Felig, *et al*, Pozefsky, *et al* and Owen, *et al.*

166

pyruvate release by muscle remained relatively constant throughout a 24-day fasting study. We were somewhat surprised to learn how much glucose the forearm muscle extracted after the overnight fast. Some of the extracted glucose (6-carbon compound) was broken down and released as lactate and pyruvate (two 3-carbon compounds). Nonetheless, even after correcting for lactate and pyruvate release from glucose, about one-half of the oxygen consumed after an overnight fast was used to oxidize glucose to carbon dioxide and water. Thus, glucose was a major and valuable fuel for muscle metabolism after an overnight fast. Glucose consumption fell during starvation, but some net extraction and oxygenation persisted even after correcting for the release of lactate and pyruvate. In essence, muscle always consumed a quantity of glucose, even after prolonged starvation. Perhaps a small quantity of glucose may be essential to promote muscle consumption of ketone bodies and free fatty acids. Nonetheless, the supply of glucose for muscle metabolism during prolonged starvation is limited, and this organ must derive most of its energy from other fuels as starvation progresses.

Our studies revealed that after an overnight fast, when ketone body concentrations in arterial blood were low, only small quantities of AcAc and ß-OHB were extracted by muscle from the arterial blood. With the progression of starvation, the ketone body concentrations rose, and forearm muscle extracted a greater quantity of AcAc and ß-OHB. By 3 days of starvation, muscle derived about 50% of energy requirements from ketone body oxidation. As the days of starvation increased and ketone body concentrations rose to higher values, there was a paradoxical decline in ketone body extraction by muscle. AcAc was preferentially extracted over ß-OHB, but in 5 of 8 patient-volunteers, AcAc was extracted and converted into and released as ß-OHB. Thus, AcAc was taken up by muscle, and in the majority of the patient-volunteers, it was reduced to its partner, ß-OHB, and released into the venous blood. Thus, very little net utilization of ketone bodies occurred in muscle after prolonged starvation.

167

AcAc and ß-OHB are produced in equal quantities by the liver. In the blood, however, during prolonged starvation, the concentration of ß-OHB is 3 to 6 times greater than the concentration of AcAc. The preferential extraction of AcAc and release of ß-OHB by muscle, at least in part, explains the high concentration of ß-OHB to AcAc concentration during the hyperketonemic state of starvation.

Free fatty acids eventually became the principal fuels extracted by the forearm muscle after prolonged starvation; the extraction of these fats from the blood (plasma) was evident at every time period studied but the quantity extracted increased with duration of starvation. Thus, muscle selected free fatty acids as the primary source of fuel for metabolism after 3 days of starvation. In doing so, muscle conserved the water-soluble ketone bodies for brain metabolism. This is another example of orchestrated interplay among organs to promote survival during prolonged starvation (Owen, O.E, G.A. Reichard Jr. Human forearm metabolism during progressive starvation. *J. Clin. Invest.* 50:1536-45, 1971).

Our studies on forearm muscle metabolism provided three important clues regarding muscle consumption of fuels during starvation. First, muscle consumed glucose at all times during starvation; however, after the overnight fasting period was extended, glucose consumption by muscle was very small. Second, ketone body consumption by muscle underwent a paradoxical decline after the arterial concentration progressively rose during starvation. The cardinal issue of muscle metabolism is its ability to selectively change its consumption of fuels. It may diminish or reverse its exchange of ß–OHB. Third, free fatty acids become the dominant fuel for muscle during starvation.

A complex system for removing the carbon skeletons and nitrogenous groups from amino acids in muscle developed during starvation. The work of others, including Felig *et al*, Pozefsky, *et al* and summarized by our group, reported that branched-chain amino acids (primarily leucine, isoleucine and valine) surrender in muscle their carbon skeletons and nitrogenous groups to alanine and glutamine for transportation to the liver and kidney (Figure 4). Some of the glutamine released from muscle is converted in the liver to glutamate, which travels back to the muscle to pick up more nitrogen from other amino acids in muscle undergoing catabolism (Owen, O.E, S.C. Kalhan and R.W. Hanson. The key role of anaplerosis and cataplerosis for citric acid cycle function. *J. Biol. Chem.* 277: 30409-12, 2002).

Muscle metabolism during starvation was not only the first organ system that we studied at Temple University's General Clinical Research Center, it was also the last we studied at Temple. In 1986-1988, we revisited muscle metabolism during prolonged starvation. This time we concentrated on measuring amino acids both in whole blood and in plasma to determine the uptake or release of amino acids across the lower extremities. We confirmed Dr. Philip Felig and colleagues' work showing that alanine (a 3-carbon skeleton with one nitrogen group) was the predominant amino acid released from muscle during starvation (Figure 4). Alanine travels in the water of plasma and whole blood to the liver where it is extracted and converted into newly synthesized glucose (gluconeogenesis) during starvation. The nitrogen originally contained in the alanine is removed from the carbon skeleton of alanine and converted into urea. This nitrogenous compound is excreted in the urine as a by-product of protein (amino acid) breakdown. We also complemented the works of Drs. Thomas Pozefsky, Errol Marliss and coworkers regarding glutamine metabolism. Glutamine is an amino acid with a 5-carbon skeleton and two nitrogen groups (amide and amino) attached to its carbon skeleton. Like alanine, glutamine is transported in the water component of plasma and red blood cells. Its related amino acid is glutamate which has a 5-carbon skeleton but only one nitrogen group (amino), and it travels primarily inside red blood cells. Glutamine has dual responsibilities, one for transporting one of its nitrogen groups (amide nitrogen) from muscle to the liver where this nitrogen group (amide group) is removed and converted into urea. Some of its carbon skeleton remains intact as glutamate. Glutamate travels primarily inside of red blood cells and returns to muscle

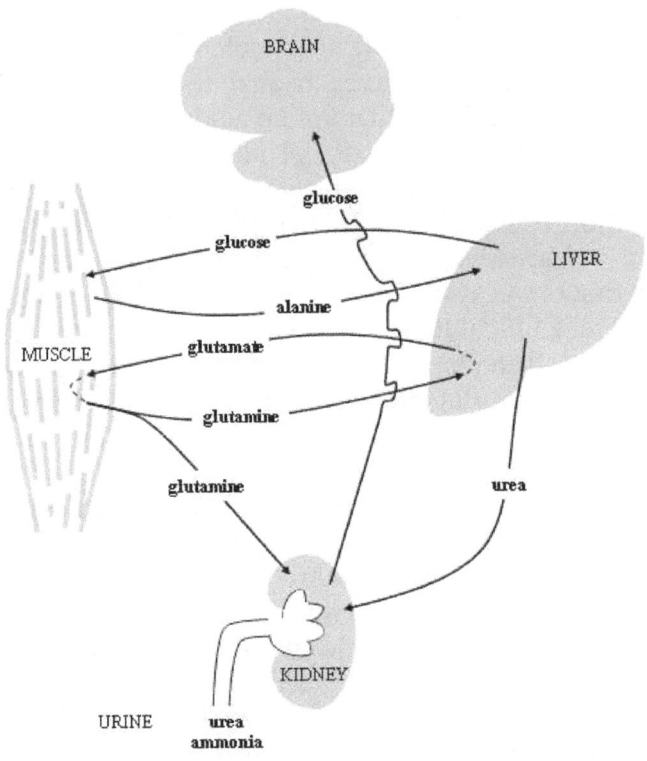

Figure 4. The predominant interrelationships among glucose, alanine, glutamine and glutamate and muscle, liver, kidney and brain metabolism. Not shown is the possible interplay between branched-chain amino acids and glutamine in the brain.

where it is extracted and reconverted to glutamine. Thus, glutamine and glutamate have different roles as vehicles for transporting nitrogen between muscle and liver. Most of the glutamine formed in muscle travels in equal concentration in the water of plasma and red blood cells to the kidney, rather than the liver. In the kidney, glutamine is extracted from the water of plasma and red blood cells and converted into ammonia and glucose. Therefore, glutamine travels to the kidney where its nitrogens are used to form ammonia (NH_3) which is excreted as ammonium (NH_4^+) in the urine (and maybe the gut), and its carbon skeleton enters the citric acid cycle as alpha-ketoglutarate, and it is converted into glucose

170

and released into the blood. Thus, not only do glutamine and glutamate carbon skeletons travel in opposite directions between liver and muscle, they also travel to different organs and are metabolized differently.

Sir Arthur Conan Doyle was the author who created the fictitious character, Sherlock Holmes, a British detective who solved many murder mysteries. Sir Doyle was a physician, and he believed that medical ailments were mysteries that could be solved by employing the same insightful techniques used by police detectives. As a clinical investigator, we used the investigative approaches advocated by Sir Doyle to solve the mysteries of how the body managed to survive during prolonged starvation (when only water was available). Step by step we detected what fuels were consumed by the brain, how they were produced by the liver, and how they were spared by muscle and conserved by the kidney so life could persist. In addition, we eventually demonstrated the dominant role of adipose tissue in providing free fatty acids as the major fuel for overall body metabolism during starvation.

The results from brain, liver, kidney, muscle and adipose tissue metabolism were complementary: the pieces of research data fitted together. They solved the mysteries of how humans tolerated total starvation for prolonged periods of time. They also showed that ketone bodies in healthy humans served as valuable fuels.

Chapter IX. Liver and Kidney Metabolism in Patients with Alcoholic Cirrhosis

Very few physicians or surgeons anticipate medical mysteries they eventually want to solve. Instead, diseases in their field(s) of expertise are encountered for which there are inadequate treatments. The lack of knowledge motivates them to become engaged in doing clinical research to uncover the causes and/or cures of those diseases.

In the United States of America, the two most common causes of cirrhosis are excessive alcoholic intake and a viral infection causing chronic hepatitis C. In the 1970's, about one-half of all patients hospitalized in large urban areas had alcohol-related diseases. The enormity of the health care costs associated with liver disease, especially alcoholic cirrhosis, was evident. In urban states, cirrhosis of the liver was ranked third as cause of death in active individuals between 25 and 65 years of age. In this chapter, the emphasis is placed on the devastating disease, alcoholic cirrhosis.

Synonyms for alcoholic cirrhosis are "Laennec's," "portal," "nutritional" and "micronodular" cirrhosis. More men than women have alcoholic cirrhosis, but women have a greater predisposition for developing cirrhosis; and if women consume alcoholic drinks, they are more likely to develop cirrhosis even though they consume less alcohol than men.

Many alcoholic patients are unkempt with poor hygiene. Often the body habitus of patients with liver cirrhosis is characterized by wasted extremities and a pot-belly due to the accumulation of large quantities of fluid (ascites). This spider-like form is usually easy to recognize when a patient is standing in the nude. Often the palms of their hands have an unusual redness. The breath of men and women who consume large quantities of ethanol (alcohol) frequently has a characteristic chemical smell of acetaldehyde. Among those acutely ill from alcoholism, there may be, in addition, a unique musty odor (fetorhepaticus) from the breath and urine in the hospital rooms occupied by them. Men usually have small soft testicles and breast enlargement. In both men and women, the livers are frequently enlarged, sometimes enormously so, and both the livers and spleens may be easily felt through the abdominal wall.

Small veins draining blood from the lower esophagus, stomach, pancreas, small and large intestines, and spleen join to form a large portal vessel (vein) that flows into the liver. Within the liver, this vessel branches into a multitude of small vessels which rejoin to exit the liver via the hepatic vein. Alcoholic cirrhosis scars the liver and blocks the free passage of blood through this organ, resulting in an increase in blood pressure in the portal vein. A normal portal venous pressure of 5-10 mmHg rises to 15-40 mmHg. This increase defines portal hypertension, which causes the venous system to become engorged.

The blood in the portal vein is forced to become rerouted around the liver. The exit routes dilate venous bypasses around the liver. These bypass routes become varicose veins and may envelop the stomach, esophagus and lower bowel (with hemorrhoids). These veins have thin walls that might rupture, creating life-threatening hemorrhage. When this occurs, patients are usually brought to the hospital emergency rooms vomiting blood, and complex efforts are used to salvage their lives.

The struggle to save the life of a patient vomiting blood and/or passing blood in the feces is intense. Most of these poor, miserable souls are prevented from dying during their first episode of massive gastrointestinal hemorrhage. (Survival rate decreases if a second episode occurs.) Upon arrival at the hospital emergency room, a quick assessment of the patient is made. Blood is drawn and sent to the clinical laboratories for chemical analysis and cross-matched for blood transfusions. Characteristic laboratory results reflect severe liver damage and usual abnormalities revealing malnutrition. Fresh blood, plasma, platelets and intravenous fluids containing glucose, vitamins, minerals and albumin are given as soon as possible. Other medicinal agents and physical tools are used to stop hemorrhage from the upper and lower gastrointestinal tract. These efforts may be somewhat chaotic but are frequently successful in maintaining the patient's life. Nonetheless, they are messy and always costly medical practices.

Emergency surgery to shunt all of the portal venous blood away from the liver into the inferior vena cava (major vein draining blood from all tissues below the diaphragm) can be used to control gastrointestinal bleeding and prevent recurrent bleeding. However, physicians and surgeons throughout the medical profession knew that most patients' health deteriorated after using this method (*total portasystemic shunt*) to lower the portal blood pressure and stop the hemorrhage. The patients developed liver failure, manifested by brain dysfunction. It was realized that total portal venous shunts should be limited to life-threatening bleeding. Therefore, alternate shunting methods were sought.

As doctors, we questioned whether or not the deterioration of the health of patients who had undergone total portasystemic shunts was related to the inability of the liver to assist in maintaining the overall energy requirements to meet the body's metabolic needs. Among these needs is the primary responsibility of the liver to maintain a sufficient supply of glucose and/or ketone bodies (fuels) to meet the energy requirements of the brain. Therefore, we thought it would be beneficial and wise to measure the total energy requirements of patients with alcoholic cirrhosis who had bled from gastroesophageal varices and were candidates for some kind of portasystemic shunt to decompress portal venous pressure. This would let us know if the overall energy requirements of patients with liver cirrhosis were normal. In addition, we wanted to measure liver metabolism before and after surgical shunts were performed to learn whether or not surgical decompression of the portal venous system was beneficial or detrimental to liver metabolism in patients with portal hypertension. We thought if hepatic compromise was induced by any form of surgical shunt, maybe the amount of glucose (and ketone bodies) synthesized and released into the blood was inadequate to provide glucose (and ketone bodies) for brain and other tissue metabolism. The lack of fuel production by the cirrhotic liver could be the cause for some of the deterioration in mental function known to be present in patients who have had surgical shunts. On the other hand, it was conceivable that portal venous decompression without shunting all of the venous blood away from the liver could improve hepatic functions. It was important to know the general behavior of the liver before and after "limited portal venous shunts" were surgically done.

It was known that the liver released glucose by two processes: newly synthesized glucose from lactate-pyruvate, amino acids and glycerol, and from stored glycogen. Thus, we needed to know how much glucose was synthesized and released and how much glucose was stored as glycogen and released between meals. We stepped back and asked 1) was the enzymatic activity in the cirrhotic liver for glucose synthesis adequate to form new glucose from precursors (e.g. amino acids, lactate, pyruvate, glycerol) that were funneled into it from the periphery and the gut; and 2) was there enough glucose stored in the cirrhotic liver as glycogen to contribute substantial amounts of glucose to the blood? We also knew that ketone bodies could substitute as a fuel for brain metabolism when glucose production was low. Therefore, we had to evaluate ketone body formation and release by the cirrhotic livers in addition to glucose storage and release by the same livers to determine if they provided enough water-soluble fuels (glucose and ketone bodies) for the brains and other tissues that needed them during the fasted state.

Even at this early stage of investigating liver metabolism in patients with alcoholic cirrhosis, we knew that the kidney had the potential to share the role in producing glucose for brain and other tissues under certain circumstances. Patients with alcoholic cirrhosis were often known to have high levels of ammonia in the blood. Renal ammoniagenesis and renal gluconeogenesis were known to be coupled. Thus, it was conceivable that some of the

175

ammonia produced was from the kidneys. Maybe ammonia released into the blood was the consequence of kidneys synthesizing glucose. Therefore, we reasoned that we needed to evaluate not only the liver's production of glucose and ketone bodies but also the kidney's production of glucose and perhaps ketone bodies. (Later, it was recognized that ammonia production originated primarily from gut bacteria rather than the kidney in patients with alcoholic cirrhosis.)

We had many questions that needed to be answered in order to develop and report in the medical literature the best surgical shunt for protecting patients with cirrhosis of the liver from further gastrointestinal hemorrhage or metabolic compromise after their portal hypertension had been reduced with portasystemic shunts.

The clinical investigators who used the General Clinical Research Center (GCRC) at Temple University Hospital became heavily engaged in studying the effects of different portasystemic shunts (mesocaval or distal splenorenal shunts) to divert blood away from the liver for treatment of hepatic cirrhosis, particularly those of ethanol-induced Laennec's cirrhosis, between 1970 and 1985. During that period, a great deal of the research efforts were driven by Dr. F. A. Reichle, an international scholar on blood flow rates through the gastrointestinal tract, including the liver and its portal system. (In addition, he was widely recognized as a surgeon for treating peripheral vascular abnormalities.) He was a tireless surgeon, operating day and night to salvage the livers (and the legs), and save the lives and promote the comfort of critically ill patients. It was not unusual for Dr. Reichle to find an empty bed during the middle of the night on the GCRC, fall into it, and briefly sleep before going back to work. He was the primary force that pushed us to gain knowledge about the hemodynamic and metabolic effects of liver cirrhosis. He was specifically interested in controlling portal hypertension which led to massive gastrointestinal hemorrhage with a high mortality rate. He wanted to determine which surgical operation produced the best result in reducing portal venous blood pressure and stopping gastrointestinal hemorrhage while maintaining the best liver function possible.

Before Dr. Reichle's surgical interventions were considered, various surgical procedures by other doctors had been used to reduce portal blood pressure and diminish the incidence of severe gastrointestinal hemorrhage. However, the outcome of these procedures on metabolism was not clearly defined. With Dr. Reichle's persistent encouragement, we on the GCRC all accepted the challenges and research efforts associated with caring for patients acutely ill from alcoholic cirrhosis.

The initial phase of therapy for patients with severe gastrointestinal bleeding is geared toward stopping the hemorrhage, usually from the upper gastrointestinal tract, and avoiding precipitation of liver failure. Numerous first-phase therapies are used to stop hemorrhage and resuscitate the patient. If emergency surgery is required, it is done. However, in the studies included in this chapter, surgery was delayed until fresh blood and plasma transfusions were given and hemorrhage stopped, and patients supplemented with vitamins and nutrients. Thereafter, the patients were relatively stable before being transferred to the GCRC.

The personnel of Temple's GCRC had very little prior involvement with patients who were subjected to emergency shunting of total portal blood flow into the inferior vena cava. As a cooperative group (the surgeons, myself and other GCRC staff), we began focusing on studying the outcomes of patients who were slated to undergo selective variceal decompression: *mesocaval shunt* (diversion of blood draining the small intestinal or large intestine or both by shunting the blood into the inferior vena cava); or *distal splenorenal shunt* (diversion of gastroesophageal and splenic blood into the renal vein which subsequently drains into the inferior vena cava).[14]

---

[14] Diverting blood from any major tributary to portal venous blood decompresses portal blood pressure. This diversion of blood flow away from the portal vein to diminish blood flow toward the liver can be likened to diverting river water flow in a tributary around a town to diminish the flow of water through the town.

Following a patient's admission to the GCRC, attending personnel would begin a watch for signs of alcohol or drug withdrawal – delirium tremens. Delirium tremens is an excited state and, rarely, may be complicated by seizures. With "D.T.'s" the patients frequently hallucinate and are often extremely frightened. They fear the presence of an imaginary threat, like an attacking mad dog in their environs. They are often highly suggestive, agreeing to the possibility expressed by an examiner that there is the existence of someone or something in the room who (that) is not present. For example, the examiner may ask the patient, "Do you see that old man sitting in the corner watching us?" The patient may say, "Yes, I do." Their clinically evident anxiety may be accompanied by a fast heart rate and sometimes a tremor. In addition, when their hands are held out in front of them and extended backwards, they frequently flap (asterixis). If they are able to walk, their gait may be broad-based because of nerve disease secondary to prolonged periods of malnutrition with vitamin deficiencies. Evidence of beriberi, scurvy and other skin diseases, dementia and diarrhea may be manifested. Able people must extend helping hands to save their lives.

I have largely forgotten my experiences related to dealing with the gastroenterologists or other specialists involved with controlling acute bleeding from the esophagus, stomach and/or rectum in patients with hepatic cirrhosis. Therefore, no comments in regard to their roles are given in this chapter. However, I do remember the gruesome, old-fashioned experiences using the cumbersome balloon tamponade technique to temporarily control bleeding from the esophagus and gastroesophageal junction while other arrangements were being considered. (Outcomes from stopping hemorrhage with various techniques are not presented here.)

When we began our studies, there were relatively few reports in the literature on the metabolic effects of liver cirrhosis (induced by alcohol) on individual organs or on overall body metabolism. We tackled these problems to gain knowledge pertaining to the hemodynamic and metabolic consequences of cirrhosis and elevated portal venous pressure. My role was to help by measuring total body energy requirements and to delineate hepatic and renal metabolism, and to determine if the liver was enhanced or compromised by different portasystemic shunts.

The question was, "How do investigators measure the changes in liver function before and after surgical intervention?" We knew that blood flow and liver metabolism in patients with cirrhosis before surgery had a multitude of abnormalities. Whether or not surgical shunting caused further liver compromise or aided hepatic function was unknown. We knew we would be more confident about our assessment of the results of therapy if we studied liver (and body) blood flow and metabolism from several different perspectives. Therefore, we wanted to combine a variety of research tools that would produce results that were complementary. A research protocol was designed to get the most information possible while minimizing the risk of complications to patients with liver cirrhosis or normal controls. Our aggressive research objectives had to be cautiously executed because only well-informed and mentally competent patients and volunteers could be studied. Our research protocol was approved by the Scientific Advisory Committee and the Institutional Review Board.

We decided that liver function had to be related to total body function. We had methods to measure the production of energy-yielding fuels by the liver that could be related to total energy requirements of the body in our ill and emaciated patients as well as in "healthy" volunteers. We could use indirect calorimetry to measure total body energy requirements of cirrhotic patients and normal controls, both groups corrected to 70 kg or to body size of 1.73 m^2 body surface area. The results could be used to compare patients with cirrhosis to normal adults. We could measure the differences in the quantities of blood pumped (cardiac output) by the hearts of normal and cirrhotic patients, corrected for body size, to determine if some stress was placed on the cardiovascular system by liver cirrhosis. We could measure the blood flow rates to individual organs in

179

normal adults and in cirrhotic patients. We could measure the amount of glycogen stored in normal and cirrhotic livers; further, we could determine the enzyme activity for synthesizing glucose in the livers of normal controls and compare the results with values obtained from cirrhotic patients. In addition, we could measure and compare the production of fuels, e.g. glucose and ketone bodies, by normal and cirrhotic livers during varying periods of fasting, corrected for body size. Therefore, we could determine the impact of cirrhosis and the effects of limited surgical portacaval shunts on the blood flow throughout the body and on the metabolism of the liver (and kidney) in these morbid patients. Thus, by using several measuring techniques, we could develop metabolic and hemodynamic profiles of patients with liver cirrhosis and normal controls.

We studied 28 patients (16 males and 12 females) who presented with catastrophic upper gastroesophageal hemorrhage secondary to severe hepatic cirrhosis (25 of whom had alcoholic cirrhosis). The patients were divided into two groups, determined by how long they fasted before undergoing investigational catheterization studies. Sixteen were studied after an overnight fast and 9 after a 3-day fast. Their kidney functions were normal. Our control group consisted of 22 patient-volunteers, some of whom required diagnostic cardiac catheterization studies to determine the extent of their coronary artery disease, and others taken from the literature. These controls had normal liver and kidney functions.

After a 10-12 hour overnight fast, we measured the patients' and volunteers' consumption of O_2 and production of CO_2 combined with urinary excretion rate of nitrogen. This is an accurate but indirect way of determining the heat production or the caloric requirements (indirect calorimetry) of humans. The results from indirect calorimetry showed us that, in cirrhotic patients, the total energy requirements corrected for body size were indistinguishable from normal people. Thus, the energy requirements of patients with cirrhosis of the liver can be estimated by the same equations used for healthy controls. However, from the cardiac output data we learned that the hearts were working harder in patients with cirrhosis than the hearts of normal people. We also recognized that the muscles in the extremities of patients with cirrhosis were wasted, and we assumed that the energy requirements of muscles in cirrhotic patients needed less energy than those of normal people. Nonetheless, on balance, the measured energy requirements corrected for body size were indistinguishable from normal people. However, the mix of carbohydrate, protein and fat that provided the energy requirements was different. After an overnight fast, patients with cirrhosis got relatively more energy from fat and less from carbohydrates than did healthy people (Figure 1). This occurred in spite of the fact that cirrhotic patients were emaciated and their body fat stores were somewhat depleted. This bit of information was not fully appreciated when it first became available.

A patient with cirrhosis of the liver has a metabolic profile, as reflected by indirect calorimetry, that resembles that of a normal individual who has fasted for 2-3 days. Cirrhosis of the liver induces an accelerated state of starvation. This finding made more sense as the data from cirrhotic patients accumulated.

After the indirect calorimetry studies were completed in the patients with cirrhosis, an umbilicoportal cannula was inserted through the falciform ligament (vestige of umbilical vein) into the portal venous system to measure the blood pressure and to do angiographic studies of the portal venous system and its collateral circulation. (See Figure 2.) The portal venous angiograms showed us which veins had become varicosities, and how the blood was shunted around the liver. These shunt vessels were the veins with relatively high blood pressure. This preliminary knowledge aided Dr. Reichle in selecting what type of portasystemic shunt he thought would be best suited to the individual patient to 1) prevent recurrent, life threatening hemorrhage from gastroesophageal varices, and 2) avoid hepatic failure.

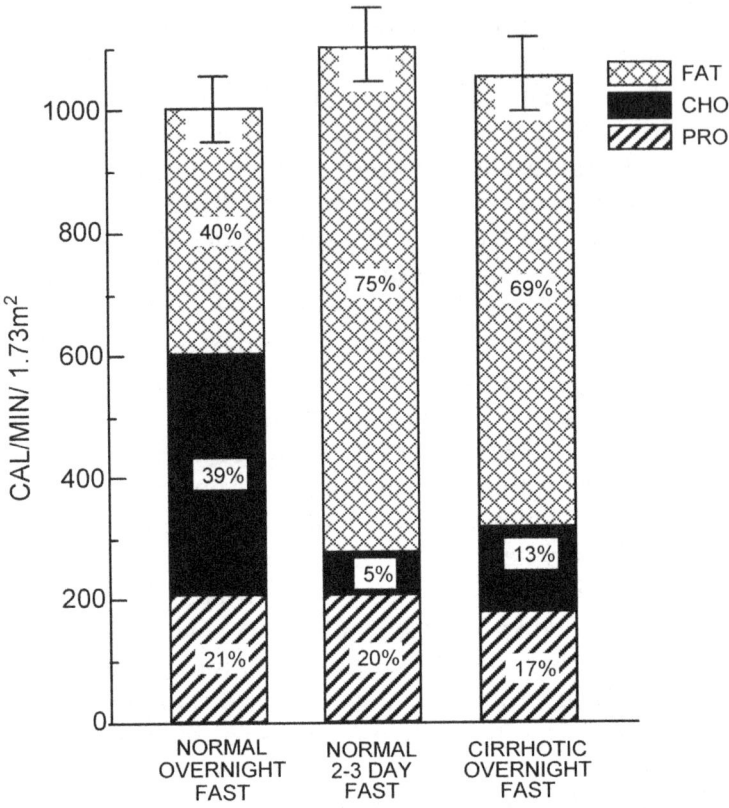

Figure 1. The heights of the bars show the caloric requirements of overnight and 2-3 day fasted normal controls contrasted with cirrhotic patients after an overnight fast. Note the difference in the quantities of carbohydrate and fat oxidized in cirrhotic patients after an overnight fast compared to normal controls. This figure depicts the fact that after an overnight fast, cirrhotic patients more closely resemble normal individuals who have fasted for 2-3 days. Cirrhosis of the liver induces an accelerated state of starvation. To convert cal/min to kcal/24 h multiply by 1.440

During the surgical procedure used to measure portal venous blood pressure, a small piece of the liver was removed and cut into three fragments. (Liver biopsies were performed on patients with cirrhosis and in a few consenting normal controls who had to undergo abdominal surgery, e.g. gall bladder removal.) These tissue fragments were used to

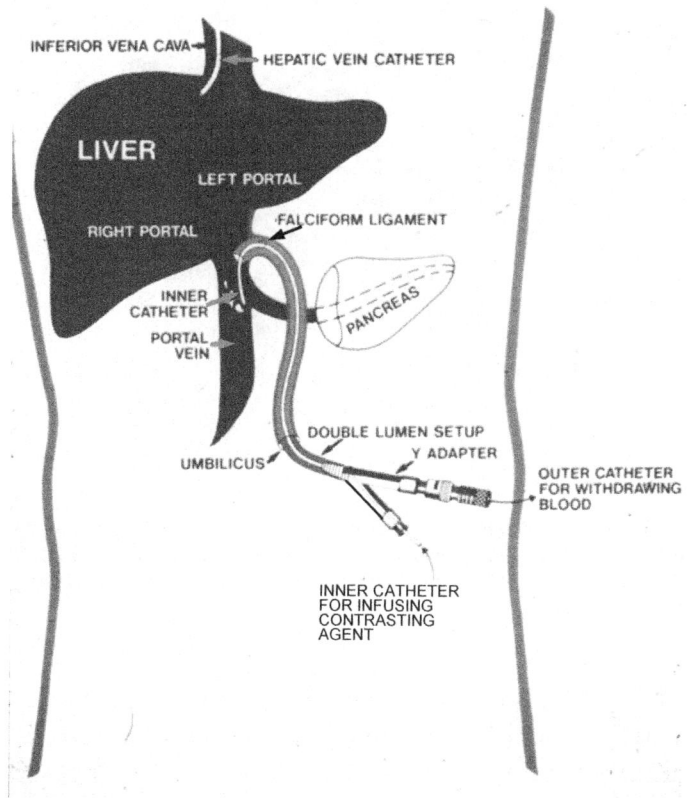

Figure 2. A schematic drawing showing the falciform ligament which has been pried open from the umbilicus to the portal vein and a double lumen device inserted through the falciform ligament.

1) evaluate how much of the liver tissue was replaced by scar (cirrhotic) tissue (See Figure 3), 2) determine the glycogen content, and 3) measure the enzymatic activity for synthesizing glucose in cirrhotic patients and normal controls. In the cirrhotic patients, subsequent catheterization studies were done for measuring portal blood flow rates (from the gut and spleen and leading into blood perfusing and bypassing the liver).

After an overnight or 3-day fast, the patients (those with alcoholic cirrhosis, and also control volunteers, some

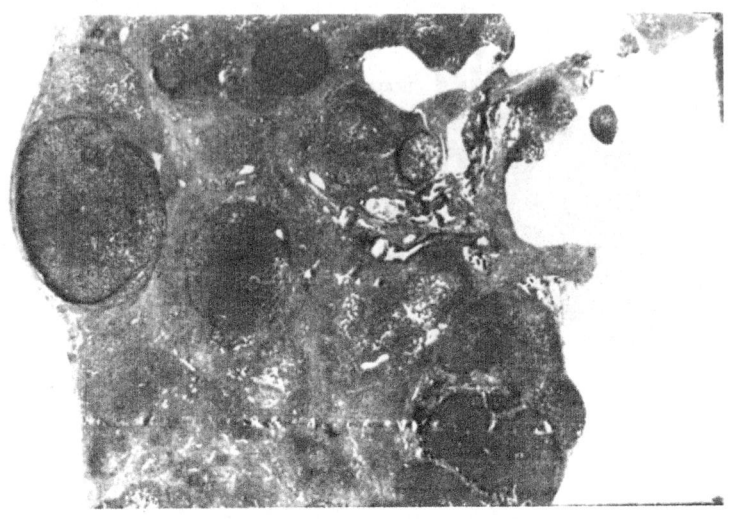

Figure 3. Biopsy of cirrhotic liver showing deranged nodules (darker color) of normal appearing liver cells and fibrous tissue (lighter color). Note that about one-half of the liver tissue is replaced by scar (lighter color).

with stab wounds of the abdomen and others with minimal or no heart disease that affected energy requirements or liver function) were taken to the cardiovascular catheterization laboratory and studied during the resting state. In the patients with cirrhosis of the liver and control volunteers, a venipuncture in the left upper extremity was made for giving specific materials used to measure liver flow rates. Patients with cirrhosis also had kidney blood flow rates measured. In all patients and volunteers, another catheter was inserted into the right superficial vein located in front of the elbow and advanced to the right hepatic vein under fluoroscopic guidance. In patients with cirrhosis, a femoral vein in the groin area was catheterized through the skin and advanced to the right renal vein. Lastly, in all patients and volunteers, arterial blood was obtained from a needle inserted through the skin into either brachial artery near the elbow. Thus, we had a setup for obtaining arterial blood supplying and venous blood draining the gut (portal vein) and liver in normal

184

people and patients with cirrhosis. In addition, we could measure kidney metabolism in patients with liver cirrhosis. After all the catheters were in place and the patients and volunteers were resting comfortably, blood was collected simultaneously at 10-minute intervals from the brachial artery and the portal (and gut) and hepatic veins in normal people and cirrhotic patients. Arterial and renal venous blood was also obtained from patients with cirrhosis. Equal quantities of normal saline with 5% human albumin were infused through various catheters to each patient or volunteer to replace the blood drawn during the study. This was done to minimize the effect of withdrawing blood from a human. The location of each catheter was checked radiologically and chemically before and after each blood sample.

At the conclusion of the blood-sampling period for determining net extraction of substrates or production of glucose and ketone bodies, the diagnostic studies needed to best delineate the abnormalities in patients with hepatic cirrhosis (and in control volunteers with possible ischemic heart disease) were completed.

Cardiac output and liver blood flow rates were normal in our controls. (In these controls, renal blood flow was not measured.) In contrast, cardiac output was high in patients with alcoholic cirrhosis of the liver. This was not surprising because the shunting of blood from the arterial system through the venous system in many conditions causes the output of blood by the heart to be high. Total blood flow through and shunted around the liver caused the high output in patients with hepatic cirrhosis. Kidney flow rates were normal in patients with alcoholic liver disease. We expected this finding because there was no reason to think that there was abnormal blood flow to kidneys in patients with alcoholic cirrhosis.

Results from the catheterization studies were complementary with the results obtained from indirect calorimetry, hepatic glycogen content and liver enzymatic activities. The results from the liver biopsies showed that 15-85% of the normal liver tissue was replaced by scar tissue in patients with cirrhosis. The average glycogen content of

185

the liver was only 50% of the normal amount. We knew that low glycogen content was also found in individuals with normal liver function but who had starved for 2-3 days and experienced some hepatic glycogen depletion. However, the enzymatic activity of the cirrhotic liver for synthesizing glucose was adequate. Thus, space in the cirrhotic liver to store glycogen was low because liver cells were replaced with scar tissue; however, the enzymatic machinery for synthesizing glucose from precursors delivered to the liver from peripheral tissues (e.g. muscle) was sufficient in spite of scar tissue.

After an overnight or 2-3 day fast it was known that the liver contributed fuels to the blood by 1) breaking down a small quantity of glycogen stored in the liver, 2) synthesizing new glucose from compounds funneled into the liver from peripheral tissues such as muscles, and 3) generating large quantities of ketone bodies primarily from free fatty acids derived from adipose (fat) tissue. At the time we began the studies on patients with alcoholic cirrhosis, we did not know how the aforementioned processes (gluconeogenesis, glycogenolysis and ketogenesis) were related in patients with liver cirrhosis. As time progressed and we completed a mixture of studies regarding liver metabolism in normal and cirrhotic patients, our view of liver metabolism and the effects of starvation began to emerge. Figure 4 shows the production rates of glucose (from gluconeogenesis and glycogenolysis) and ketone bodies (ketogenesis) in overnight and 3-day fasted normal controls and patients with cirrhosis of the liver. (See Chapter VII, Liver and Kidney Metabolism in 'Normal' Adults.)

The total glucose output by the normal liver after an *overnight fast* is about 0.86 mmol/min/1.73 m^2 (155 mg/min which extrapolates to 223 g/day/1.73 m^2). About 80% of the glucose output is derived from glycogen breakdown and about 20% comes from newly synthesized glucose. (More recent studies suggest slight, but not medically significant, differences in distinguishing the quantities of glucose derived from glycogenolysis and gluconeogenesis.) In

186

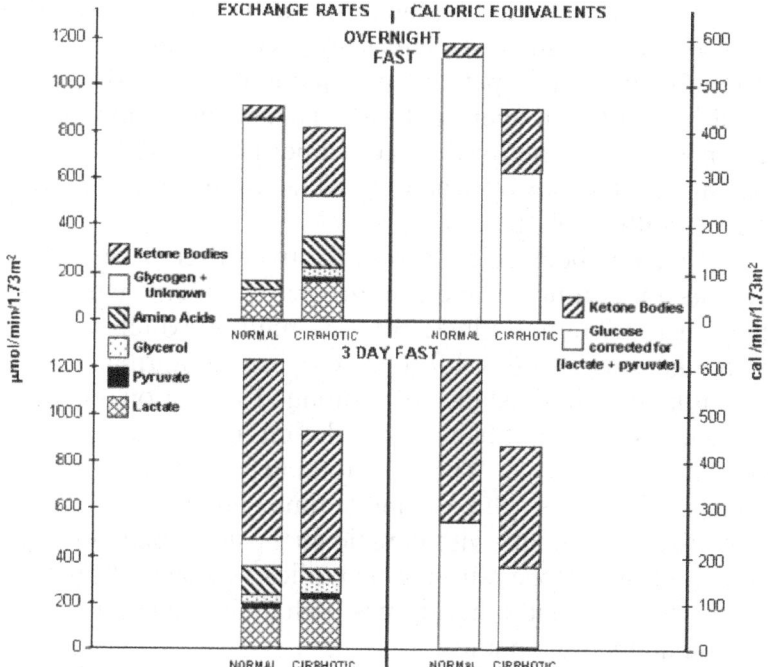

Figure 4. Indirect calorimetry measured by exchange rates of respiratory oxygen and carbon dioxide coupled to urinary nitrogen excretion. The exchange rates are expressed as caloric equivalents. The values for normal controls are slightly less than those displayed in the previous chapter because the caloric equivalents for glucose production were corrected for recycled lactate and pyruvate. However, the difference is trivial. The energy equivalents of normal controls are compared with patients suffering from hepatic cirrhosis. The values represent overnight and 3 day fasts.

contrast, glucose output from patients with cirrhosis is curtailed to 0.53 mmol/min/1.73 m^2 (95 mg/min which extrapolates to 137 g/day/1.73 m^2). Thus, glucose output in cirrhotic patients is only 62% of the normal rate after an overnight fast (Figure 4). This is due to a diminished contribution of glucose from glycogen. Newly synthesized glucose after an overnight fast comprises 67% of net glucose output, but the contribution of glucose from gluconeogenesis is insignificant to make up the loss from glycogenolysis. Another unexpected finding was the increased quantity of alanine (amino acid from muscle protein breakdown) removed from the blood by the cirrhotic liver to synthesize glucose (data not shown). This suggested that muscle protein breakdown in patients with alcoholic cirrhosis is accelerated after an overnight fast. This phenomenon may be partly responsible for the marked peripheral muscle wasting (spider-like arms and legs) known to be present in patients with alcoholic cirrhosis.

Ketone body release from the liver after an *overnight fast* was about four- to five-fold greater in patients with cirrhosis (0.39 mmol/min/1.73m^2: 41 mg/min which extrapolates to 59 g/day/1.73m^2) compared to normal people, but unlike the circumstance of prolonged starvation, hepatic ketogenesis could not balance the deficit in glucose production (Figure 4). Thus, the total hepatic release of water-soluble fuels (glucose and ketone bodies) was suppressed in patients with hepatic cirrhosis. Nonetheless, the output of glucose plus ketone bodies was enough fuel to supply the brain and other tissues with their needs for glucose and ketone bodies.

After *3 days of fasting* hepatic glucose production in patients with cirrhosis decreased to a value of 0.34 mmol/min/1.73 m^2 (61 mg/min which extrapolates to 88 g/day/1.73 m^2). The quantity of glucose produced after a 3 day fast is only 64% of that observed after an overnight fast in cirrhotic patients. Further, all of the glucose released could be accounted for by hepatic gluconeogenesis. Thus, the alcoholic patient cannot mobilize any more glucose from the liver by glycogen breakdown. This lack of hepatic glycogenolysis after 3 days of starvation is not much different from normal people, but it compounds the difficulty presented by the shortfall in hepatic ketogenesis by the cirrhotic livers. The ketone body production in cirrhotic patients is greater after 3 days of starvation than after an overnight fast (0.57 mmol/min/1.73 m^2 or 59 mg/min which extrapolates to 85 g/day/1.75 m^2); but ketone body production in patients with cirrhosis is less than the 115 g/day/1.73 m^2 in normal controls fasted for 3 days (Figure 4). The low output of acetoacetate and beta-hydroxybutyrate (ketone bodies) by cirrhotic livers was accompanied by low levels of these fuels in the blood of cirrhotic patients. The combination of diminished hepatic glucose output (64% of normal control value) and diminished hepatic ketone body output (74% of normal control value) after 3 days of fasting might compromise whole body metabolism among cirrhotic patients missing meals or undergoing longer periods of food deprivation. However, we saw no gross evidence of fuel deficiency in our cirrhotic patients, but that does not mean it may be lurking in the background in some patients with cirrhosis of the liver. Nonetheless, the blood glucose concentrations after an overnight or 3 day fast are greater, not less, than the concentrations observed in normal people fasted the same periods of time. The blood concentration of glucose reflects the rate of entry and rate of exit of glucose. There is no evidence from the blood that the supply of glucose was inadequate to meet the metabolic requirement for glucose in patients with hepatic cirrhosis. On the other hand, blood ketone body concentrations were low in the 3 day fasted cirrhotic patients. Further, the total number of caloric equivalents derived from glucose and ketone bodies added to the blood by the livers of patients with cirrhosis that could be terminally oxidized (to CO_2 and H_2O) by tissues outside the liver (e.g. brain) was less than the contributions made by normal livers after both an overnight and 3 day fast.

We initially thought the shortfall in liver glucose (and ketone bodies) production would be met by the kidney producing glucose (and/or ketone bodies). However, the kidney exchange rates (production or consumption) of glucose (or ketone bodies) after overnight and 3 day fasts were trivial. This unexpected finding should not have amazed us as it did. In retrospect, we failed to remember or grasp the fact that renal ammonia production and urinary ammonium excretion were not elevated by 3 days of starvation. The indirect calorimetry data which reflected not only the energy requirements of these patients with alcoholic cirrhosis, but also the nature (carbohydrate, protein and fat) and quantity of fuels burned (oxidized) suggested that fat provided the energy source not provided by glucose (carbohydrate) or protein (amino acids) (Figure 1).

189

We measured and reported the results from studying patients with liver cirrhosis before (Owen, O.E., F.A. Reichle, M.A. Mozzoli, *et al*. *J. Clin. Invest.* 68:240-52, 1981) and after (Owen, O.E., M.A. Mozzoli, F.A. Reichle, *et al. J. Clin. Invest.* 76:1209-17, 1985) subjecting them to limited (splenorenal or mesocaval) surgical shunting. The mental states of the patients subjected to limited shunts showed no signs of deterioration. In fact, stopping the gastrointestinal loss of blood and providing good nutrition with the absence of alcohol improved the patients.

Cardiac output increased significantly (P<0.05) as a consequence of the limited portacaval shunts. Blood flow through the liver remained practically identical, but some of the blood in the portal vein mixed with arterial blood normally directed through the liver, reversed its direction of flow. Some of the blood apparently flowed back out of the liver (retrograde flow), bypassing the veins that normally drain the liver (hepatic veins), before flowing into the mesocaval shunts and then into the inferior vena cava (Figure 5). Post-shunt liver glucose production was 0.70 mmol/min/1.73 m^2 (126 mg/min or 181 g/day/1.73 m^2). Extraction and conversion of gluconeogenic precursors accounted for 62% of the glucose released from the liver. Post-shunt liver ketone body production was 0.58 mmol/min/1.73 m^2 (60 mg/min or 86 g/day/1.73 m^2). Although the post-shunt calculated values for glucose and ketone bodies, and their respective caloric values, were greater than the pre-shunt values both after overnight and 3 day fasts, these increased values are not statistically significant. Nonetheless, fuel delivery by the liver to the blood was not compromised further by limited surgical shunts to reduce portal venous blood pressure and salvage the lives of patients with massive gastrointestinal hemorrhage. Our post-shunt study clearly showed that the ability of the liver to continue its important role in maintaining a supply of water-soluble fuels by adding glucose and ketone bodies to the blood was not adversely

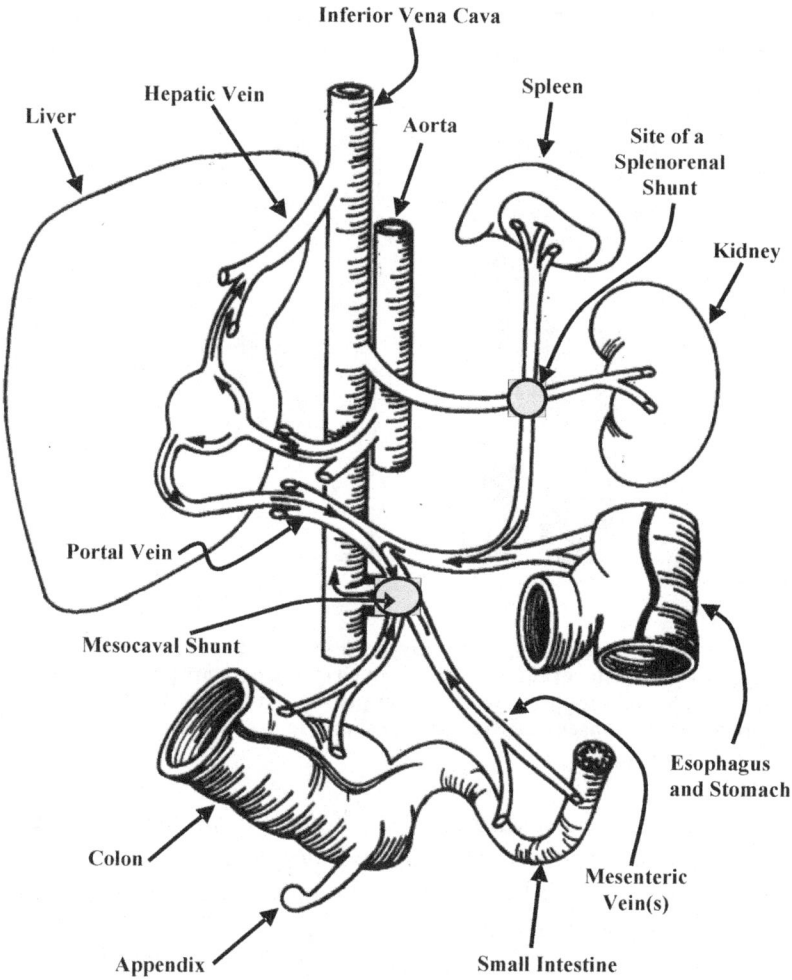

Figure 5. The mesocaval shunt allows arterial blood flow to the liver to mix with hepatic venous blood before undergoing retrograde blood flow into the portal vein and exiting through a surgically created mesocaval shunt.

191

affected by either a distal splenorenal or mesocaval shunt (Figure 6). Fortunately, the portal venous pressures were

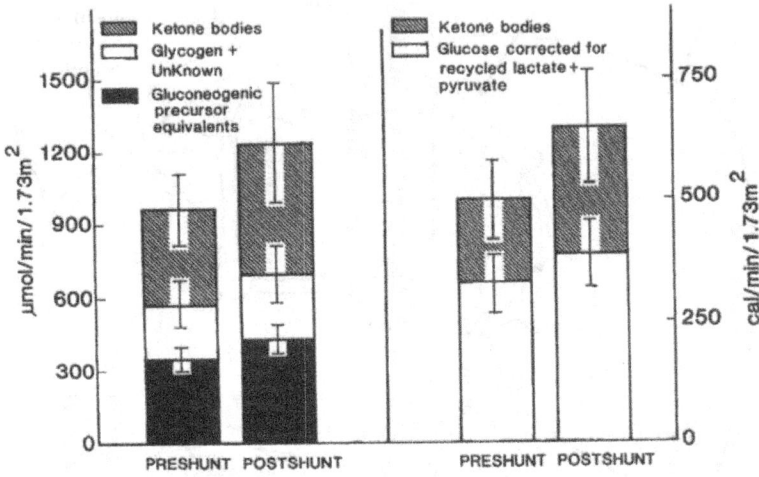

Figure 6. Liver gluconeogenesis, glycogenolysis and ketogenesis, and caloric equivalents of these processes in cirrhotic patients pre- and post-shunt. The data suggests, but does not prove, that hepatic function improves as a consequence of surgical shunting decompressing the portal-venous system.

reduced to normal values. The chances of recurrent bleeding were clearly diminished provided the patients did not add subsequent alcoholic insults to the liver (and portal system).

We studied patients with hepatic cirrhosis and massive gastroesophageal hemorrhage before and after limited mesocaval or distal splenorenal portasystemic shunts were done. Cardiac output and hepatic, portal and kidney blood flow rates were measured and combined with arteriovenous concentration differences across the liver, gut and kidney to calculate flux rates of glucose, ketone bodies and various other biochemical compounds. We gained knowledge about abnormal organ behavior and what the effects were of trying to reduce the high portal blood pressure and potential for gastroesophageal hemorrhage. The results of clinical investigations pertaining to the catheterization and indirect calorimetry studies were

192

integrated with microscopic anatomy of the liver, glycogen content and enzymes involved in synthesizing new glucose. The data obtained from our patients with cirrhosis were compared with the data from "normal" controls. The combined effort of patients, surgeons and physicians, complemented by nursing, dietary and technical staff, saved lives and advanced the practices of health care.

Dr. Reichle learned that limited portasystemic shunts were equally good and the best way to reduce portal venous pressure. Collectively, we learned that liver function was not compromised by limited portasystemic shunts used in patients likely to die if surgeries were not used to save their lives. We helped these patients to have another chance at life.

The quantity and types of fuels released into the blood by normal and diseased (cirrhotic) livers were different. Further, the total caloric equivalents of fuels produced by the cirrhotic livers were deficient (Figures 4 and 6). We studied people who were defective in liver production of fuels but who were able to maintain normal energy requirements. What was/were the mechanism(s) for compensating deficit fuel production in patients with liver disease? The kidneys were not supplying either glucose or ketone bodies to the bloodstream. What was the source for maintaining energy needs in patients with alcoholic cirrhosis?

As is usually the case, our research provided new information but not the whole picture of how sick patients with liver disease maintained their energy requirements (fuel homeostasis).

We knew that free fatty acids from adipose tissue stores were strangely elevated in blood of patients with cirrhosis. Maybe there was a clue in this fact to explain survival mechanisms in patients with liver disease. Another clue was provided from the data derived from indirect calorimetry that suggested fat provided more of the total energy requirements and glucose less in patients with cirrhosis than in normal adults after an overnight fast. Could it be that the fat stores, as limited as they were, had heightened activity to provide the energy requirements not supplied by the failing liver?

When one organ fails, maybe another one tries to pick up the slack. It is interesting how this exists. Human societies seem to function in the same way.

Twenty years after we studied our last patient vomiting blood and in a state of shock with liver cirrhosis and gastroesophageal hemorrhage, I am still haunted but strangely pleased by the mental images that pop into my mind. These desperate people were suffering and on the edge of death. Their eyes reflected fear as they searched for relief. Only fragmented, mental images of faces and bodies attached to life-supporting devices are now conjured up in my consciousness. I can no longer remember most of their names, but some of their images are encased in the steel traps of my memory.

One man, about 50 years of age, reverberates in my mind. He was dying from the consequences of alcoholic cirrhosis of the liver plus severe malnutrition. He had a large, bony frame, but his muscle mass had wasted away. His liver was big, and the white of his eyes and his brown skin were jaundiced. His blackened legs were swollen and darker than his genetic expression should have warranted. He was anxious and had a twitch. Blood loss from his gastroesophageal tract had stopped. Initially he was able to walk with a broad-based gait reflective of nerve damage in the lower extremities. After several days of supportive therapy and baseline studies, including catheterization studies, he was taken to the operating room where Dr. Reichle performed a portasystemic shunt. Repeated catheterization studies were done. Good nutrition was initiated and continued. Subsequently, he began gaining weight and was grateful for the health care he received. Laboratory studies became near normal. His muscle mass began to increase. His gait became normal as the nerves in his legs and feet regenerated. After three months of continuous hospitalization he was discharged home. Dr. Reichle oversaw his outpatient management. When the patient returned to the hospital outpatient clinic for follow-up visits, he would frequently come by the General Clinical Research Center to visit with the nursing, dietary and laboratory personnel. He would also visit me. He returned to a large, muscular man with a pleasing smile and pleasant behavior. I do not know whether or not he returned to work, but I do know that for many years he maintained abstinence from alcohol consumption and was a grateful person.

This is a good place to review the behavior of a "clinical investigator": If a "medical detective" fails in an attempt to solve a mystery, he/she should review the data looking for clues that might lead in another direction. In our case, we found the answer that clearly explains what mechanism(s) a patient population uses to obtain energy which is essential for the survival of patients with severe alcoholic cirrhosis.

Chapter X. Nature and Quantity of Fuels Consumed in Patients with Alcoholic Cirrhosis

When food is eaten in overabundance, it is primarily converted into fat (triglycerides) and stored in adipose tissue. The fat mass of the adipose tissue of humans can vary from about 3% to 50% of body weight. Because fat is stored in adipose tissue as an oily material inside a membranous casing, this fuel tank has the highest caloric value of any tissue in the body. In emaciated people, skin sometimes hangs over the bones with practically no fat stored under the skin or in the abdominal cavity. In contrast, huge people weighing approximately 400 pounds (182 kg) have about one-half of their body weight stored as fat housed in the adipose tissue. This white tissue mass is distributed throughout the body but mostly concentrated under the skin or in the abdominal cavity and in the buttocks. After an overnight fast and more protracted periods of food deprivation, the adipose tissue releases free fatty acids (FFA) into the fluid surrounding fat cells. The FFA become immediately attached to protein (albumin) in the body fluids and are eventually transported throughout the body in plasma (cell-free component of blood). Over the first 2-3 days of total starvation the concentration of plasma FFA increases 2- to 3-fold. As the circulating concentration of FFA increases, the rate of FFA oxidation increases. After about 3 days of starvation FFA oxidation contributes over 90% of the body's total energy requirements. The oxidation of FFA curtails the consumption of both glucose and amino acids as sources of fuels for the body. Elevated plasma FFA induce a natural and desirable form of insulin resistance to suppress glucose oxidation when this carbohydrate is in short supply.

Some of the FFA released from the adipose tissue are channeled through the liver where they are broken down from 14- to 20-carbon length chains into 2-carbon fragments before being used to synthesize 4-carbon fuels, ketone bodies: acetoacetate and beta-hydroxybutyrate. In this process, ketogenesis, about one-half the energy content of the FFA is released to the liver to support hepatic functions.

The remaining energy content resides in the water-soluble ketone bodies released from the liver. (See Chapter IV, Nutrition, Biochemistry and Physiology.)

The human liver has a central role in providing water-soluble fuels for energy consumption. In normal adults, after an overnight or several days of fasting, the liver contributes about one-half of the total caloric requirements. (See Chapter VII, Liver and Kidney Metabolism in "Normal" Adults.) This task is accomplished by liver releasing both glucose and ketone bodies into the blood. In patients with alcoholic cirrhosis, however, the total number of caloric equivalents derived from glucose plus ketone bodies added to the bloodstream by the livers that can be terminally oxidized is less than that made by normal livers after both an overnight and 3 day fast. Further, there is no renal glucose contribution to the blood: the kidneys do not compensate for observed deficiency in liver fuel production. We measured total body energy requirements and found them to be normal in patients with cirrhosis of the liver. However, the nature of the fuels oxidized was different between normal controls and patients with cirrhosis. The latter group oxidized more fat and less glucose than did normal controls. In addition, we found the well recognized elevation of plasma FFA in patients with liver cirrhosis. It was reasonable to assume that augmented mobilization and oxidation of FFA occurred more quickly during food deprivation in patients suffering from cirrhosis of the liver. However, no one had ever investigated this possibility.

The most practical method available for determining total body energy requirements and the quantities of carbohydrate, fat and protein oxidized is indirect calorimetry. More direct information regarding the release of FFA (fat) from adipose tissue and the oxidation of these fuels can be obtained by giving a commercially available "tracer amount" of radioactive free fatty acid and measuring its rate of FFA entrance into the bloodstream and rate of FFA oxidation to carbon dioxide (CO_2) and water (H_2O). The CO_2 derived from the radioactive FFA is exhaled in the breath.[15]

We used the techniques of indirect calorimetry simultaneously with tracer analysis of a radioactive fatty acid [^{14}C] palmitate to measure the quantity of fuels consumed by patients with biopsy-proven alcoholic cirrhosis. First, we compared the results of indirect calorimetry with the results from tracer analysis. Second, we compared the results from patients with alcoholic cirrhosis with values obtained from healthy humans.

Nine patients with histories of excessive alcohol consumption and biopsy-proven cirrhosis of the liver were selected from inpatient and outpatient populations of Temple University Hospital. Fifteen volunteers served as normal controls. The patients were transferred or admitted to the General Clinical Research Center (GCRC). All patients and volunteers were informed of the nature, purpose and possible risk involved before obtaining their volunteered and signed consent to participate in the study. The values obtained in the study were standardized to 1.73 m^2 body surface area.

Several patients deserve special comment. Four of them had been previously hospitalized and treated for massive gastroesophageal variceal hemorrhage secondary to portal hypertension. Three of the patients had undergone portacaval anastamosis before the ^{14}C studies were done.

For the study, a plastic hood with a polyethylene curtain was placed over the heads of patients and volunteers, and the airflow through the hood was measured. Cirrhotic

---

[15] The rate that a fuel (FFA) is released into the blood and the rate it is converted (oxidized) to carbon dioxide and exhaled in the breath can be measured by infusing a small amount (tracer amount) of a radioactive material which contains carbon atoms emitting detectable radiation in the breath ($^{14}CO_2$). The rate of infusion and dilution of the radioactive material in the plasma by FFA entering the circulation allows for the calculation of the production rate. If the concentration of the radioactive material is constant over several timed intervals, the production rate is equal to the removal rate. If the material is oxidized to CO_2 (and water) and excreted in the breath, the ratio of radioactive $^{14}CO_2$ to total CO_2 permits the calculation of relative amount of material (fuel) contributing to CO_2 production.

patients and healthy volunteers were studied in air-conditioned rooms equipped with efficient ventilation systems to exhaust the exhaled radioactive carbon dioxide ($^{14}CO_2$) to maintain normal room air content. At timed intervals, samples of the expired air were collected and analyzed for oxygen (O_2) and CO_2 and for $^{14}CO_2$. Immediately after collecting the respiratory gas samples, blood was withdrawn from the patients and volunteers, placed in test tubes, and treated appropriately so the samples could be used for determining plasma FFA and labeled FFA (^{14}C FFA) along with the glucose and ketone body concentrations. The relative amount of expired $^{14}CO_2$ (radioactivity) to total CO_2 was calculated to estimate how much fatty acid oxidation contributed to CO_2 production. In addition, the radioactivity per volume in the plasma FFA was compared to the radioactivity per volume in the solution containing the ^{14}C FFA infused into the bloodstream. Urine excretion was timed and analyzed for nitrogenous excretion so protein oxidation could be calculated. From the respiratory exchange rates of O_2 and CO_2, the amount of CO_2 that was labeled with ^{14}C, and urinary excretion rate of nitrogen, we could determine the total resting energy requirements and the contributions of fat, carbohydrate and protein. In essence, we determined the rate of FFA release from storage sites and the oxidation of these fats by the body in cirrhotic patients after an overnight fast and in normal volunteers fasted for 36-72 hours. Therefore, the contribution of FFA oxidation to total energy requirement could be calculated by two different methods, indirect calorimetry and tracer analysis of radioactive FFA oxidation.

There are 9 major FFA found in venous plasma, with 4 of them composing 80%. Most venous plasma FFA vary from 14-20 carbons in length. The FFA labeled with ^{14}C that we chose to use to represent FFA release from adipose tissue and oxidation throughout the body, [1-^{14}C] palmitic acid, turned out to be an excellent selection.

Prior to fasting, the compositions of FFA in the venous plasma of alcoholics and normal subjects were approximately the same. However, the FFA concentration in venous plasma in the overnight fasted cirrhotic patients (934 µmol/liter) was about 2 times greater than that found in normal volunteers (487 µmol/liter) after an overnight fast. After 36 to 72 hours of fasting, normal individuals had plasma FFA (905 µmol/liter), comparable to cirrhotic patients after an overnight fast.

Elevated plasma FFA concentrations in patients with cirrhosis after an overnight fast had been previously demonstrated by other clinical investigators. Our study showed this elevation was due to enhanced mobilization of FFA from adipose tissue. We also showed that heightened FFA release from fat stores was accompanied by heightened oxidation (burning) rate of FFA (Figure 1). Our tracer study

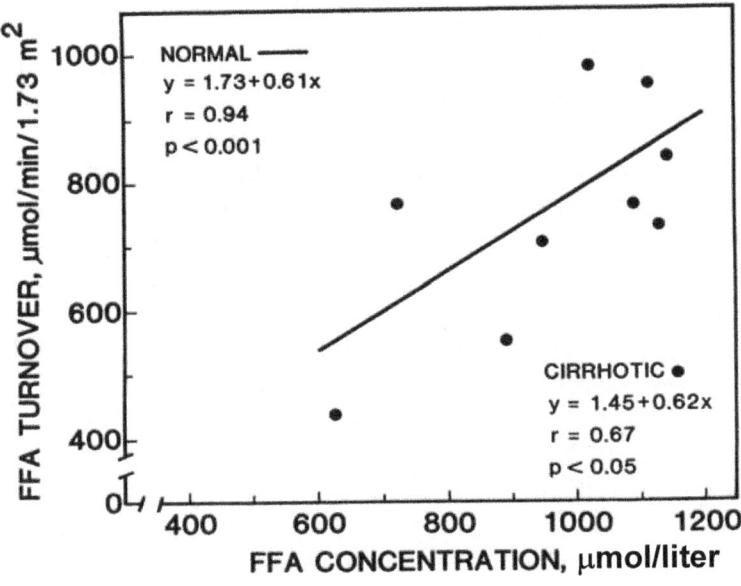

Figure 1. Relationship between FFA concentrations and FFA turnover rates. The solid line represents results obtained from normal individuals undergoing various durations of starvation, and the individual dots represent the nine overnight fasted cirrhotic patients.

(^{14}C FFA) revealed that augmented fat breakdown after an overnight fast and FFA oxidation are the primary mechanisms for maintaining the delivery of needed fuels when liver production of glucose and ketone bodies is abnormally low.

We demonstrated that in cirrhotic patients there was a direct relationship between plasma FFA concentrations and the rate of release of FFA from adipose tissue and the oxidation of these fuels to carbon dioxide and water: The higher the plasma FFA concentration, the greater the rate of oxidation in cirrhotic patients, just like normal people. Our results from the use of radioactive materials showed that the increase in fat breakdown was the primary cause for the elevated plasma FFA concentration in patients with alcoholic cirrhosis (Figure 1). Further, our data revealed that this increase in fat breakdown and subsequent fatty acid oxidation are the backup mechanisms for maintaining the delivery of fuel to the body when glucose (and ketone body) production by the liver is abnormally low. Our previous catheterization studies revealed that after an overnight fast the livers in patients with alcoholic cirrhosis contributed less glucose (about 0.53 mmol/min/1.73m^2) to the blood than do the livers in healthy patients (0.86 mmol/min/1.73m^2). A major portion of the glucose produced by the cirrhotic liver is derived from recycled lactate and pyruvate. This simply means that glucose released from the liver circulates in the blood to the periphery and is incompletely broken down into lactate and pyruvate, which are subsequently returned to the liver in the blood and converted back into glucose (Cori cycle). Very little energy for peripheral (extrahepatic) tissue use is derived from recycled lactate and pyruvate. It is only the glucose produced mostly from amino acids and some of the glycerol from triglycerides (gluconeogenesis) that are completely oxidized (burned) to CO_2 and H_2O. These sources for glucose formation are usable for energy. In patients with cirrhosis, the quantity of glucose available for complete oxidation after an overnight fast is limited and amounts to only 0.22 mmol/min/1.73m^2. This provides an equivalent of about 0.16 Kcal/min/1.73m^2. The catheterization technique used to measure the liver production of glucose for terminal oxidation is in excellent agreement (0.13 kg/min/$1.73m^2$) with a completely different method (indirect calorimetry) for estimating glucose contribution to energy requirements for the entire body (Figure 2).

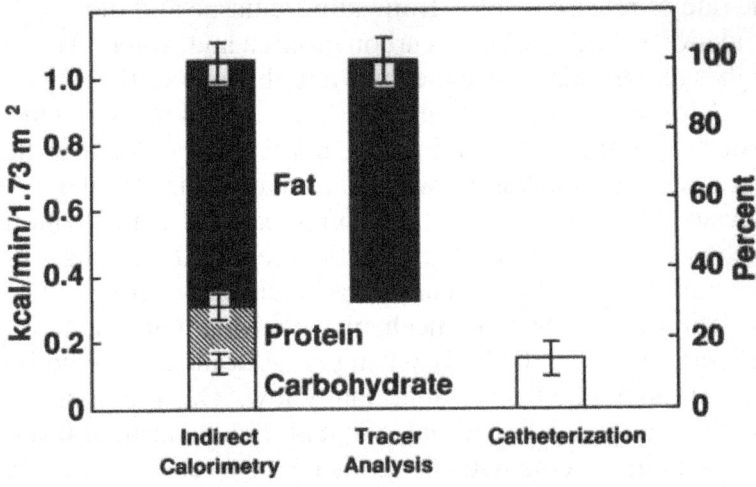

Figure 2. The integrated results obtained from studying patients with alcoholic cirrhosis and comparing indirect calorimetry, tracer analysis (^{14}C FFA), and catheterization techniques. These 3 methods complement and confirm the accuracy of these divergent methods for evaluating human metabolism.

Indirect calorimetry, analysis of ^{14}C tracers and catheterization techniques are old but classic methods to determine the nature and quantities of fuels oxidized in a variety of health and diseased states. In the current world of molecular biology these three techniques may be considered to be primitive by some clinical investigators. Nonetheless, they still provide solid, fundamental information. Further, the validity of the results obtained with indirect calorimetry, ^{14}C tracer analysis and catheterization techniques and how they relate to each other had not been demonstrated until we used them simultaneously to study fat metabolism in patients with alcoholic cirrhosis. Figure 2 shows the relationship obtained from indirect calorimetry, catheterization techniques and analysis of radioactive tracers to delineate metabolism (energy requirements) in patients with cirrhosis of the liver. These three widely diverse techniques complement each other and show a remarkable agreement for quantitating the amount of glucose (carbohydrate), protein (amino acids) and fat (FFA) released and oxidized in cirrhotic patients after an overnight fast. Moreover, the indirect calorimetry shows that patients with alcoholic cirrhosis have normal overnight resting metabolic requirements. Unlike healthy adults who receive about 40% of energy requirements from fat after an overnight fast, in these cirrhotic patients, fat furnishes about two-thirds, and glucose and amino acids each furnish only one-sixth of the total energy requirements. Tracer analysis of radioactive FFA also showed that fat oxidation contributed about 67% of the energy requirements after an overnight fast in cirrhotic patients. Catheterization results also complement indirect calorimetry and showed that glucose delivered about one-sixth of the total resting metabolic rate. Collectively, the results showed clear evidence that indirect calorimetry, radioactive (^{14}C) tracer techniques and catheterization methods complemented each other and truly reflected the nature and quantity of fuels oxidized during resting and fasting states.

To reiterate, our studies showed that patients with chronic alcoholism and cirrhosis of the liver who were hospitalized before being studied and fed adequate and balanced meals had resting energy requirements that were indistinguishable from normal humans. However, the quantities of carbohydrates, fat and protein oxidized by cirrhotic patients after an overnight fast were different from normal adults. After an overnight fast, patients with cirrhosis had the same metabolic profile found in normal humans who had fasted for 36-72 hours. The time needed to develop a catabolic state of starvation was much shorter in patients with alcoholic cirrhosis than normal humans. This accelerated state of starvation in patients with cirrhosis is probably due to the diminished quantity of glucose stored as glycogen in the cirrhotic livers. Although energy yield from amino acid (protein) oxidation is approximately equal among overnight fasted cirrhotic patients and normal controls after an overnight fast and after 36-72 hours, it should be recognized that patients with cirrhosis are often emaciated. Their lean body mass (e.g. muscle) is depleted. Cirrhotic patients lose more nitrogen during a 24-hour fast than expected considering they are usually emaciated. Perhaps persistent mobilization of amino acids from lean tissues aids in the maintenance of blood glucose, but the cost of this accelerated protein breakdown may be reflected in the extensive muscle wasting observed in patients with liver cirrhosis.

One of the patient-volunteers presented an unusual personality. He was the 53 year old father of one of the nurses that worked in the cardiovascular laboratory where the catheterization studies relating to cirrhosis of the liver were done. He had biopsy-proven alcoholic cirrhosis and hepatitis, and learned that I was looking for volunteers to study the aftermath of alcoholic cirrhosis. When he came to see me, I explained to him the details of the study and the risk involved. He agreed to arrive after an overnight fast at the GCRC on the morning the study was scheduled. When he showed up for the study, it was obvious that he was inebriated from drinking alcohol (ethanol) during the night before the study was planned. In fact, he began consuming 4/5 of a quart of whiskey nine hours before the study was to be initiated. After his daughter consented, we initiated the planned protocol. His blood alcohol concentration was high. The respiratory uptake of O_2 was high and out of proportion to the amount of CO_2 produced. Thus, his ratio of O_2 consumption to CO_2 production reflected that the majority of his energy requirements were being met by the oxidation of ethanol. It was a surprise to learn that a drunk patient received the majority of his energy requirements from the oxidation of ethanol. Like the other volunteers, his expiratory exchange of O_2 and CO_2 was determined at 0, 1, 2, 3, 4, 5 and 6 hours. Over a 6-8 hour study, the alcohol content of his blood decreased. At the termination of the study, his O_2 consumption and CO_2 production corrected to body surface area was normal. Thus, at the end of the study his O_2 consumption and CO_2 production were similar to the other patients. However, his $^{14}CO_2$ production from ^{14}C FFA was abnormally low, not high as it was in other cirrhotic patients who were sober. Through serendipity we had the opportunity to study a patient inebriated from drinking whiskey. The results from this study showed us that alcohol was the preferential fuel oxidized by the body when it is present in the bloodstream. Ethanol suppressed the oxidation of FFA (and glucose). Ethanol reigned sovereign over fat, glucose and amino acids in providing a source of energy for this man's body. In general, it was recognized that when FFA are elevated in the plasma, they are preferentially selected over glucose and amino acids. In this single patient, it was evident that alcohol reigned supreme over all fuels including fat as well as glucose and amino acids. This pick-up on the selectivity and priority of fuels when alcohol is present in high concentrations in the bloodstream was a fortuitous but a valuable discovery. I doubt that we could have designed a better study to delineate the hierarchy of fuel utilization by the body.

It was disappointing for me to learn that 2 of the 8 cirrhotic patients studied after an overnight fast were individuals who had undergone limited portasystemic shunts (splenorenal shunts) 3-4 years earlier. However, recidivism is not that unusual. Maybe this is not totally disastrous because 75% of patients who suffer from massive gastroesophageal hemorrhage are dead within one year of the bleeding events if no medical interventions are employed. The overall benefit from the medical and surgical support given to patients dying from massive gastroesophageal hemorrhage because of alcoholic cirrhosis of the liver has to be questioned. Many of those resuscitated and given the opportunity to regain compensated health relapse into habitual abuse of alcoholic drinks. But physicians' and surgeons' responsibilities are to help the suffering and not to judge.[16]

Most of the biomedical science articles focus on the hell and damnation created by diseases. Yet the human population of the world has had an exponential growth rate, and people in general are better fed and housed now than anytime before in the history of mankind. Maybe clinical investigators see their "jar of water" half empty rather than half full. Nonetheless, voluntary repetitive behavior that destroys the health of the body is an insult to society.

In summary, our studies showed that the nature and quantities of fuels oxidized are modified in patients with alcoholic cirrhosis. Their metabolic profiles are similar to those found in normal adults after 2-3 days of starvation. The diminished delivery of glucose (and ketone bodies) to the blood by the liver of patients with cirrhosis is

---

[16] There is a railroad that runs between Philadelphia and Chicago. Homes built in the suburbs along that railroad track are referred to as houses "on the Main Line." Most of the families who live in the Main Line area are socially and financially secure. Many of the individuals serve in some capacity to benefit those less fortunate. One of my friends is a retired executive who is heavily engaged in meeting the aims of the Rotary Club. He drives into the inner urban ghettoes around Temple University's main campus and hospital. The Rotary organization provides money for books and other educational materials for the inner city children and adolescents. My friend is there to maximize the gifts.

Although it appears that alcohol consumption among teenagers may have decreased, it has not disappeared. In some cases it has been replaced by narcotic use. Nonetheless, during a recent visit by my friend from the Rotary Club to a grade school near Temple University, a 13 year old boy was sent to the principal's office because he was found to have a bottle of gin. The purpose was to provide alcoholic drinks for himself and classmates.

As physicians and surgeons, we can treat patients with alcoholic cirrhosis and get some of them through an acute medical emergency. However, the much more daunting problem is how to prevent someone from being placed in a downtrodden position in his/her society. How do "altruistic missionaries" get a community to employ healthy habits and lead productive lives? A change comes from "intra-personal" recognition that the successful route to an enriched life comes from aspirations of decency with its good return on healthy and benevolent behavior.

complemented by an augmented supply of FFA in the bloodstream which compensates for the deficiency of the liver in fuel delivery.

The healthy organs of the body (e.g. adipose tissue) shift their metabolic behavior to aid another failing organ (e.g. liver) in times of need so the energy requirements for life can be maintained. It is this organ cross-talk that appears to be essential for survival.

Chapter XI. Impact of Insulin on Liver Metabolism

Insulin is the major fuel-regulating hormone in humans. Its failure is usually recognized by a high blood glucose concentration, but abnormalities in blood lipids and amino acids are also present. Insulin is formed in the Islets of Langerhans in the pancreas and secreted into the blood, primarily in response to a rise in concentration of glucose in the blood. Other fuels may also stimulate insulin secretion. Diabetes mellitus is a disease in which the quantities of available insulin and the actions of insulin are deficient. In patients with type 1 diabetes, the pancreas is incapable of making an adequate amount of insulin; therefore, insulin injections are required for survival. In patients with type 2 diabetes, the body does not produce enough insulin in response to the blood glucose concentration, and the cells of much of the body ignore the presence of insulin; these patients can usually survive without the immediate supplementation of insulin injections.

Six to seven percent of Americans have diabetes mellitus. This percentage can be broken down into categories based on age and body fat. Approximately 0.25% of the population under 20 years of age has insulin dependent, or type 1, diabetes. With the surge of obesity in children and adolescents, the prevalence of non-insulin dependent, or type 2, diabetes in this population is increasing rapidly, but the overall incidence of type 2 diabetes in young people to date is unknown. Of individuals 20 years and older, 8.7% have diabetes. About 18-19% of Americans over 60 years of age have this disease. Thus, the prevalence of diabetes significantly increases with age. As people increase their body fat mass, the discrepancy between body adipose tissue and insulin-producing pancreatic islets tissue increases. Therefore, the incidence of diabetes is also increased as body weight (fat) increases. Among individuals who are grossly or morbidly obese, the incidence of diabetes is about 50%.

Temple University Hospital is an inner urban institution situated in the northern ghettoes of Philadelphia. Although this population is mostly composed of fine, grateful people, there is also a violent element within the community. Cuts from knives are common, and stab wounds in the abdomen are so frequent during the weekends that the vernacular of the "Saturday Night Knife and Gun Club" is frequently used to describe injuries encountered in this ghetto population. When a physician/surgeon asks a patient what has happened to him or her, the reply is frequently, "My friend cut me." Most of these patients are young, relatively healthy adults who may or may not have been involved in consuming alcoholic beverages or drugs at the time of the knife fight.

As physicians and surgeons at Temple University Hospital delivering health care to patients with diabetes mellitus and other diseases, we envisioned an opportunity not only to give immediate medical help to those suffering from acute injury but to also study relatively healthy patient-volunteers with abdominal stab wounds. Knowledge regarding metabolism of the livers (and the kidneys) with normal blood flow rates could be gained once the acute insults were properly managed. When a knife wound penetrates the abdominal wall, an exploration of the inner abdominal contents is usually needed to determine whether or not the gut, liver, spleen, bladder or another organ has been lacerated so it can be repaired and serious hemorrhage and/or abdominal infections can be avoided or controlled.

Diabetes mellitus is prevalent among the ghetto population surrounding Temple University Hospital, and the physicians/surgeons at this institution served these patients with the greatest integrity possible. When patients with stab wounds were asked if they would participate in research activities relating to the impact of hormones (insulin) on liver metabolism, some of them would readily agree because "sugar diabetes" was a disease within their families, especially their grandmothers.

When we decided in the early 1970's to study the impact of alanine and hormones (insulin and glucagon) on liver metabolism, the knowledge was sparse. Ample evidence existed that the uptake of free fatty acids (FFA) from plasma by various tissues was proportional to the FFA concentrations in the plasma, and this led to the suggestion that the rate of ketone body synthesis by the liver was largely dependent upon the concentration of plasma FFA. Support for this contention was provided by experiments showing parallelism between the concentrations of plasma FFA and ketone bodies. However, increasing evidence appeared which indicated that the metabolic behavior of the liver in regards to producing ketone bodies (and glucose) was influenced by hormones as well as by the supply of FFA (and glucose) precursors.

Ketone body production by perfused rat livers was augmented when the FFA concentrations in the perfusates were increased, but the increments of ketone body production due to changes in FFA concentrations were less in livers derived from fed rats [with high blood (serum) insulin concentrations] than from those derived from fasted rats [with low blood (serum) insulin concentration]. Further, ketogenesis in perfused livers of diabetic animals exceeded that of normal animals. Thus, bits of evidence were appearing that factors other than the concentration of FFA perfused in the liver had roles in modifying hepatic metabolism. For example, high concentration of ketone bodies in the blood did not develop in dogs when their plasma FFA were elevated by infusing FFA into their bloodstream. Further, by administering exogenous insulin to ketotic rats, Dr. Dan Foster and colleagues at the University of Texas, Southwestern, also noted a dissociation between plasma FFA and ketone body levels in the plasma and blood. Subsequently, more investigations showed that in rats the availability of plasma FFA to the liver was not the sole determinant of the blood concentration of ketone bodies. Data showed that insulin could suppress hepatic ketone body production by means other than lowering the delivery of FFA to the liver. Similarly, Dr. Felig at Yale University School of Medicine and Dr. Wahren at the Karolinska Institute in Sweden, demonstrated in humans that insulin inhibited the formation of new glucose in the liver and thus dissociated the supply of precursors to the liver from the production of glucose. Thus, in rats, insulin appeared to have a direct regulatory role on hepatic ketone body formation. In humans, insulin influenced hepatic glucose formation. However, the role of insulin on hepatic synthesis of ketone bodies in humans, the most ketotic prone animal, had not been demonstrated. After all, clinical investigators (and, obviously, patients) are interested in human metabolism.

The published information on the impact of hormones, specifically insulin and glucagon, and other key modifiers of hepatic behavior needed to be advanced. All of us clinical investigators knew that the concentration values of glucose, ketone bodies and FFA in blood and/or plasma were not clearly defined. The many factors influencing the mobilization of precursors and the behavior of the liver needed to be delineated.

We theorized that if we could keep hormones (specifically insulin and glucagon) and precursors (especially the key gluconeogenic amino acid, alanine) constant in the general bloodstream, we could evaluate both the influence of hormones (insulin and glucagon) and precursors (alanine) on hepatic behavior in relatively healthy people.

Although the availability of precursors that could be converted into glucose and ketone bodies and the impact of hormones may each have independent effects on liver metabolism, another important regulatory factor was raised by J. P. Flatt, Ph.D. of the Massachusetts Institute of Technology. Perhaps he was the first to recognize the multiplicity of factors controlling metabolism. More recently, Richard Strohman, Ph.D. of the University of California at Berkeley has conveyed the message that all metabolic processes are multifactorial and much more complex than investigators envisioned in the 1970's. Nonetheless, with a lot of enthusiasm and some of the ignorance present in the early 1970's, we undertook the task of trying to measure hepatic extraction of precursors and production rates of ketone bodies and glucose before and after infusing insulin, glucagon or alanine in patients with abdominal stab wounds who were deprived of caloric intake for about 72 hours. We thought that the roles of hormones (specifically insulin and glucagon) and precursors on ketone body formation and glucose synthesis could be determined. Further, the quantitative relationship between hepatic ketone body and glucose synthesis could be investigated.

Approximately 20 patients per month entered the Temple University Hospital Emergency Room with penetrating wounds of the abdomen. An exploratory laparotomy was essential in a large proportion of these patients. Those presenting with suspected penetrating abdominal wounds who showed no clinical signs of inflammation in the abdominal cavity and whose heart rates and blood pressures were stable were selected as possible candidates for placement of an umbilicoportal vein catheter (cannula) during the period when the exploratory operation was performed.

We submitted a protocol to the Scientific Advisory Committee and the Institutional Review Board for evaluation and approval of our proposed studies to measure blood flow rates and metabolism in well compensated adult males with stab wounds of the abdomen. Safeguards to protect the individual's welfare were clearly emphasized. The surgeon, Dr. F.A. Reichle, and I were called before the committee members to testify about the safety of catheterizing the umbilicoportal venous system before they approved the research proposal. Dr. Reichle had developed a safe and useful technique for catheterizing the umbilical vein which had undergone a normal occlusion during the postpartum period (falciform ligament). He had catheterized over 100 patients with liver diseases and encountered no complications from placing a catheter into the portal vein via the umbilical vein to measure blood pressure and blood flow in this vessel. This vestige vessel could provide access to portal venous blood from the gut that perfused the liver (Figure 1). There were standard techniques available for obtaining blood from the arteries and from the hepatic and renal veins. Complications from obtaining blood

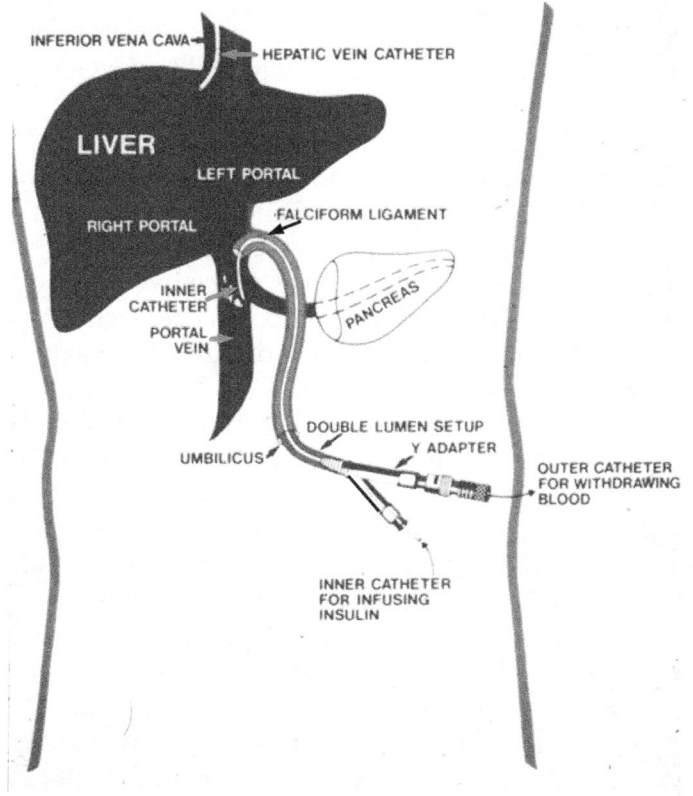

Figure 1. A graphic display of a double lumen set-up placing catheters into the portal vein for infusing insulin and measuring its impact by sampling blood across the liver via portal venous and hepatic venous blood.

from these vessels were rare. The uptake of O_2 and the production of CO_2 along with exchange rates of glucose, ketone bodies, amino acids, fatty acids, and other fuels across the gut, liver and kidney could be measured in compensated adult patient-volunteers.

Patients were fully informed of the nature, purpose and risk involved relating to umbilicoportal vein cannulation. In those that consented, Dr. Reichle first performed the necessary abdominal exploration and then the investigational umbilicoportal vein cannulation. Oral feedings are usually withheld after abdominal surgery. Several days after the operation, patients with normal liver function studies and free of intra-abdominal infections and whose heart rates and blood pressures were stable, were admitted to the General Clinical Research Center and placed on a calorie-free regimen for about 72 hours. The umbilicoportal cannulae were kept open with a solution that prevents blood from clotting (0.5% sodium citrate and isotonic saline). As noted above, over 100 umbilicoportal vein cannulations for diagnostic (in patients with cirrhosis of the liver and portal hypertension) and for treatment purposes had been performed with no major complications directly due to this procedure.

Figure 1 shows the physical arrangements for doing research on patients with catheters in the umbilicoportal vein and another catheter in the hepatic vein. (The arterial catheter is not shown.) A smaller catheter was inserted through the umbilicoportal cannula and rested in a position away from the liver but in the portal vein supplying a majority of the blood to the liver. The catheterization technique we used involved a double lumen device. In the figure, note that the inner catheter for infusing insulin is pointing away from the liver, but the blood flow is toward the liver. Dr. Reichle had to employ his extraordinary dexterity to insert and guide this catheter into the position needed to perform this intensive and delicate operation for the research experiment. The inner catheter had to be directed upstream in the portal vein. In essence, a "shepherd's hook" was formed by turning and placing the inner catheter away from the liver. Through the smaller, inner catheter, insulin, glucagon or alanine could be infused. Through the outer lumen closer to the liver, portal blood samples could be obtained. Another catheter was inserted in a large (antecubital) vein at the crease of the elbow and advanced to a hepatic vein draining the liver. Another needle was placed into a peripheral artery (not shown in figure). After catheters were in place and patient-volunteers were stable, total blood flow to the liver (portal plus arterial blood) was measured. In addition, portal blood flow was measured with a radiographic technique developed by Dr. Reichle and colleagues. Thus, a safe but tedious and dainty experimental setup was developed that could be used for measuring hepatic extraction of precursors (free fatty acids, lactate, pyruvate, glycerol and amino acids), and the hepatic production of ketone bodies and glucose before and after insulin (or glucagon) or precursors were infused locally into the portal vein. The quantities of blood removed from the portal venous and arterial blood entering the liver, and the hepatic venous blood leaving the liver, were known and could be replaced volume-for-volume with human albumin in saline.

Figure 2 shows the hepatic venous ketone body

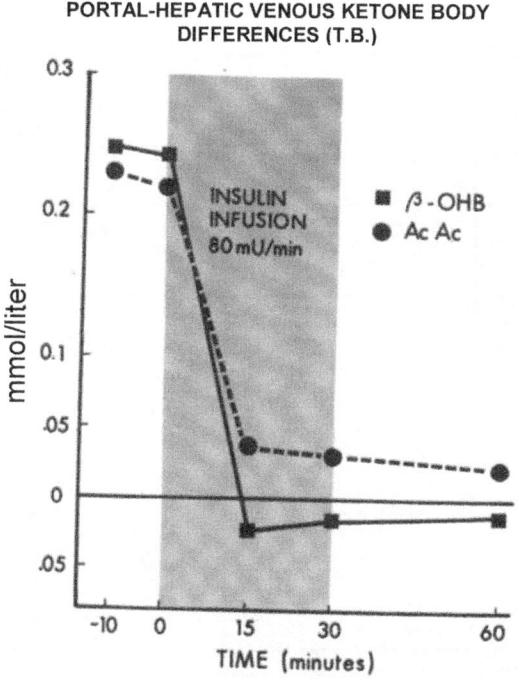

Figure 2. Infusing insulin directly into the portal vein supplying most of the blood to the liver inhibited hepatic ketone body production without significantly altering the availability of FFA. Note the liver uptake of ß–OHB with a small but significant release of AcAc.

concentration differences. The production of beta-hydroxybutyrate was completely stopped by the infusion of insulin into the portal blood. However, a minute amount of acetoacetate production persisted. It is conceivable that a small amount of beta-hydroxybutyrate may have been converted into acetoacetate. The delivery of FFA (not shown) to the liver was not significantly modified by the small amount of insulin infused directly into the portal vein supplying the liver. Thus, insulin had a regulatory effect on hepatic ketone body formation that was independent of the delivery of precursors (free fatty acids) to the liver for ketogenesis.

Figure 3 shows the direct impact of infusing insulin

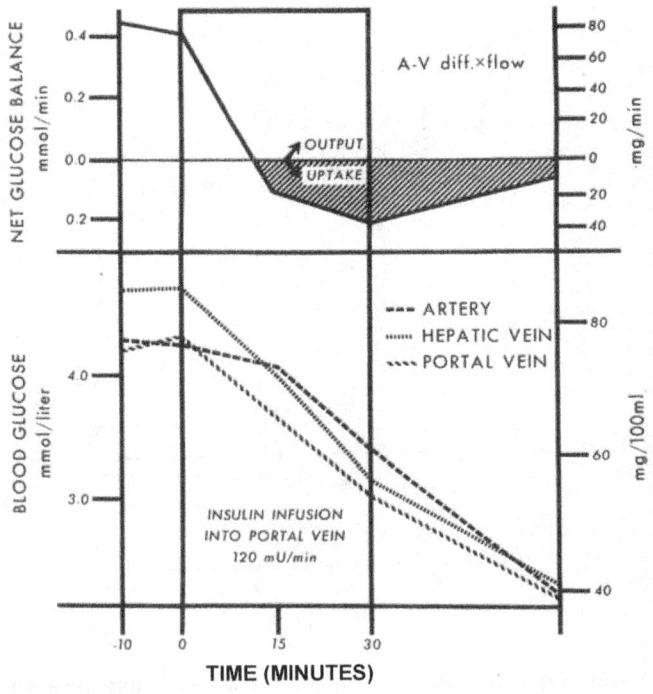

DIRECT EFFECT OF INSULIN ON HEPATIC GLUCOSE BALANCE

Figure 3. Direct effects of insulin infusion into the portal vein on hepatic glucose exchange and on blood glucose concentrations in a normal man after a 3 day fast.

216

into the portal system on liver of a fasting man. During starvation, the liver normally adds glucose to the bloodstream, but when insulin is infused into the portal blood, the liver reverses its behavior and extracts glucose from the bloodstream. Alanine, the key glucogenic amino acid, remained relatively constant in the arterial and peripheral venous blood, but hepatic extraction was converted into hepatic release of alanine. This implies that the impact of infusing insulin into the portal vein was dissipated before it reached the periphery. The liver may have extracted the infused insulin, or the concentration of insulin in the peripheral arterial system was not significantly increased but it was diluted in the large quantity of blood beyond the liver. In addition, it may be other body tissues (muscle) stopped releasing or began extracting alanine when small quantities of insulin entered the blood that may have passed through the liver. The extraction by the liver of lactate, the dominant carbohydrate converted into glucose, was markedly curtailed. Thus, with this infusion of insulin the liver reversed its metabolic profile from being the dominant organ that *released* glucose into the bloodstream to an organ that *extracted* glucose from the blood, and the extraction of alanine and lactate was modified.[17]

After a study was completed, the umbilical vein catheter was cautiously removed and the patient-volunteer closely observed for any bleeding tendencies. (Incidentally, we observed no complications from studying these patients.) After a few pilot studies were done, a grant request for money to continue to investigate the impact of hormones

---

[17] An editorial comment made by Dr. George F. Cahill, Jr. after reviewing Figures 2 and 3: "The insulin effects of changing glucose output into glucose uptake associated with a decrease in ketogenesis shows to me the dominant role that energy plays on gluconeogenesis: no gluconeogenesis $\cong$ no ketogenesis *a la* J.P. Flatt. Hepatic extraction of beta-hydroxybutyrate and release of acetoacetate coupled with the hepatic release of alanine are in agreement with this hypothesis." I believe the importance of energy in controlling body (and organ) metabolism has not received proper emphasis.

217

(and substrates) on regional hepatic metabolism was submitted in 1971 to the National Institutes of Health (NIH).[18] Although the NIH Study Section members approved the application, a memo from overview (Council) members stated that we could not study stab wound patients. Some Council members believed that an individual with a stab wound could not freely give his/her consent for research purposes because the injured patient was under duress and would be reluctant to deny the doctors treating him/her the opportunity to catheterize his/her portal vein for research purposes. The Study Section at NIH approves and recommends that a grant be paid, but only the Council has the legal right to approve funding. The law says that without Council approval, the grant cannot be made. We did not challenge the Council's decision. After the pilot studies were completed, no other patients were studied. The data presented in this chapter reveal the selected and incomplete information derived from the pilot studies. Other than a brief mention in a textbook[19], it should be noted that the results of our studies remained buried in a 1971 NIH grant application.

Under normal circumstances insulin is released from the Islets of Langerhans into the portal blood. This arrangement has an important influence on the concentration of glucose in blood beyond the boundaries of the liver. Obviously, an insulin delivery system that adds insulin

---

[18] Investigator-initiated grants submitted to the NIH for funding were allegedly confidential information. Eventually, the enforcement and amendments of the Freedom of Information Act overturned the confidentiality restriction on grants submitted to the NIH. Nonetheless, while this restriction was in effect, I received a telephone call from a clinical investigator working at a research-intense university in New York before our grant had been reviewed by the Study Section. He told me that he was interested in how we catheterized the umbilical vein to gain access to the portal circulation and asked how we made the calculations to arrive at the insulin concentrations we proposed to use for perfusing the liver. So much for confidentiality!

[19] Owen, O.E., M.S. Patel, B.S.B. Block, T.H. Kreulen, F.A. Reichle, and M.A. Mozzoli. Gluconeogenesis in normal, cirrhotic and diabetic humans. Gluconeogenesis. Its Regulation in Mammalian Species. Edited by R.W. Hanson and M.A. Mehlman. John Wiley, New York, Chapter 15, 1976, pp. 533-558

directly into the portal blood creates a more normal situation than injecting insulin under the skin and would have enormous benefit to the diabetic population. In addition, under the usual circumstances, the liver is the primary source of blood glucose, and the regulation of liver production of glucose has a marked impact on the glucose concentration in peripheral blood that flows throughout the body (e.g. eyes, kidneys, nerves, muscles, etc.)

The knowledge gained from our research pertaining to the direct influence of insulin on hepatic metabolism did not benefit patients. It was two decades later when similar data obtained from dogs was published in the literature! What a waste of human effort to advance biomedical science. Admittedly, reviewers did (and do) the best they could (can) to protect the welfare of patients, but sometimes overzealous individuals run the risk of impeding medical progress.

With the thankless opportunity of reviewers to critique and approve or block research efforts comes responsibility: be careful about stopping medical progress that may benefit the welfare of many patients.

Chapter XII. Diabetic Ketoacidosis: Catastrophic Fuel Mobilization

In a period of rush when there is no time to think, busy doctors want solutions, not explanations. Here, I provide explanations and some story-telling!

Over the years I have treated a large number of patients with diabetic ketoacidosis (DKA). I wanted to study some of them to gain understanding of the fundamental abnormalities (pathophysiology) of this devastating disease. Getting patients to volunteer to undergo research studies when they were dying from DKA was a difficult process. First, a physician, usually working in his office or in the emergency room and who was independent of the research team, had to refer the patient for study so there was no conflict of interest between the patient's welfare and the research personnel. This was a delicate matter and not always possible. Some of the sick patients knew of the integrity of their physicians and the researchers and wanted to aid in advancement of knowledge regarding DKA, especially the mechanisms responsible for the development of their severely elevated blood glucose (and ketone bodies).

I wrote protocols for studying diabetic patients suffering from DKA. The protocols were approved by the Institutional Review Board and the Institutional Advisory Committee. The substance of the protocols was this: Diabetic patients in moderate to severe ketoacidosis needed to be studied, providing their clinical situation was stable and they could understand and sign the consent form. We screened about 4 patients in DKA for each one studied. This was laborious and time-consuming but necessary in order to assure that the patients selected for the studies were 1) in DKA; 2) clinically stable, and 3) able to comprehend the nature of the research project. A patient could withdraw at any time from the study. It was stated that the benefits

220

to be gained by each individual were minimal. However, it seemed equally true that the benefits to be gained from the knowledge obtained from these studies should help other diabetic patients, and perhaps society in general.

Histories and physical examinations were done and routine blood, urine, electrocardiographic and roentgenographic studies requested. Of those patient-volunteers selected, their clinical courses were monitored by blood pressure, pulse, respiratory rates and mental alertness; stat laboratory tests for blood electrolytes, glucose and acid-base measurements were used to evaluate stability. Results from arterial blood gases and pH were obtained within 5 minutes.

We had learned that the patient's welfare was protected if a physician divorced himself from the research project and devoted his efforts toward taking care of the patient. Therefore, one physician managed the patient's diabetic condition while another physician-scientist team carried out the investigative studies. The individual research protocols varied as the aim of the research changed.

Our patients previously studied using non-invasive techniques had fewer complications than those admitted to the general hospital for treatment of DKA. I can honestly write that I cannot remember any patient that we studied during DKA and subsequently treated that had an adverse outcome as a consequence of the research. The situation is so stressful and attention is so great when a patient-volunteer is being studied, the research team is unlikely to overlook a pending dangerous sign. Patient-volunteers undergoing a research protocol were more closely watched than other patients.

In this chapter I focus on the results obtained from studying varying groups of diabetic patients who were experiencing DKA. In addition, I also describe some

221

interesting patients that simply popped into my mind while writing about DKA.

DKA is a catastrophic, complex, medical emergency that leads to death if not treated with insulin and fluids containing salts (electrolytes) and eventually sugar (glucose). It is one of few diseases for which a doctor can rescue a dying patient within an 8 to 24 hour period with appropriate therapy. This horrific disease can be rapidly reversed and the patient resuscitated. The reversal of the dying process in a patient to a compensated state is one of the most dramatic and gratifying experiences a doctor can have.

During the 1960's and 1970's, metabolic mechanisms operating in patients dying of DKA were poorly understood. At that time, physicians knew that when the body had an inadequate amount of insulin in the blood, the blood glucose became dangerously elevated (severe hyperglycemia). The primary hormonal abnormality was a deficiency of insulin. Many of the tissues of the body became deranged. The hyperglycemia led to profuse urination causing the body to become dehydrated and the blood volume and pressure to fall. Other hormones that regulate the fuels that move through the blood were identified and more hormones that respond to dehydration were found. Eventually, elevated blood concentrations of several hormones (glucagon, epinephrine, norepinephrine, growth hormone, cortisol and other regulatory hormones) accompanying the diabetic state, which further augmented the mobilization of free fatty acids (FFA) and affected the mobilization of amino acids, were detected by investigators. Substrates flowing to the liver were under hormonal influences which aided in the conversion of amino acids, glycerol, lactate and pyruvate into glucose, and FFA into ketone bodies. For each ketone body synthesized in the liver and released in the blood an ion of hydrogen (H+ or hydronium) was formed and released into the blood. Thereby, liver synthesis of ketone bodies generated a metabolic acidosis. (See Chapter VII, Liver and Kidney Metabolism in "Normal" Adults.)

The diagnostic criteria for DKA include a high blood glucose concentration (hyperglycemia), high ketone body concentration (hyperketonemia) and high hydrogen ion concentration (metabolic acidosis). The criteria must be broadly interpreted because a variety of clinical situations can modify the degree of hyperglycemia, hyperketonemia and metabolic acidosis.

Sometimes DKA develops in an undiagnosed or newly diagnosed diabetic patient. However, the most frequent causes of DKA include inadvertent or intentional discontinuation of insulin injections. Strokes or heart attacks can precipitate DKA. Pneumonia or other infections are frequent causes. Trauma from automobile accidents or other forceful events can initiate DKA. Insulin requirements are increased during pregnancy, and this state may induce DKA. "Excessive" alcohol consumption is associated with DKA. However, nothing obvious may be the case in a patient presenting for acute medical care for DKA.

The diagnosis may be hampered by the heterogeneity of the patient population that suffers from DKA. Individuals may be lean or obese; young to old; male or female. Conscious patients can relate a history of passing large amounts of urine; excessive thirst not quenched by drinking great quantities of fluids; eating more food but still losing weight. There are numerous other complaints, including abdominal pain.

A physical examination of a patient reveals rapid respirations, dry skin with the loss of elasticity or loss of turgor (from dehydration), a fruity breath smell (acetone halitosis), mental dullness (20% confused and drowsy; 10% comatosed, manifested by no purposeful eye movement, no meaningful verbal responses, and absent response to pain), wide variations in body temperature (92-106°F), a rapid heart rate (>100/min), and frequently a low blood pressure (<120/80).

Analysis of blood in the clinical laboratory usually reveals grossly elevated blood glucose (>250 mg/dl) and ketone body (>6.0 mmol/l) concentrations and low arterial blood pH (<7.3) and bicarbonate (<19 mEq/l) concentrations. A urine analysis usually shows a loss of glucose and ketone bodies in the urine. In addition, urine analysis is needed to detect renal disease, including infection. An electrocardiogram aids to evaluate the heart. A chest x-ray or other radiological studies help to detect precipitating causes of DKA, especially pneumonia.

Findings associated with fatalities caused by DKA are blood pressure less than 90 mmHg (systemic hypotension), body temperature below 92° F (hypothermia), severely elevated hydrogen concentrations (acidemia with arterial pH < 7.0), and grossly elevated blood glucose (>1000 mg/dl), urea, and electrolyte concentrations (hyperosmolarity).

Clinicians across the world knew the history, physical findings and laboratory data associated with the development of DKA long before they had an in-depth understanding of the causes for the elevated blood glucose, ketone bodies, acidemia and dehydration in patients dying from DKA. Of course, clinicians knew the blood of patients with DKA suffered from a lack of insulin, but the mechanisms responsible for flooding the bloodstream with an overabundance of fuels and the metabolic acidosis had not been defined. Further, how the kidney handled glucose, ketone bodies and fluids during DKA was blurred. It was generally assumed that the liver overproduced glucose and ketone bodies, but how hepatic glucose and ketone body production rates were interrelated during DKA was unknown. Further, in the early 1970's when we began to investigate the causes of abnormal blood glucose and ketone body concentrations and accompanying acidosis, there was no or very little human data available on mechanisms causing this dire clinical situation.

Between 1970-1985, about 40-50 adult patients per year presented to the Temple University Hospital emergency room in DKA. (St. Christopher's Hospital for Children provided pediatric medical services needed by the community.) About 80% of the Temple Hospital patients suffering from DKA were older than 20 years of age. Five to eight percent were patients who had previously been treated for DKA. They had the spectrum of hyperglycemic-ketotic syndromes. Over a period of 3 years, several patients agreed

224

to undergo studies to delineate the abnormalities of DKA. Selection of the patients was based on their clinical stability and willingness to participate in the research study. The nature of the study and the associated risk of the research protocol were fully explained to each patient before the planned study was initiated. Treatment was never delayed if it was anticipated that the patient's health and response to therapy would be jeopardized. We had learned that patients could usually be stabilized by giving them intravenous fluids with electrolytes to replace the volume of fluid loss in the urine.

Nine patient-volunteers participated in our initial studies to measure the liver production rates of glucose and ketone bodies. Their arterial blood glucose concentration (234-954 mg/dl or 13-53 mmol/liter); ketone body concentration (acetoacetate 1.4-3.8 mmol/liter and beta-hydroxybutyrate 5.6-12.0 mmol/liter); arterial pH (7.09-7.36), and plasma bicarbonate (3-11 mEq/liter) met the criteria for moderate to severe DKA. It should be noted that patients suffering from DKA have a broad range of blood chemical abnormalities. We restricted our investigations by not studying the most severely compromised patients.

The patient-volunteers were taken to the catheterization laboratory. A catheter was inserted in the large vein in front of the elbow and advanced to the main vein draining the right lobe of the liver. A needle was inserted into the artery in front of the elbow in the opposite arm. Another venous avenue was used to infuse a dye needed to measure the blood flow through the liver. After all catheters and needles were placed, we paused for a few minutes to make sure the patient was stable and was in no accelerated rate of decompensation. Arterial and liver venous bloods were drawn simultaneously and placed in appropriate containers (e.g. test tubes) for subsequent analysis. Two sets of these samples were drawn at about 10 minute intervals. After the research component of blood sampling was completed, insulin and fluids with electrolytes (salts) and, later, glucose (sugar), were given intravenously.

225

The analyses of the blood samples took top priority in our laboratories.

All patient-volunteers had complete recovery from their DKA with no complications from the catheterization.

Of the nine patients who volunteered to undergo catheterization studies to define liver metabolism during DKA, eight patients completed the study. The ninth patient brought a peculiar sense of humor to mind. She was a middle-aged woman who presented to the Temple Hospital Emergency Room in DKA. After her baseline laboratory and clinical measurements were completed, and she was found to be in a manageable state, she was asked, and she agreed, to participate in a research study to gain knowledge about her diabetic state. She was taken to the catheterization laboratory where her artery and hepatic veins were catheterized and dye was infused to measure liver blood flow. All procedures were set up to measure her liver function during DKA. We paused for a few minutes to monitor her stability. She looked at me and asked what we were doing. I said, "We are making sure you are stable before we draw any blood from you." She asked, "Why are you withdrawing blood from me?" I responded, "To measure metabolic behavior of your liver while you are in this sick state of diabetic ketoacidosis." She asked, "Why are you doing this to me?" I answered, "We are trying to do some research so we can better understand how the body develops diabetic ketoacidosis." She responded, "Don't do any research on me." All the personnel in the catheterization laboratory looked at her with great wonderment. We had gotten up in the middle of the night, rushed to the hospital, got her voluntary consent after a detailed explanation, and had the arterial needle and hepatic vein catheter in place. It would only take about 15 minutes more time to complete the research endeavors. Nonetheless, we stopped the research activities and pulled the catheter out of the hepatic vein but left it in the arm so it could be used to infuse insulin and fluids with electrolytes first, and glucose later. The patient recovered completely from DKA after an additional 8-10 hours of closely monitored therapy throughout the rest of the night. So be the disappointments, futility, trials and tribulations of clinical research efforts.

I want to give a brief account of another young woman who was a patient of Dr. Charles Shuman, a noted diabetic specialist at Temple University Hospital. She telephoned Dr. Shuman and told him she was becoming progressively more ill from her uncontrolled diabetes, passing copious amounts of urine and experiencing rapid respirations. Her mouth was dry and she was thirsty. Dr. Shuman was familiar with this patient and over the telephone he prescribed a dose of rapid acting insulin. He told her to inject the insulin under the skin into the fat and come to the emergency room. When she arrived, she was found to have the classic criteria of DKA. She was dehydrated, breathing rapidly and had a fruity halitosis, a typical smell of acetone (a ketone body exhaled in the breath). Her heart rate was fast and her blood pressure was low. Her blood glucose and ketone body concentrations were markedly elevated and her arterial pH reflected a severe acidosis. Her laboratory data confirmed the diagnosis of DKA. She agreed to be studied while her deranged metabolism was corrected. She was taken to the cardiac catheterization laboratory. A large bore needle for giving intravenous fluids was placed in her left forearm. A trocar was placed in a peripheral artery, and a hepatic vein catheter was advanced to the right lobe of the liver. Blood samples were being drawn to measure her response to the insulin dose she had taken before arriving at the hospital. Intravenous fluids were being appropriately administered.

Although she had been fighting for her life, breathing forcefully, she slowly began to recover from her catastrophic state of DKA. With her arms stretched out at her sides, with needles stuck into the vessels of these extremities, and with a hepatic vein catheter in place, she looked at me and asked for a cigarette. Damn! She would not benefit from smoking a cigarette, especially at this moment in time. Nonetheless, I hustled around the immediate environment and found her a cigarette and a match. The cigarette was placed between her lips and it was lit. She held it in place with her lips as she smoked it. In spite of being in a precarious and dangerous situation, she was regaining peace of mind. Shortly thereafter the hepatic vein catheter was removed and she was given more insulin and more fluids and electrolytes into her vein. Eventually, intravenous glucose was added at the appropriate time in therapy. She underwent complete recovery from her DKA.

Because she had taken insulin before arriving at the hospital, her results were not included with those of the other patient-volunteers. Her data showed that the plasma free fatty acid (FFA) concentrations were falling during the catheterization study. More important, the liver was extracting, not producing, beta-hydroxybutyrate and was releasing acetoacetate. As clinicians, we knew that during the therapeutic period for treating DKA, about half of the patients exhibited a precipitous fall in blood beta-hydroxybutyrate and a small and transient rise in blood acetoacetate. This study provided an explanation for these clinical findings (Figure 1).

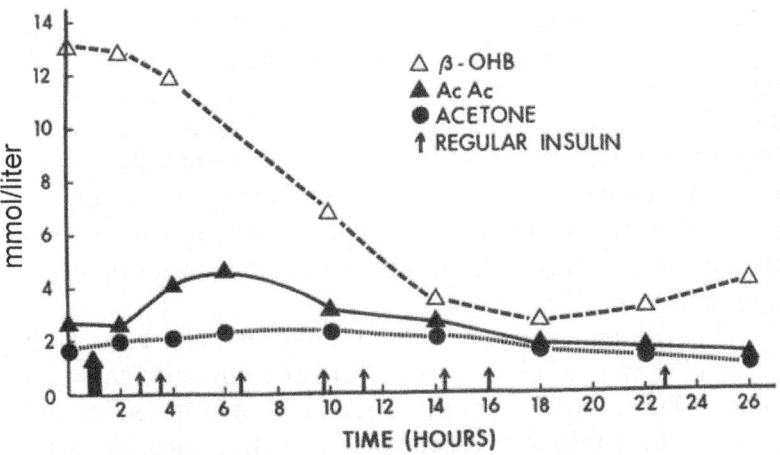

Figure 1. Displayed are the changes in blood ketone body concentrations during therapy for DKA. Beta-hydroxybutyrate falls precipitously while acetoacetate undergoes a transient rise before decreasing in blood concentration. Acetone blood concentrations respond more slowly to treatment.

When the nine patients were initially interviewed for catheterization studies, we had no information suggesting that any of them consumed excessive quantities of alcohol. Recognition of alcohol abuse became apparent either during the catheterization study, after further questioning the family, or from old hospital records of three of the patient-volunteers.

The data we accumulated from normal adult-volunteers over the years became most useful for comparison with data derived from patient-volunteers during DKA.

Normal liver metabolism after an overnight and more protracted periods of starvation are described (see Chapter VII, Liver and Kidney Metabolism in "Normal" Adults). Here, liver metabolism in "healthy" states after an overnight and 3 day fast is briefly reviewed.

After an overnight fast, the liver contributes about 0.86 mmol/min/1.73m^2 of glucose to the bloodstream. The simultaneous quantity of ketone bodies is small. After fasting for 3 days the glucose contribution falls to about 0.42 mmol/min/1.73 m^2. Much of this glucose is derived from recycled lactate and pyruvate. The shortfall in contribution of glucose is compensated by large contributions of ketone bodies to the blood. Therefore, the total delivery of fuels to the bloodstream by the liver is approximately equal after overnight and 3 day fasts (Figure 2). In contrast, the livers of diabetic patients suffering from DKA contribute about the same amount of glucose to the bloodstream as do normal people after an overnight fast. Concurrently, they add about the same amount of ketone bodies to the bloodstream as normal adults do after a 3 day fast. There is a lack of reciprocal interplay between the amount of glucose and the amount of ketone bodies contributed to the blood by the livers of diabetic patients suffering from DKA. In addition, the diabetic patients in severe catabolic states with a deficiency in insulin also release an excessive quantity of FFA into the bloodstream. Virtually all tissues dump their fuels into the blood. These fuels all compete for utilization. The simultaneous release of FFA, glucose and ketone bodies into the bloodstream during the severe insulin-deficient state

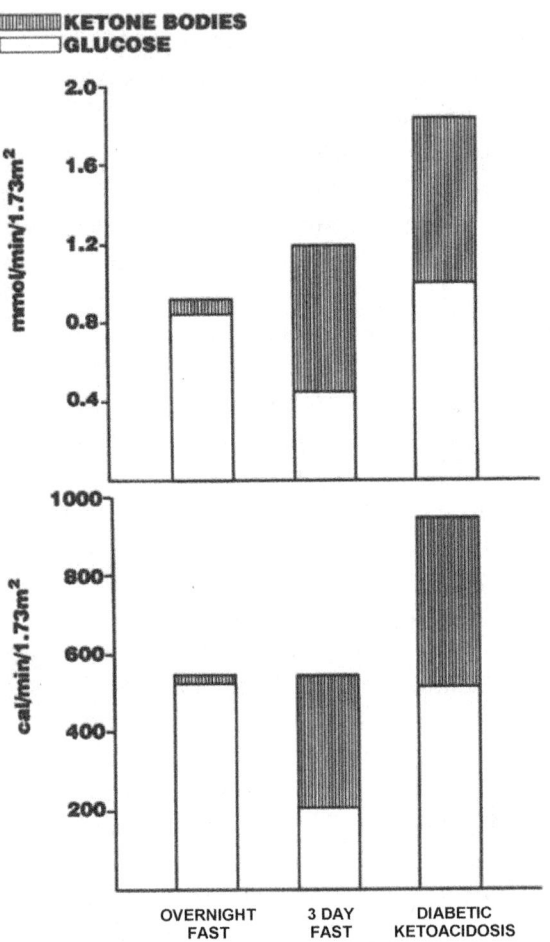

Figure 2. The top part of the figure displays the glucose and ketone bodies delivered by the liver in mmol/min/1.73 m². The bottom part expresses the delivery of ketone bodies and glucose to the bloodstream in cal/min/1.73 m².

of DKA progressively floods the body with an overabundance of fuels. When ketone body oxidation is curtailed, hydrogen ion accumulates. The combined effect of simultaneous release of FFA and the production of glucose and ketone bodies leads to severe hyperglycemia and hyperketonemia, and a subsequent acidosis.

The kidneys excrete large quantities of glucose and ketone bodies along with body fluid in the urine. This creates voluminous excretion of water and salts coupled to an acidosis which leads to dehydration and to vascular collapse and death.

The major hormonal abnormality in DKA is an insufficient quantity of circulating insulin to restrain unwarranted breakdown of body stores that can serve as fuels. The increased quantities of glucagon, catecholamines and other hormones in the blood that exhibit anti-insulin activity aggravate the catastrophic state.

We researchers asked, "What are the roles of the kidney in mitigating the disastrous effects of altered liver behavior (metabolism)? Is there a cross-talk between the liver and the kidney aimed at trying to compensate the body for the liver's over-production of water-soluble fuels by excreting some of the blood glucose and ketone bodies in the urine?" In the absence of sufficient amounts of insulin, cross-talk appears to be inadequate to maintain metabolic compensation.

During medical school I was taught that when the concentrations of glucose and ketone bodies reached critical levels in the blood, these fuels were "spilled in the urine." The concept of a renal threshold for glucose and ketone bodies was taught throughout the medical community. These teachings were erroneous! It is true that practically no glucose or ketone bodies are found in the urine when the blood concentrations of the fuels are low. Nonetheless, the handling of glucose and ketone bodies by the kidney is more complex than a simple renal threshold.

Drs. D.G. Sapir and J.H. Licht from Johns Hopkins Hospital helped me to study renal function in 10 diabetic patients suffering from moderate to severe DKA. The patient-volunteers were hospitalized on the General Clinical Research Centers in Temple University and Johns Hopkins Hospitals. Admission blood glucose and ketone bodies were high and the arterial pH's were low. The patient-volunteers were partially rehydrated with intravenous salt water (0.45% saline in water) but no insulin was given until the studies

231

were completed. Partial rehydration reduced the blood (plasma) glucose, but had no effect on blood ketone body concentration or on the metabolic acidosis.

Our studies showed that the kidney's reabsorption of glucose and ketone bodies increased linearly (directly) with the quantities of glucose and ketone bodies filtered by the kidney (through the glomerulus) (see chapter VII, Liver and Kidney Metabolism in "Normal" Adults). We found no maximal rate for the reabsorption of either glucose or ketone bodies. Because renal reabsorption of ketone bodies was less than 100%, ketone body loss in urine increased as the filtered load from the blood (plasma) increased (Figure 3). Glucose reabsorption rate was directly related to the quantity of glucose filtered (data not shown). Thus, there are no renal thresholds for ketone bodies (or for glucose) (Figure 3). The wide range of the data reveals how heterogeneous the patients in DKA were. (Owen, O.E., J.H. Licht and D.G. Sapir. Renal function and effects of partial rehydration during diabetic ketoacidosis. *Diabetes* 30:510-518, 1981.)

A large amount of nitrogen was excreted as ammonium during DKA. Ammonium loss in the urine is coupled to the synthesis of glucose by the kidneys. However, the net effect of the kidneys on blood glucose is to lower blood glucose concentration because the amount of glucose excreted (lost) in the urine far exceeds any glucose synthesized and added to the blood by the kidney.

The fact that most of the glucose and ketone bodies filtered out of the blood by the kidney (glomeruli) is reabsorbed by the kidney (tubules) protects the body from experiencing even greater dehydration, vascular collapse, and death. Greater losses of glucose and ketone bodies in the urine would be accompanied by larger losses of body water and minerals (sodium, potassium, phosphate, ammonium and other ions) in the urine. Greater losses of water and minerals would hasten cardiovascular failure and death during DKA.

Thus, the teachers who taught us as students that there were "renal (kidney) thresholds" for glucose and ketone bodies simply lacked the correct information. It took

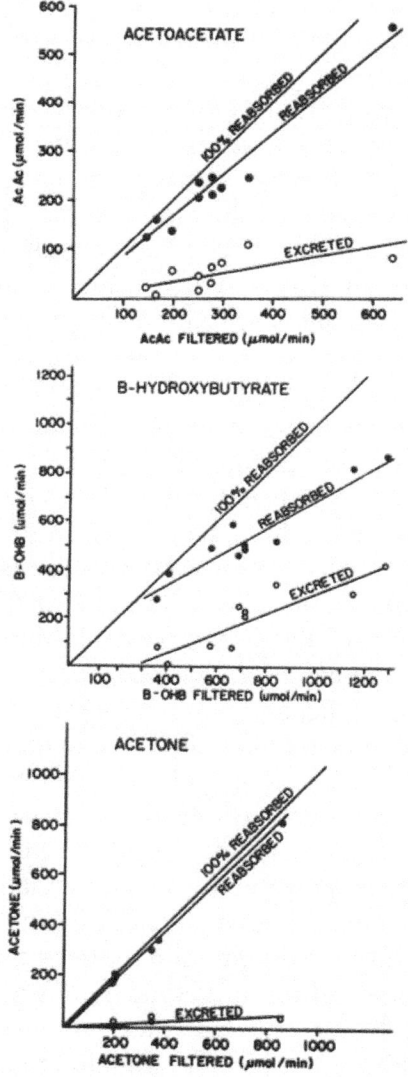

Figure 3. This figure shows the kidney's handling of ketone bodies. The greater the filtered load of AcAc, ß-OHB and acetone, the greater the tubular reabsorption of these ketone bodies. Reabsorption is not 100%; therefore all 3 ketone bodies are excreted in the urine. Acetone is a neutral compound; it freely diffuses across all kidney tissues and, therefore, has a very low excretion rate.

233

clinical investigators to correct these erroneous concepts and teachings. There are no other professions that are as dedicated to correcting mistakes, advancing biomedical sciences and spreading new information comparable to the medical profession.

After catheterization studies showed ketone body production rates by the liver during DKA, we began to realize that markedly elevated concentrations of ketone bodies in the blood had to be due to impaired ketone body oxidation as well as inappropriate ketone body production rates. We shifted our efforts to measuring ketone body oxidation rates simultaneously with measuring ketone body production rates. Over the years we had learned that multiple factors determined the ketone body concentration in blood. Specifically, factors other than production rates influence the blood concentrations of acetoacetate and beta-hydroxybutyrate. We had shown that there was a linear relationship between production and concentration up to 2-4 mmol/L, a value usually obtained after 2-3 days of fasting. At higher concentrations, such as those observed during more prolonged starvation, blood concentrations do not reflect production rates. From our catheterization studies the dissociation between hepatic production rate of ketone bodies and blood concentrations became evident. There was a dissociation between ketone body production rates and ketone body blood concentrations after prolonged starvation and during DKA (Figure 4). We began to realize that several mechanisms were responsible for this dissociation. One of these factors, which has not been discussed in this book, is the restricted volume of distribution in the body for ketone bodies. The concentrations of ketone bodies in blood and extracellular fluids were much greater than that found in intracellular fluids. For a given production rate of ketone bodies a restricted volume of distribution heightens the concentrations of ketone bodies measured in the blood. Further, we had demonstrated that the renal retrieval of ketone bodies contributed to a high blood concentration of ketone bodies in both starvation and DKA (Figure 3). We

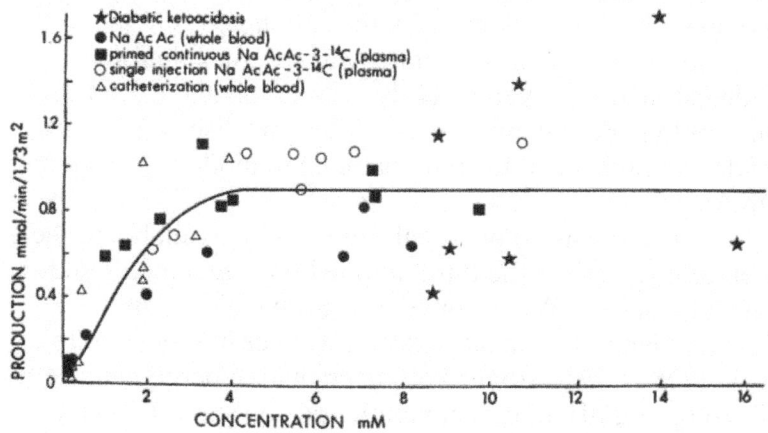

Figure 4. Displays the dissociation between the production rate of ketone bodies and the concentration of ketone bodies after the blood concentration exceeds 4 mmol/liter.

knew that in starvation, ketone body production and removal rates did not equilibrate until high blood ketone concentrations were reached after about 2-3 weeks of starvation. Maybe death from progressive ketoacidosis during DKA was in part due to impaired ketone body removal by tissue oxidation. Several other investigators did report impaired ketone body oxidation rates in diabetic animals during DKA. We had enough experience to know that such patients could be maintained in the steady-state condition for about 4-6 hours by giving intravenous fluids with salt (saline). Rehydration with saline reduced the blood glucose concentration but had no effect on acetoacetate, beta-hydroxybutyrate or acetone concentrations, and no effect on arterial pH. By choosing the proper dose of (3-^{14}C)-acetoacetate, rapid steady-states for labeling ketone bodies could be obtained and total ketone body production and oxidation rates could be measured. The analysis of tracer techniques to determine the production and oxidation of ketone bodies in diabetic patients suffering from ketoacidosis showed impaired ketone body oxidation rates.

In the process of developing methods to measure ketone body production and oxidation rates in diabetic patients in DKA, we learned that a third ketone body, acetone, which is derived from the spontaneous decarboxylation of acetoacetate, was responsible for the underestimation of ketone body production and oxidation rates in hyperketonemic states. After this discovery was made, we proceeded to study patients in moderate to severe DKA.

There was no practical information available in the literature regarding the third ketone body, acetone, found in catabolic states. We hospitalized seven patients on the Temple General Clinical Research Center in moderate to severe DKA. All patient-volunteers had hyperglycemia (241-603 mg/dl), hyperketonemia (acetoacetate 1.71-4.4 mmol/l, beta-hydroxybutyrate 3.8-13.4 mmol/l, acetone 0.5-6.0 mmol/l), and acidosis (pH 7.25-7.33). We found that a significant quantity of acetoacetate had probably undergone spontaneous decarboxylation to form acetone. In this process, for each molecule of acetone formed from acetoacetate, a cation of hydrogen (hydrogen ion, hydronium) is removed from the body fluids, and this negates the acidosis produced when acetoacetate is synthesized. Contrary to some modern scientific teachings, we found acetone, derived from endogenous fat stores via acetoacetate, can be converted into glucose. Using $(2-^{14}C)$-acetone we found that acetone contributed about 2% of the average amount of glucose formed during DKA. A 2% net gain in new glucose formation from fat during DKA is not a small quantity of glucose. It amounts to about 50% as much glucose as alanine contributes during DKA (Reichard, G.A., Jr., C.L. Skutches, R.D. Hoeldtke and O.E. Owen. *Diabetes* 35:668-674, 1986). We found that breath and urine excretion of acetone accounted for 2-30% of the body's production rate of acetone. In essence, our pioneer research work revolving around acetone (derived from spontaneous decarboxylation of acetoacetate) showed it could be converted into glucose. Thus, a small amount of glucose formed during starvation as well as during DKA was derived from acetone, a product of fatty acid breakdown. The discovery that one of the ketone bodies, acetone, could be

236

converted into glucose was a novel finding that needed to be pursued in more detail to have a greater grasp on survival during starvation.

After the completion of the mental exercises needed to understand and evaluate the patient suffering from DKA, treatment must be initiated. The patient must be constantly monitored and data maintained on a flow sheet until compensation is regained. Rapid acting insulin must be administered and accompanied by intravenous fluids, electrolytes, minerals and vitamin replacement, and eventually, glucose supplementation (Figure 5). Metabolic control should be accomplished within 12-24 hours after initiating therapy. If possible, the doctor should identify the cause for the DKA. Education has to be provided to the patient and assured outpatient care arranged for the patient.

I lectured to medical students and taught residents and other physicians on the causes and the treatments of DKA. Frequently I was contacted and told that my services were needed to provide health care to a patient suffering from DKA. When junior members of a healthcare team are providing directions for treatment, sometimes they need a consultant and would ask me for assistance. I relate the clinical story of a 13 year old girl brought to the emergency room in St. Christopher's Hospital for Children by her mother and father. When the young medical team opened the curtains surrounding the patient, they noticed an unusual fruity smell of fingernail polish remover (acetone) in the air. The patient was apprehensive, breathing hard and looking for help. They vaguely remembered the teachings on fuel homeostasis in health and disease that I had provided in months past. They tried to reflect on the significance of smelling a fruity halitosis emitted by a patient. This was one of their first encounters of this type of forced respiration. The patient was obviously very sick, and there was no history that her rapid respirations were due to exercising. She had no cough yet she was forcefully breathing 40 times a minute. Her mouth was dry and she was severely dehydrated. She was thirsty. Her pulse was rapid and her

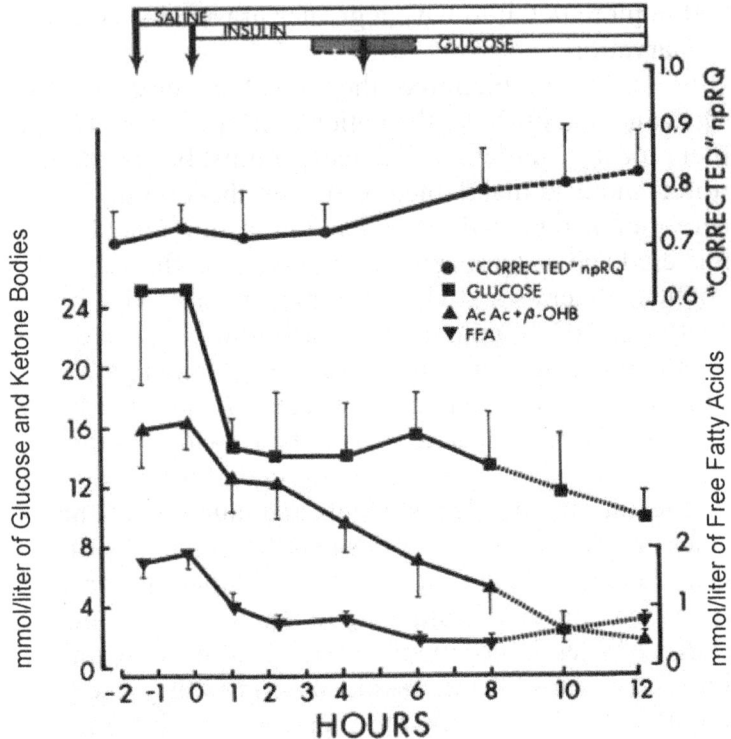

Figure 5. The impact of intravenous saline and insulin therapy and glucose administration in diabetic patients suffering from severe diabetic ketoacidosis is displayed. Insulin was delayed until the first 2 measurements were made to comply with the experimental protocol. Note the prompt decline in blood glucose, ketone bodies and free fatty acids following rehydration and insulin administration. The corrected non-protein respiratory quotient (npRQ) progressively increases during therapy. The rising npRQ reflects increased glucose oxidation.

blood pressure was low. Her eyesight was not adequately evaluated.

A quick digression from the patient to medical history may be of interest. "On May 19, 1873, Professor Dr. Kussmaul in Germany described a 35 year old woman with dry skin and great shortness of breath and uneasiness, throwing herself here and there and begging for help because she feared she was dying. Her breathing was loud and rapid, and the respiratory movement of her chest strikingly large.

Powerful costal abdominal inspirations alternated with powerful expirations. She was disturbed by great thirst and drank a great deal of spring water. She urinated much and her straw colored urine contained much sugar. She sank soon afterwards into a stuporous condition in which the loud breathing continued until just before her death that night."

The young patient in front of the junior care team had a dry mouth and kept asking for water. In spite of being dehydrated, she needed to urinate. Those former lectures and discussions regarding diabetic ketoacidosis may have been meaningful. This patient appeared to have seriously uncontrolled diabetes mellitus, and she was in the process of dying from ketoacidosis. They realized that they were observing a dying patient and needed a little advice on how to handle this medical emergency. I was called in as a consultant.

This 13 year old patient was resuscitated with intravenous insulin, fluids, electrolytes and later with glucose. Her grossly abnormal concentrations of glucose and ketone bodies in her blood and her metabolic acidosis were corrected. However, the circulation to her brain had been transiently inadequate during the latter stages of her decompensation. This caused a deficient amount of oxygen reaching the occipital cortex of the brain, the area that processes conscious vision. The patient had developed "cortical blindness." Thank God, her vision slowly began to improve over the ensuing days. She subsequently sought my care as an outpatient. I reviewed her history which revealed the horrible and inconsistent way she was eating, exercising and taking her prescribed insulin doses. After counseling her on several occasions, I harshly scolded her one day during an outpatient visit. She got up from her chair, walked out of the door between my inner office and my secretary's office and walked through the hallway before reentering my office through a side door. She screamed at me, "You old gripe!"

We worked together several years trying to develop the best regimen for managing her diabetes. Over the years she gave me pieces of her artwork; I gave her my affection and professional help.

Another, but unsubstantiated, recollection regarding DKA, is that it seemed to me that adult men and women slipping deeper into diabetic ketoacidosis came to the emergency room late in the day or near nightfall. Maybe they believed if they went to bed in a severe, decompensated state, they might die during the night. Most of our studies were done late in the day or during the night.

Sometimes it was difficult to round up the team needed to do a safe and comprehensive study. Once assembled in the catheterization laboratory, every member of the research team was tense and anxiety pervaded the surroundings. Some facial expressions reflected discontent. "Why was I called to return to work during non-scheduled hours?"

The movements of personnel in the catheterization laboratory during the studies were intentional. There were very few lighthearted comments. The patient-volunteers were closely monitored: were the blood pressure and heart rate constant and acceptable for the clinical condition of the patient? Was the patient-volunteer passing urine? Was the body temperature acceptable? The patient-volunteers were all in jeopardy. Sick patients are always in jeopardy.

Did the results of our grueling studies add to better understanding and treatment of DKA? I think so, but I don't know. However, I do know that our metabolic studies showed that the differences among normal individuals subjected to starvation and patients dying from DKA are surprisingly small. Starvation is tolerated for weeks to months because the *production* of fuels matches the *utilization* of fuels, and homeostasis (balance) is obtained. In contrast, DKA causes death in days, if not in hours; there is a mismatch of production and utilization of fuels, and death from this imbalance occurs. The combined effect of various metabolic deviations sucks the life from human beings suffering from DKA.

Some might have asked if it really mattered *how* the behavior of the body organs was deranged when the methods for reversing this acute diseased state were known? Get on with treating the lack of insulin and the dehydration. To hell with the cause. "Treat now and worry about the cause later." Unfortunately, maybe this attitude has contributed to lack of knowledge regarding the fundamental cause of insulin dependent diabetes.

Disregarding who gets credit for what, in 1959, 50% of the patients who presented to hospital emergency rooms in DKA died. In 1985 and thereafter, about 5% of the patients who entered the emergency rooms in DKA died, not from DKA, but from overwhelming complications like heart attacks, strokes or severe infections associated with DKA. Dr. Abbas Kitabchi and coworkers at the University of Tennessee in Memphis have developed detailed and superb methods for treating patients suffering from DKA. We clearly have learned how to correct the metabolic derangements causing the "hyperglycemia, hyperketonemia and metabolic acidosis."

Chapter XIII. Obesity, Energy Requirements and Body Composition

Obesity (increased body fat content) is the natural consequence of living in a society where food of high caloric content (energy) is available in overabundance. Exercise helps to lose weight, but the answer to obesity is eating fewer calories. It should be noted, however, that obese humans consume food in a manner similar, but not identical, to patients with substance dependence disorder, e.g. narcotic addiction. There are no periods of insane behavior (acute psychosis) during the first days of food withdrawal. However, there is incessant craving of food during semi or total prolonged starvation periods. The cause for this behavior regarding food consumption is simply unknown, but it is related to brain alterations that drive overeating and can be demonstrated with functional brain imaging techniques. We need devoted clinical investigators to unravel this dilemma and offer useful information to overcome this human malady. In the meantime, humans have to accept personal responsibility to avoid obesity or reduce body fat when significantly overweight.

This chapter is written with the belief that people can understand most of what is known about the energy requirements and body compositions of adults. Specifically, the average person can understand the underlying cause of obesity or why people get fat. Hopefully, it will convey my observation to the learned and novice, all kinds of people with far-reaching backgrounds and interests. Data are presented for your analyses. Truth is really easy to understand, and it brings pleasure. I have tried to remove the murk and show the uncamouflaged results. Although it may be "tough to accept," finding the truth provides incomparable gratification.

If the reader has the misfortune of being heavier than desired, maybe the information given in this book will drive away the melancholy and delight the senses. Let me drag into light the propensity for Americans (all people) to be fat, so they can decide if they want to do anything about obesity.

Obesity is not a problem of poor people. It is a problem for people of all financial classes. Obesity may be a problem in the USA that is beyond the point of no return – beyond where the U.S. populous can return to a state in which body composition of most people no longer reflects an excessive amount of body fat. Most people who are grossly obese fail to lose a significant amount of fat and keep it off their bodies. Their weights go down and up, and billions of dollars are wasted on dietary products. Nonetheless, I hope that some intelligent people will recognize the burden excess fat places on the body and reduce their caloric intake or increase their caloric expenditure, or both, to become or remain lean. There is a subset of humans in which this may be practically impossible in a society where food is readily available.

When most adults begin to gain more weight than they want, some simply reduce their food intake and/or exercise to lose weight. Others, however, begin to look for an excuse for their obesity. Often their initial question is whether or not their metabolism is slow (low) like that observed with failing thyroid gland (hypothyroidism) rather than the lack of exercise or excessive food intake. The possibility of hypothyroidism is relatively easy to rule out by measuring the thyroid stimulating hormone and/or the thyroid hormones in the blood. Denial may take hold and other faults are entertained to delay doing what is needed. Certainly, genetics can play a major role, but a person cannot become grossly overweight unless there is a significant imbalance between nutrients eaten and energy expended. Nonetheless, the role of environmental influences on genetic expression needs much more evaluation.

It is interesting and pertinent what a small number of volunteers did for the USA, if not for the world, by undergoing closely monitored studies so factual information regarding metabolism could be provided. They dismissed the fabrication that "healthy" individuals could get fat on a low caloric intake. The fattest country in the world, USA, finally recognized the reality that eating more food (calories) than you use to meet your energy requirements results in obesity. Now the USA population has to realize that obesity during pregnancy programs the offspring to be obese. Thus, a fetus, living in the abdominal environment created by a fat mother, may have had imposed upon him/her genetic alterations that program him/her to become a fat adult with diabetes mellitus. This is known as an "epigenetic phenomenon." Recent reports suggest that obesity rivals smoking tobacco products as the leading cause of death among USA citizens. As a population, let's hope we are not beyond the point of no return with the epidemic of obesity and diabetes. Parents must stop compounding the predisposition to develop obesity. The food industry must find a way to be profitable without suggesting that the USA public should eat or drink something every 3-4 hours. Maybe we can export more food and cut the trade deficit. This is probably a silly recommendation because hungry people (nations) don't have any money.

The United States of America has more fat people than any other nation. According to the Centers for Disease Control and Prevention, 64 percent of Americans are overweight. This is significant because obesity is associated with diabetes mellitus, high blood pressure, heart attacks and strokes and some cancers. In the 1930's, Dr. E.P. Joslin described obesity as the most important contributing factor to the precipitation of diabetes mellitus. "For this," he stated, "we should be grateful because obesity is preventable." Of course, obesity is preventable, but it is against natural tendencies. When food is available in overabundance and is cheap to buy, the natural reaction of people is to eat more nutrients than needed and to gain weight. Obesity is not a doctor's problem or the fault of the food industry. It is a personal problem. Maybe professional help is warranted, but without a personal desire to lose weight, no one will be successful in shedding pounds of unwanted fat. People on diets are hungry, and they seek food.

During the Great Depression and during World War II when food was scarce or rationed, there were few fat people in the USA. Standard clothing sizes for men were established in 1941 during World War II so uniforms could be made. After 1945, more food has become available in the advanced nations. With the ready supply of food during the last 50-60 years, men and women have become rounded with subcutaneous fat centered in the abdomen. Obesity has become the more usual and natural state of USA adults. Unfortunately, it is fraught with dire complications. Even children are developing type 2 diabetes mellitus. Nonetheless, we must distinguish between morbidly obese patients with a two-fold death rate and healthy overweight people. We need to stop lumping all people together who are overweight.

We all are sometimes dishonest with ourselves. However, most people are recognizing and admitting that their obesity is secondary to eating more food than needed and exercising less than is necessary to remain healthy and have the desired body weight.

The common person is able to understand the language and interpret the figures in this chapter. I hope the writing in this chapter will not only entertain you but also give you wisdom. Let the data refresh the minds of the readers and cause them to reflect on the facts with pleasure. Lean and obese men and women are encouraged to review this monograph to seek the pleasure that comes from gaining knowledge.

Hopefully, these writings are simple in design and devoid of superfluous complexities and claims. They are to the point, and the assertions are published in top tier medical journals. The tale of obesity is not a mystery. It is straight forward and based on factual data gathered from patients through clinical investigations. On the other hand, there is a mystery: what to do once you have become fat and your body weight has stabilized. In a practical sense, you may be beyond the point of no return! For some people, it may take radical intervention to permanently reduce the body fat content.

All obese people can recount their misfortune of having too much fat. However, there is no reason to disparage yourself for being overweight because you may do something about it.

Those with the genetic predisposition for obesity and who live in a society where food is plentiful and lack the judgment, or the desire, or the control to handle the internal signals to consume more calories than are optimal for their best body composition, so be it. Food is pleasant to the sight, smell and taste. On the other hand, if normal people do not want to become overweight, they must restrict their caloric consumption. There should be no doubt that obesity among humans has a genetic basis. Selective breeding among animals for meat and fat production is clearly established. We all see family likeness for body type. Everyone recognizes that skin color, height, foot size, etc. are largely determined by genes. Obese mothers and obese fathers have obese children. Of course there is a genetic predisposition for obesity. In addition, normal weight people have innate capacities to store excessive fat in adipose tissue and develop various degrees of obesity or fatness. Otherwise, how could 64% of USA adults and 13% of children and adolescents be overweight and/or obese? It has become obvious that obesity is natural in an environment with more foods, especially cheap carbohydrates, than are needed to provide the body with energy requirements. Nonetheless, overeating, even gluttony, must be recognized as the major contributor to obesity. The human body is designed to take in and store nutrients when food is in overabundance. The genetic makeup of humans lacks physical comprehensive gauges of excessive eating. This has become the job of the mental consciousness: to recognize that any normal person who eats more food than needed to meet his/her metabolic requirements will become fat. This maxim has only come before us during the last century. Environmental influences have been more important for the development of obesity than are genetic influences.

Dorland's medical dictionary defines addiction as "the state of being given up to some habit, especially strong dependence on a drug etc.; a detrimental effect on the individual and on society." The question I pose: "Are people addicted to food?" It is clear that the success rate of treating obesity is comparable to the success rate of treating narcotic addiction. Nonetheless, people do "kick the habit."

If a narcotic addict is locked up in a jail room and left there without any medical support, about one-half of the victims will die during the withdrawal period. In contrast, if morbidly obese patients continue to consume excessive quantities of food, about one-half of the patients will die prematurely. Both narcotic and food addiction kill patients.

Brain functional studies done long after my time as a clinical investigator have shown some interesting results. Mark S. Gold, M.D. of the University of Florida claims that altered brain activity associated with obesity can be measured with radiologic techniques. *Functional* magnetic resonance imaging and positron emission tomography support the hypothesis that "there are important similarities between overeating highly palatable and hedonic foods and the classic addictions." Researchers have shown that overfed animals limit their self-administration of drugs, and starved animals increase their self-administration of drugs. Gene-Jack Wang, M.D. and coworkers of the Brookhaven National Laboratory have reported that the brain circuits of fat people have few dopamine receptors, the neurotransmitters associated with pleasure and satisfaction. This finding is similar to that found among drug addicts. Researchers have also found that the brain areas associated with the mouth and eating are larger in obese people than normal weight people.

Sitting at a table and watching most grossly obese people freely eat, it becomes evident that they consume a lot of food. Neuroimaging studies showed that the sensory perception regions in the brain are more intense for the mouth, lips and tongue in obese humans.

Prior to specific neuroimaging techniques it was difficult to pinpoint brain activity. Now with new techniques to focus on areas of the brain known to relate to various areas of the body and behavioral activities, it has become evident that brain function is altered by obesity. Specifically, positron emission tomography reveals that the sight of food causes increase in whole-brain activity as well as volunteers expressing greater desire for food and hunger compared to other types of mental stimulation.

On the other hand, a lack of self-discipline regarding the ingestion of high caloric foods plays a role in the development of obesity. Hunger may be a natural phenomenon. Eating to relieve the discomfort from hunger may be expected. However, looking into the mirror or standing on weight scales can subvert appetite and food consumption in some, but not all, people.

There is ample evidence that genetics (and epigenetic factors induced during pregnancy) and environment (presence of high caloric foods in overabundance) have strong roles for inducing obesity. However, self-discipline, or the lack thereof, has a role that cannot be denied. The attitude of those who remain lean by eating good nutritious meals without excessive calories and participating in physical activity can do more to control the obesity epidemic than changes in health procedures and medications.

Obesity is a worldwide problem, and its accompanying diseases of diabetes and heart diseases will bankrupt the healthcare systems.

Exercise helps the body expend stored fat, but the primary method of avoiding obesity is to eat less food. As a physician, I always hate it when I make a dogmatic statement like this because I realize some psychologically imbalanced person is likely to develop anorexia. However, no statement can be made that is foolproof. Some people need a shepherd to oversee their health and welfare. Let's hope there will always be enough guardians to protect mankind.

Throughout my first 12 years of schooling, 1941-1953, very few classmates were overweight and none were grossly obese. Food was not plentiful through World War II, and many of those who prepared the meals in Roswell, New Mexico, were not particularly gifted chefs. Most of the food types were rationed, especially butter and meats. However, malnutrition from food rationing was unknown.

Since the end of food rationing after World War II, alarm bells have been ringing. For the last five decades citizens in the USA are getting to be more and more obese.

Among the physiologic states that are known to influence energy expenditure is that associated with eating food. Chewing, digesting, absorbing and storing or oxidizing (burning) nutrients are associated with increasing the energy requirements to accomplish these tasks. Eating proteins causes a greater expenditure of energy than eating fats or carbohydrates. However, there are no differences in the cost of energy for these tasks between lean and obese people if the food challenge per weight of lean body mass is equal. When lean and obese people eat meals with the caloric contents that are multiples of their lean body mass (fat-free mass), the rise in energy expenditure is indistinguishable. Fat people do not have a more efficient system of metabolism than lean people. Fat people do not oxidize a smaller content of the food they ingest and store more of the nutrients in adipose tissue. There are variations in metabolic efficiency, e.g., the amount of food oxidized or stored; however, this efficiency is independent of leanness or obesity (body size or composition). The more a person eats the more nutrients are oxidized (burned) and the more nutrients are stored, primarily as fat. However, one of the most remarkable findings from studying a range of lean to obese volunteers is the individuality of peoples' responses to metabolize ingested food. A human being has the functional equivalent of a "metabolic fingerprint." An individual with a low metabolic rate for body size has a low thermic (energy) response to food ingestion; in contrast, a person with a high metabolic rate for body size has a high thermic response to food ingestion. Individuals are unique; that is why they are individuals. Their uniqueness is independent of leanness or obesity just like fingerprints are independent of body composition.

Hunger sensation between meals is not pain. Hunger is normal. People of past generations recognized and tolerated hunger. It is a symptom that the stomach can take in more food. Hunger can be, but is not likely to be, a signal that impending nutritional deficiency is present. In contrast, eating induces a mild euphoria.

One reason people want to know their metabolic requirement is because of the obesity epidemic; many people recognize that they need to lose weight. Therefore, they want to know not only the energy requirements of their bodies but also the energy value of tissue associated with weight gain or weight loss.

When I was studying starving obese volunteers and training under the direction of Dr. George F. Cahill, Jr. at Harvard, the questions arose regarding the caloric value of adipose (fat) tissue. We made arrangements with Dr. Francis Moore, Professor and Chair, Surgery, at the Peter Bent Brigham to provide us with small fragments of abdominal fat tissue obtained at the time of abdominal operations. This was approved, and we analyzed the adipose tissue for caloric content. Dr. Cahill participated in a live radio talk show in Boston. He said the caloric value of adipose tissue was about 3500 Kcal/pound (7700 Kcal/kg). This value spread across the nation faster than any of our carefully defined scientific facts did. It was, however, not an accurate caloric value for a pound (or kg) of gained or lost body weight.

Changes in total body fat mass are accompanied by changes in total body lean mass. Thus, changes in gains or losses of obesity tissue are different from isolated adipose tissue. During weight gain, more lean body mass (muscle, blood, extracellular fluid, connective tissue and skin) is needed to support and maintain the accumulated adipose tissue. Obesity tissue is about 14 percent fluid, 62 percent fat (triglycerides) and 24 percent active protoplasmic tissue. This latter mass is mostly water: 80 percent water which contains primarily proteins suspended in a salt solution. Thus, the energy equivalent of obesity tissue is not equal to that of fat under the skin. Instead, obesity tissue is only about 2600 Kcal/pound (5720 Kcal/kg). The lower caloric equivalent of a pound (or kg) of weight gain or weight loss tissue is surprisingly balanced by the fact that recent evidence shows that the classic prediction equations (Harris-Benedict and others) overestimate the resting energy requirements of young men and women: thus, overestimation of caloric value of tissue is offset by overestimate of caloric requirements. The purpose of research (look again) is to "get it right."

Before the reader gets engaged in learning or predicting his/her energy requirement, please recognize that there is wide variation in the energy requirement of humans who are similar in age, sex and body weight. If someone wants to pretend that he/she is a special case with a low caloric requirement and cannot lose weight, there is certainly the opportunity to make such an argument even if it is usually false. This situation is rare and does not account for the huge number of fat people in America.

There is some lack of knowledge among people of normal intelligence regarding the cause of obesity. The U.S. population needs to know more about energy requirements and, thus, obesity. Humans must have the intellectual machinery to deal with obesity. Knowledge can be a powerful tool. It can bring obesity out of the shadow of ignorance. It is possible that ignorance about the imbalance between caloric intake and caloric expenditure may be contributing to the incidence of obesity in the USA. It is more likely that natural gluttony and low physical activity compound the development of obesity. Let's face it. Eating and drinking are enjoyable. Humans desire that their appetites be satisfied.

These comments should not be misconstrued that I do not recognize the importance of genetics in influencing obesity. Instead, I simply do not believe that someone can become overweight without eating more food than he/she needs to maintain healthy body weight. Numerous patients have come to me stating they could not lose weight on the low caloric diet prescribed for them. Few individuals recognize that people can eat in a minute about 150 times their resting minute energy requirements. The caloric content in food eaten on Saturday and Sunday may be enough to meet their caloric requirements for a week. On the other hand, walking 3 miles per hour up a 5% grade only increases the caloric expenditure about 5-7 times over the resting energy requirements. This is a moderate amount of physical exertion. The following writings will present data to confirm these claims.

Knowledge regarding energy requirements of human beings has accumulated mostly over the last century. Daily or seasonal food consumption by an individual varies widely, but the utilization of energy by a specific body is more constant. Therefore, the Expert Consultation (FAO/WHO/UNU, 1985) recommended that if estimates of energy requirements are needed it is easier to measure energy expenditure than energy intake from food eaten.

My colleagues and I gathered and interpreted information regarding the energy (caloric) requirements of men and women. We studied in detail the energy requirements of well over 1000 individuals, including normal volunteers, obese, athletic, dwarf, and diabetic people and patients with alcoholic liver cirrhosis. In addition, we determined the body composition of many of these lean and obese volunteers.

Let's review energy expenditure. The resting energy requirements of lean and obese humans are displayed first. The energy consumed and stored after eating a large meal is described second. The energy consumed during exercise and its relationship to food intake is presented third. The lowest rate of energy requirement is described last. It occurs during deep sleep. The impact of sleeping is only briefly described because of limited information and because of its probably obvious influence (Figure 1).

Among healthy adult human beings, energy requirements are *primarily* dependent upon body size and physical activity, with energy requirements increasing as body weight and physical activity increase. Strenuous exercise impacts metabolic requirements more than all other factors combined. *Secondary* variables affecting energy requirements are gender and inheritance. In general, men have greater metabolic energy requirements than non-

252

pregnant non-lactating women, even if their body weights are similar. However, this gender difference is mostly

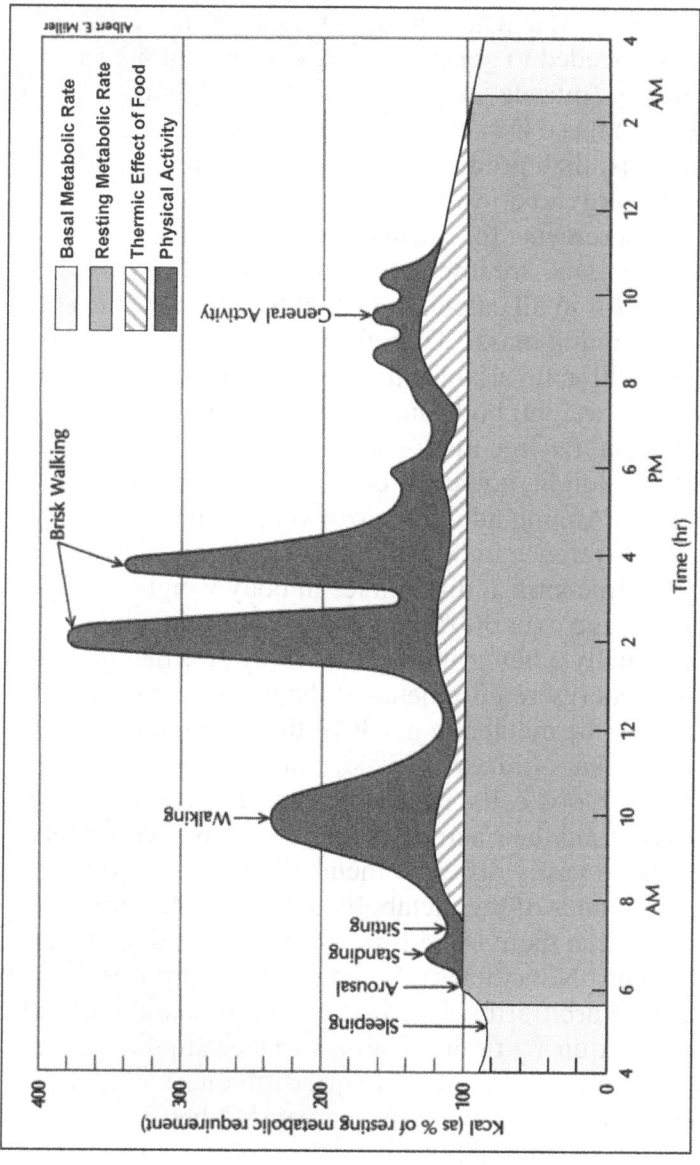

Figure 1. The metabolic rates for various activity states are schematized here. The basal metabolic rate (BMR) occurs in the early morning hours during deep sleep. After arousal, with the individual still in the supine position, resting and fasting, metabolism increases to the resting metabolic rate (RMR). The thermic effect of food (TEF) occurs postprandially, and the thermic effect of exercise, or exercise-induced thermogenesis, occurs with any kind of physical activity and is the most variable state of energy expenditure.

eliminated when energy requirements are calculated on the basis of lean body tissue (fat-free mass). Rates of energy expenditure also show strong familial aggregations. *Tertiary*

253

influences are age and environment, with a trivial, inverse relationship between age and resting metabolic rate and between environmental temperature and metabolic rates.

Active protoplasmic tissue of the body has the components needed to generate energy for useful purposes. Either directly (muscle, etc.) or indirectly (red blood cells via the liver, etc.) these tissue components require oxygen and consume fuels; they produce carbon dioxide and provide sources of energy to do work, e.g. move the body.

Measurements for estimating the size of active protoplasmic tissue are imprecise, and body weight is the dominant factor in all calculations that predict estimates of oxygen consuming mass. Therefore, it is not surprising that body compositional variables that reflect active protoplasmic tissue such as weight, body surface area, lean body mass, body cell mass, fat-free mass and fat mass are all highly interrelated. Height, however, only grossly reflects body composition. Among adult men or women with normal stature, the difference in body height usually only varies about 20%. In contrast, differences in body weight commonly range over 300% or greater. Thus, in adults, weight is usually a better indicator of body size than height.

The energy requirements of the body are determined by the sum of the metabolic needs of the individual tissues (brain, liver, heart, kidney, muscle, skin, adipose tissue, spleen, white blood cells, etc.) which are dependent upon the organ masses and their activity states. The body components or organs have vastly different metabolic rates per unit weight. Estimates of the metabolic requirements per unit weight show that there is a 50- to 100-fold variation at rest among tissues. Nonetheless, for conceptual purposes, human organs can be arbitrarily classified into high, moderate, and low energy-requiring tissue. Large variances in the weights of adults occur, not because of major differences in high energy-requiring brain and liver masses, but because of large differences in the amount of moderate energy-requiring skeletal muscle mass (primarily in men and athletes) and/or huge differences in the amount of low energy-requiring adipose tissue mass.

Energy requirements and heat generation (thermogenesis) are directly related. Whole body energy requirements are measured directly by determining the amount of heat generated by the body in a calorimeter (direct calorimetry) and indirectly by measuring the respiratory exchange rates of oxygen (O_2) and carbon dioxide (CO_2) and urinary excretion rates of nitrogen (indirect calorimetry). The relationship between direct calorimetry and indirect calorimetry for measuring heat production by the human body is near perfect. Respiratory exchange rates of O_2 and CO_2 can be rapidly and accurately measured using automated O_2 and CO_2 analyzers connected to computers. The determination of urinary nitrogen excretion, which is used to measure protein metabolism, is time consuming and introduces an unwarranted time-lag and financial expense in obtaining measurement of energy requirements. However, it is generally recognized that in most cases reasonably accurate measurements of energy requirements can be obtained without measuring urinary nitrogen excretion rates.

Underwater weighing techniques (hydrodensitometry based on the Archimedes principle) are probably the best way to divide the body into two distinct components, fat mass and fat-free mass (lean body weight). Measured or predicted resting metabolic rate is frequently related to the size of the fat-free or lean body mass. There are currently numerous other methods to assess in vivo human body composition. A useful but crude way to estimate fat-free mass or lean body mass can be calculated from urinary excretion of creatinine. Muscle comprises about one-half of the lean body mass of average weight men and women. Creatinine is released from muscle and excreted in the urine. The 24 hour urinary excretion rate of creatinine is related to the muscle mass and thus to lean body mass. Since lean body mass (grossly equated to fat-free mass) is the major active protoplasmic component of the body, lean body mass is closely related to the resting metabolic rate. However, in patients with severe body wasting (cachexia), muscle mass may be depleted to a greater degree than other organs, and urinary creatinine excretion falls to a disproportionately low

255

rate. The resting energy requirements of skeletal muscle are less per unit weight than those of the brain, liver, heart and kidney. Expressing total body energy requirements per gram creatinine excretion for malnourished patients may produce distortedly high values. For an individual person, estimates of fat-free mass or lean body mass from skinfold thickness measurements are relatively imprecise, and body mass indices (frequently used) are practically worthless except at the extremes. The data show that the frequently used body mass indices based on weights and heights do not accurately diagnose leanness or obesity. Figure 2 shows the body mass index contrasted against percent body fat of 213 women and

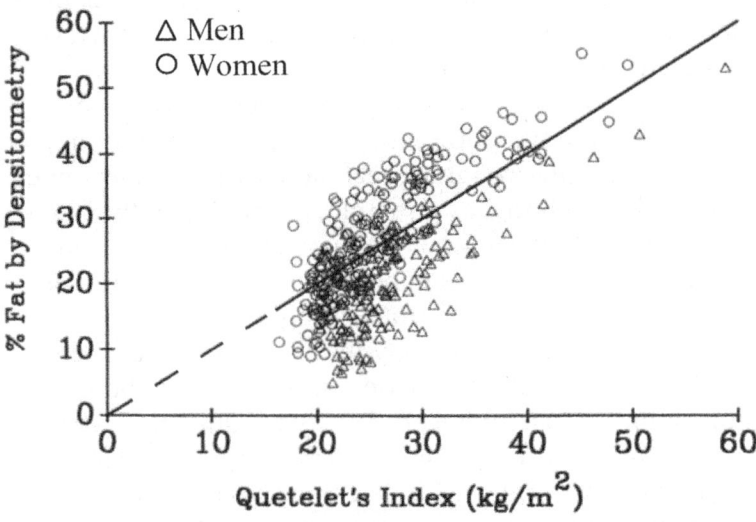

Figure 2. Percent body fat vs. Quetelet's Index. (Body mass index: BMI). Reproduced with permission from *Am. J. Clin. Nutr.*, 1990, 52:405-8.

150 men. This figure shows how poorly an individual's body mass index of Quetelet related to percent body fat.

When the French explorers were sailing around the world in search of food in the 1850's, it was recognized that when food was available in overabundance the population at these sites became overweight. In 1869, L.A.J. Quetelet developed a mathematical index that could be used to estimate the prevalence of obesity among various tribes or populations. It was simple: wt kg/ht m^2. The index maximized the impact of weight and minimized the influences of height. It was useful for population studies. Since 1869, several more indices have been developed. These indices, referred to as body mass indices, are of very limited value for a given person. It appears that researchers who refer to a number obtained from calculating the body mass index have never evaluated the merit of using indices. Except for population studies, they are nearly worthless. In fact, professional basketball players have high body mass indices. Body mass indices usually produce numbers that are no better than the naked eye in assessing obesity.

Are you fat? Look in the mirror. You decide.

Various normal physiologic states are associated with different metabolic rates (Figure 1). These metabolic states are defined slightly differently by various groups. By some groups, the basal metabolic rate is the energy expended in the basal state after a night's sleep, in the fasting state, with the subject in bed, under thermoneutral atmospheric conditions. The resting metabolic rate is the energy expended in a resting individual, at different times of the day, before or long after a meal. The resting metabolic rate may be higher than the basal metabolic rate. The resting metabolic rate is the most frequently measured metabolic state, and the resting metabolic rate is the reference metabolic rate to which other states are compared. We have strictly defined this state. The resting metabolic rate we refer to is measured in the wakened state after an overnight fast while lying supine by standardized techniques. Respiratory uptake of atmospheric oxygen and release of carbon dioxide is measured by a gas analyzing machine coupled to a computer. Urinary nitrogen excretion may also be measured during the period of determining the exchange rate of respiratory gases. The reproducibility should vary less than 5 percent for 95 percent of the measurements. Resting metabolic rate is the best predictor of overall requirements and usually relates to about 65-70 percent of the daily energy requirements of most ambulatory adults; it may also be used to reflect most of the energy requirements of bedridden patients, providing body temperature is relatively constant. Thus, the resting metabolic rate has relevance to both ambulatory and confined human beings. An overactive thyroid gland increases the resting metabolic rate and is usually associated with weight loss as well as other symptoms. Severe insulin deficiency of diabetes mellitus is associated with a normal resting metabolic rate but weight loss caused by the excretion of glucose in the urine. Glycosuria (urinary sugar loss) drains calories from the body in the form of glucose. The lowest metabolic rate occurs during deep sleep. The sleeping metabolic rate amounts to about 85 percent of the resting metabolic rate. Large meals before going to bed have a minor impact on overnight metabolic requirements, and the sleeping metabolic rate is not significantly affected by different levels of exercise on the preceding day. Eating food usually heightens the resting metabolic rate about 10 percent. (This usually amounts to about 8 percent of the caloric content of a large mixed meal.) Gorging may increase the resting metabolic rate by 30 percent. This augmented metabolic rate association with oral food or to nutrient given intravenously is referred to as the thermic effects of food. It varies with the quantity and nature (protein, carbohydrate and/or fat) of the food (macronutrient) eaten. The thermic effects of food are the greatest with protein meals. The intermittent physical activity or mild exercise usually increases the overall metabolic expenditure by about 30 percent in most sedentary individuals. However, heavy day labor can increase caloric requirements by 3-fold over daily resting metabolic requirements. Exercise thermogenesis over brief periods of time can augment resting metabolic rate 20-fold. No other states compare in capacity to expend metabolic fuels. On the other hand, as noted above, human beings can readily ingest foods at a rate of 75-150 times greater than their resting metabolic rate. These multiples of the resting metabolic rate can be likened to a motor vehicle that burns (oxidizes) gasoline. The gas tank can be filled in minutes, but it usually takes hours to consume the fuel. It should be obvious that reduction in nutrient intake is the most efficient mechanism to reduce body weight.

When food intake is below the requirements recommended for prolonged survival by the FAO/WHO/UNU Consultants, Beninese women of West Africa, from whom generalizations can probably be accurately made, spend less time working and more time resting, sitting and sleeping. Thus, when food intake becomes inadequate, physical activities are decreased. This appears to be a natural behavioral adaptation to malnutrition. Semi-starvation and total starvation states among obese volunteers confined to hospital environments during research studies are usually accompanied by definitive behavioral changes characterized by curtailing high energy-consuming activities. Changes in the resting metabolic rate occur during periods of total starvation. However, the decreased resting metabolic is less than generally touted. In fact, we found no reduction in resting metabolic rate per kg body weight in morbidly obese people subjected to prolonged and total starvation.

Among the women we studied were 8 world-class athletes. They competed in ice skating, field hockey, swimming and body building. Their body weights and energy requirements were remarkably constant, and the range in kcal/kg (kcal/lbs) body weight was unusually narrow. In essence, women world-class athletes were relatively homogeneous in body size and energy requirements.

Doctors use the aforementioned general rules for estimating the energy requirements and guessing at body composition. However, there are many exceptions to the general rules employed by physicians. The following three cases demonstrate the unexpected.

Early in my career as a physician treating obese patients, I ascribed to the concept that humans had three different body types. Ectomorphic people were thin with long, tubular bones (i.e. fingers). They never became obese.

Mesomorphic humans were the muscular athletes. They tended to maintain their body weight. Endomorphic people tended to become obese. Their body frames were relatively large; their fingers were short and stubby, and their bodies had excessive quantities of fat. Figure 3 shows the hands of an ectomorphic woman (27 years old) and an endomorphic woman (42 years old). The endomorphic woman developed diabetes mellitus and died at 70 years of age. The ectomorphic woman came to the funeral. She was so fat that I did not recognize her. The point of this clinical vignette is that even an ectomorphic person can gain enough weight to become obese.

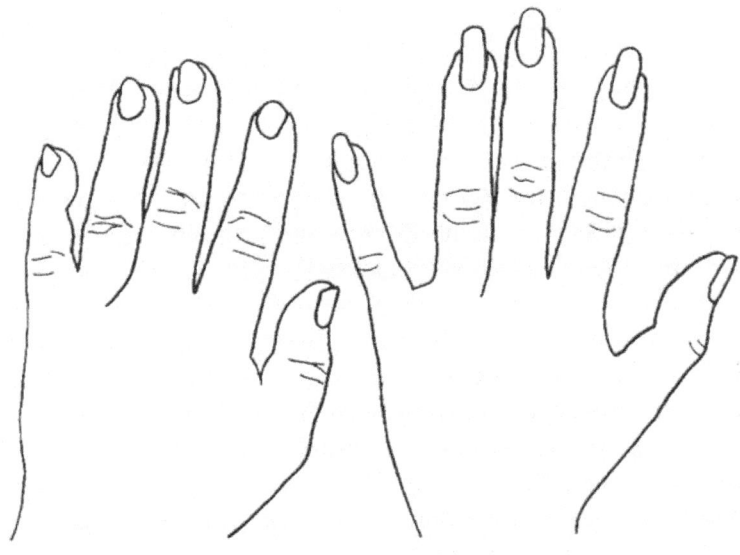

Figure 3. The drawing of the hand on the left was taken from a picture of an endomorphic (obese) female. The hand on the right is that of an ectomorphic (lean) female.

Another point I want to make before I proceed with generalization is centered on two men who are identical twins. As young men, they worked as lifeguards on the beaches of the Atlantic Ocean. They would often date the same women and would claim that the women could not or did not distinguish them. With the progression of time, one became a lawyer and sat at a desk much of the time. He dropped physical activity programs and was married to an excellent gourmet cook. His weight increased over the years I served as his physician. The twins agreed to have their pictures taken and used to demonstrate the impact of food and lack of exercise on body structure (Figure 4). The

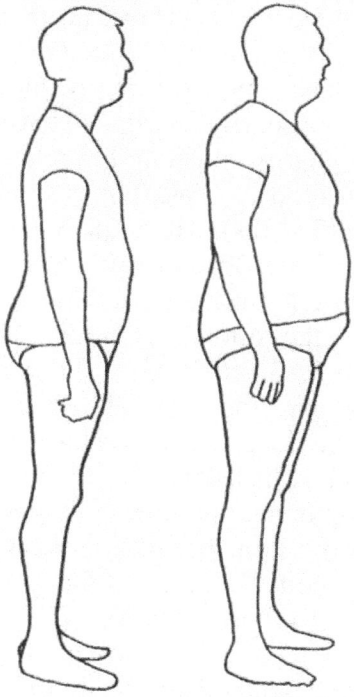

Figure 4. Identical twins confirmed by genetic analysis. The twin on the right side of the figure consumed food based on taste and gratification and initially was not guided by an attempt to restrict his body weight.

lawyer brother is about 70 pounds heavier than his twin. Genetics has an influence on the development of obesity but so do diet and exercise.

Among the three basic kinds of nutrients (carbohydrates, fats and proteins), carbohydrates (sugars and starches) taste the best to most people, and they are very cheap. The cost of a pound of refined sugar is about 35-53 cents per pound. The cost of chicken and filet mignon ranges from about 2-20 dollars per pound. Thus, the cost ratio of sugar to meat varies up to about 1:60 per pound.

After eating large quantities of bread, cakes, potatoes, corn, peas, spaghettis and syrups, they are readily absorbed from the gut. An acute and multifold rise in blood insulin occurs. This hormone is the cardinal hormone that promotes the nutrient extraction from the blood. Glucose, amino acids (proteins) and fats are removed from the blood and converted into fat and stored, primarily in adipose tissues. When we were studying the energy consumption related to eating (thermic effects of food), a typical obese male volunteer weighed 170.1 kg (374 lbs). He drank 3104 kcal of Ensure Plus (53% carbohydrate, 32% fat and 15% protein) in 10 minutes. This nutrient mixture raised his metabolic rate about 8 percent for the following 6 hours. His resting metabolic rate was 1.83 kcal/minute. Food intake increased his resting rate to an average of 1.98 kcal/minute (8%) over the next 6-hour period. Thus, during the 10 minutes he ingested the nutrients, he used a total of about 20 kcal for maintaining resting metabolic rate and ingesting, absorbing, oxidizing and storing some of the 3104 kcal he consumed. Thus, the ratio of energy in ingested food to energy expended was about 150:1. However, this estimate of intake-vs-time dependent energy utilization overlooks the fact that heightened metabolism secondary to food lasted about 6 hours. Nonetheless, the rate of caloric ingestion greatly exceeds the rate of caloric utilization. He consumed more calories in 10 minutes than he emitted the ensuing 24 hours while remaining in the hospital. Further, he ate additional calories at lunch and dinner while in the hospital research center.

In another study, we investigated the energy utilized (thermic effects) during exercise. Another representative obese male volunteer who was about the same size as the individual who underwent studies on the thermic effects of food underwent studies on the thermic effects of exercise. He was an obese male volunteer who weighed 163 kg (360 lbs). His resting metabolic rate was 2.10 kcal/minute which was high normal for his body size and greater than that of smaller volunteers. He walked on a treadmill up a 5% incline at 3 miles per hour for 10 minutes. His exercise metabolic rate increased to about 13 kcal/minute. This approximate 6-fold increase in energy expenditure was enough to make him sweat and increase his breathing rate. During the 10-minute exercise period this huge man consumed about 130 kcal. Thus, his increased expenditure during exercise was only $1/25^{th}$ as much as his energy intake can be from gorging. Admittedly, a person can only eat at the rate of about 150 times the resting metabolic rate for only a few minutes whereas an individual with good physical conditioning can exercise at a rate of 6 times their resting metabolic rate for an hour or two. Nonetheless, the point to be made from easily reproducible, experimental data is that per unit time caloric ingestion can greatly exceed caloric expenditure. Therefore, weight reduction can be more readily accomplished by cutting caloric intake rather than increasing caloric expenditure.

Numerous equations have been derived for predicting resting metabolic rate from the body composition and other measures using weight, height, fat-free mass, fat mass, age and gender as variables. The Harris-Benedict, published in 1919, is the most popular prediction equation for energy requirements. These investigators used indirect calorimetry to measure the energy consumption of factory workers who walked off the street, rested, and underwent measurements to determine the resting metabolic rate of young women and men. More recently, we showed that individuals who rested overnight in the hospital before the resting metabolic rates were measured have lower metabolic rates than those calculated from the Harris-Benedict prediction equations. Nonetheless, our newer predicted values of resting metabolic rate show no clear evidence our equations are any better than those of other investigators. The correlations among the predicted and measured resting metabolic rate from the different equations are reasonable for estimating one's caloric requirements. The resting metabolic rates calculated from prediction equations that use fat-free mass (lean body weight) correlated better with the measured resting metabolic rates than the resting metabolic rates obtained from prediction equations that use weight as the predictor. The lower correlations with the resting metabolic rate predicted only from weight may reflect the misleading contributions of adipose tissue to weight due to the low energy requirements of adipose tissue. Nevertheless, under most circumstances, weight is the most easily and accurately measured variable for estimating resting metabolic rate for both men and women. In most clinical situations, weight is appropriate to use if estimates of the metabolic rate are needed.

One of many problems readers face in trying to evaluate statements or recommendations made by some "experts" is that the authors may not provide verifiable data to support the claims. On the other hand, my colleagues and I have collected the data, and I am trying to supply the reader with results that have been verified by other clinical investigators. I emphasize the wide variation in energy requirements of people and state that the wide variations are also independent of leanness or obesity.

The purpose of Figures 5 and 6 is to caution intelligent people about accepting quantitative data from a small group of individuals as factual information readily applicable to a given patient or population of patients without careful review of data.

Figure 5 shows the wide variance in the resting metabolic rates and body sizes of 135 men and women, composed of Caucasians, Blacks, and Asians. This group of volunteers without thyroid, liver or kidney diseases and free of diabetes also included 32 dwarfs. They had broad socioeconomic, educational and employment backgrounds. They ranged in weight from 32 kg (70 lbs.) to 171 kg (376 lbs.), and are representative of the adult population of large metropolitan areas in North America. These divergent human beings provide unique data from one species whose resting metabolic rates were measured in the hospital under standardized conditions. The variance in energy requirements among individuals of identical body size is demonstrated by the results obtained from "healthy" lean and

RESTING METABOLIC RATES OF HUMANS

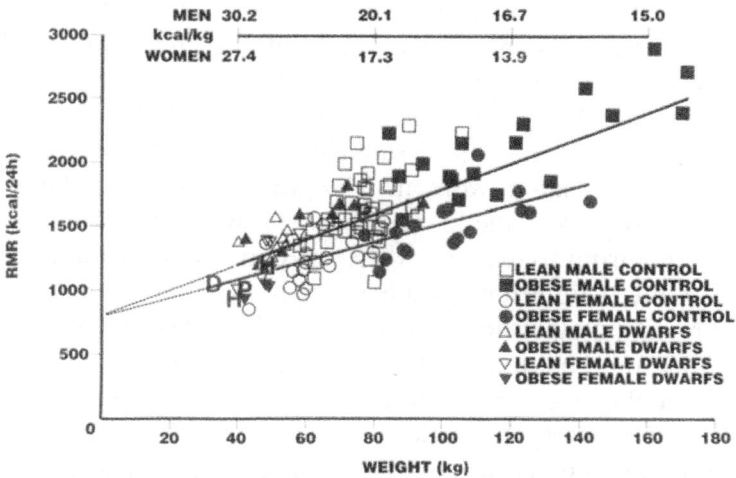

Figure 5. The resting metabolic requirements (RMR) expressed as kcal/24 h were related to body weight in kg. The regression lines for women (bottom) and men (top) include dwarfs and average-stature lean and obese humans. The caloric requirements/kg body weight are shown at the top of the figure. 1 kg = 2.2 lbs.

obese men and women combined with the results of dwarfs (Little People of America) which allows an examination of the relationship between resting metabolic rate measured after an overnight 10-12 hour fast and body size determined by weight. The results reveal some general principles of energy requirements (bioenergetics) for adult human beings with body weights (sizes) varying over a 5-fold range. The resting metabolic requirements increase as the weights (or body sizes) increase. However, the energy requirement per unit weight decreases as body weight increases. For example, as the weights of men increase from 40 kg (88 lbs.) to 160 kg (352 lbs.), the average resting metabolic rate increases from about 1300 kg/day to about 2500 kcal/day. However, the resting metabolic rate per kg body weight decreases from 30 to 15 kcal/kg/24 hour. Thus, a 4-fold increase in body weight is accompanied by a doubling of the resting metabolic rate but a 50% reduction in kcal/kg or lbs.

265

Comparable changes also occur in women. This general principle is illustrated to all of us by considering the amount of food a small person usually eats compared to a large person. A person with a body weight of 182 kg (400 lbs) usually eats only twice as much as a person whose body weight is only 45 kg (100 lbs). Note in Figure 5 that the increase in resting metabolic rate for a given body weight is greater in men than in women. The greater percentage body weight in women is due to more body fat which is a low energy requiring tissue. The difference in resting metabolic rate per unit weight for women and men is largely removed when resting metabolic rate is contrasted against fat-free mass measured by underwater weight techniques to determine the size of the lean body mass. Although men and women have nearly the same energy requirements per fat-free mass (lean body mass), the broad variance in energy requirements of the "healthy" adults remains. This finding is also independent of leanness or obesity. The caloric requirements of human beings of identical gender, age and body composition also vary over a two-fold range because human beings vary in metabolic efficiency. Data to support this claim has been published in the best peer reviewed medical journals and medical book chapters.

Figure 6 shows the resting metabolic rate extrapolated to 24 hours and contrasted against the fat-free mass (kg) or lean body mass of 771 men and women. The general principle of the greater the body weight the greater the resting metabolic rate holds true for fat-free mass (lean body mass). It should also be evident (each dot represents a person) that the enormous variation in resting metabolic rate is independent of leanness and obesity even when the amount of fat tissue is functionally excluded by body compositional determinations. Some people with fat-free masses of 50-60 kg have unusually high resting energy requirements that are equal to obese individuals with fat-free masses of 100-120 kg. (The opposite is also true.) The point to be made and repeated is that there are wide variations in energy requirements among "healthy" adult people. Superimposed on the resting energy requirements are

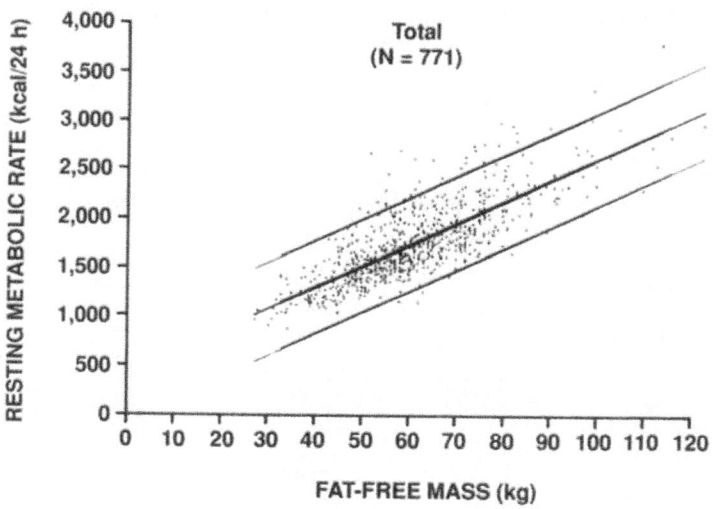

Figure 6. Resting metabolic rate (RMR) of men and women plotted against their fat-free mass determined by densitometry.

calories spent doing physical activity, creating even greater metabolic requirements among human beings. However, the author cautions the reading audience not to overlook the fact that the results shown in Figure 6 contrast the resting metabolic rate against the fat-free (lean body) mass which is less than total body mass. The fat-free mass may be only 50% of the total body mass (weight) in morbidly obese individuals. Thus, the slope of the regression line for weight is not as steep as the regression line for fat-free mass. Thus, the energy requirement per kg (or pound) of body weight is less as fat mass increases.

The primary purpose of Figure 5 is to show the general principle that energy requirements increase as body size increases, but decrease per unit of body weight. The primary purpose of Figure 6 is to show that the wide variation in energy requirements persist from small to huge adults even when the influence of the body fat has been practically eliminated.

Figure 7 displays the impact of wide variance in body weight and resting energy requirements. This situation is

267

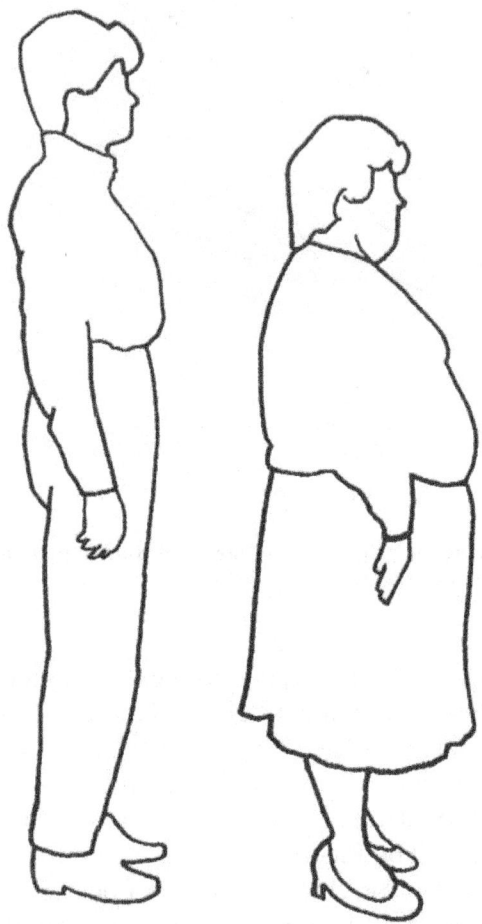

Figure 7. Outline of two women whose age in years was identical
and the resting metabolic rates were indistinguishable.
Nonetheless, the woman on the right side of the figure weighed 100
pounds more than the lean individual on the left side of the figure.

atypical but not infrequently encountered in the practice of
medicine. These two women have practically identical
resting metabolic rates, but the shorter woman weighs almost
twice as much as the tall, lean woman. This is most
unfortunate for the obese woman, but it reflects the wide
variation in energy requirements among people.

A common mistake is to express energy requirements of human beings as energy units per body weight (e.g. kcal/kg). This has the potential to give a false impression if different body sizes exist between the groups; the groups with a smaller body weight or fat-free mass will be shown as having a greater caloric requirement per kcal/kg compared to the group with a larger body weight or fat-free mass. This lack of understanding of energy requirements has led some "experts" to write/say that fat individuals have a low resting energy requirement. They don't. They have a greater energy requirement, but less per kilogram (pound) body weight.

Although there are limitations in estimating energy requirements, equations for predicting the resting metabolic rate based on gender and weight are available. Simple and practical equations for predicting the resting metabolic rate of men and women were developed which are useful in most clinical situations when metabolic requirements are not directly determined. The following equations have been "forced" into easily remembered numbers so they may be more useful.

Men resting metabolic rate = 900 + 10 (kg body weight) Kcal/24 hours[19]

Women resting metabolic rate = 800 + 7 (kg body weight) Kcal/24 hours

When using these forced prediction equations, qualifying knowledge should be kept in mind.

Ferraro *et al* recently measured 24-hour energy expenditures in 235 Caucasian men and women living in a large respiratory chamber. The 24-hour expenditure was 5-10% higher in men than women after adjusting for differences in fat-free mass and physical activity. Thus, this lower metabolic rate for women was not secondary to less physical activity. However, menstrual function, specifically the first half (luteal phase) of the menstrual cycle, was accompanied by a higher metabolic rate than the second half (follicular phase) of the cycle. Therefore, both gender and menstrual cycle have a small impact on the metabolic rate.

---

[19] One kilogram (kg) equals 2.2 pounds

This gender difference may predispose women to relative gains in adipose tissue mass.

Other studies from the metabolic ward of the National Institutes of Health, Diabetes and Nutrition Section in Phoenix, Arizona, claim that a low resting metabolic rate and a high respiratory quotient, reflecting carbohydrate oxidation are associated with weight gain over several years. Guenther Boden, M.D. and coworkers have supplemented the finding of David D'Alessio, M.D. and coworkers showing that the high-protein, high-fat, and low-carbohydrate diet of Atkins *et al* is a diet low in total calories. It is the low caloric intake of the Atkins diet that is responsible for weight reduction while consuming the low-carbohydrate diet. The foregoing is consistent with the claims of Robert C. Atkins, M.D. that a low-carbohydrate diet promotes weight reduction.

Vaughan, Zurlo, and Ravussin also studied aging and energy requirements. With aging there is a progressive loss of muscle and a concurrent increase in adipose tissue. From the second to the seventh decade, resting metabolic rate decreases 1-2% per decade. However, total daily energy requirements measured in a free living respiratory chamber reveals no difference between young and elderly individuals when the energy requirements are corrected for gender and fat-free mass. Thus, the decline in energy requirements was primarily attributed to a curtailment in physical activity as adults age.

Many patients claim they cannot lose weight on a prescribed low caloric diet. I have never encountered a healthy person confined to the hospital under continuous observation who did not lose weight on a diet that contained fewer calories than his/her measured resting metabolic rate. The grand scheme that healthy people lose weight if they eat fewer calories than they need to maintain their metabolic requirements holds true. In contrast, if healthy people eat more calories than they require, they gain weight, primarily fat.

A straight-forward summation of the foregoing information can be provided. Adult humans, other than world-class athletes, have a large range of energy requirements and body compositions. Nevertheless, if you are healthy and gaining weight, you are taking in more food than you need. You are eating too much or expending too little energy. Thus, if you want to lose weight, decrease caloric intake and/or exercise more. This is a universal axiom for human beings. Pathological denial has not reduced the incidence of obesity in the USA.

The aforementioned data came from clinical investigations. They provided fundamental information regarding obesity. Other more current research arising from animal studies suggests that the development of obesity modifies genetic expression so the predisposition to obesity may be transferred from mother to fetus. This environmental transfer of acquired obesity to an offspring is referred to as an epigenetic phenomenon. Women who become fat may transfer this epigenetic influence to their children. If this is true, the health care cost related to obesity will become enormous.

In the late 1960's and thereafter, third party payers for health benefits would not pay healthcare providers (doctors) for helping people who were believed to be obese from eating too much. This form of obesity was secondary to excessive food intake, and insurance companies and government agencies were not going to pay for something that was believed to be self-induced. This behavior by third party payers angered me. Nonetheless, I continued to provide guidance to obese patients, frequently free of charge. However, things that were free may not have been worth much. Admittedly, my efforts to reduce obesity were of only transient benefit to most obese patients and did not curtail the current epidemic of obesity. Nonetheless, something needs to be done because the USA is in a hell of a difficult situation with burgeoning obesity. Further, there is a lack of clinical investigators to begin rethinking and resolving the problems related to a fat nation. I doubt that surgical procedures for obesity will be the solution for millions of American citizens. It may decrease some of the old

271

problems associated with gross obesity, but it may create new problems.

I wrote a letter to Congressman Tom Delay on January 15, 2001, complaining that Medicare and Medicaid would not pay for services related to exogenous obesity. On July 16, 2004, Yahoo! News released a top story revealing that federal officials announced a new policy on obesity that could make weight-loss treatments eligible for Medicare coverage. Maybe I will have to "eat a little crow." Maybe this reimbursement for time and effort to treat patients 65 years and older for obesity is better than nothing. However, after 65 years of age people usually stop gaining weight. Instead, they lose weight. Sixty-five years of age is too old to begin to pay for health care. The elderly are not the primary age range to target.

I've been watching the obesity problem grow into an epidemic in the USA and becoming a problem in Europe, Asia and the Middle East. I hope this chapter on energy requirements and food consumption provides the information necessary to help the reader obtain their desired weight. Hopefully we are not beyond the point of no return in regard to obesity. For the current obese group, however, this is unknown.

In my approximate four decades of practicing medicine and doing clinical research, I've had the opportunity to treat many obese patients. Some of these individuals' obesity was complicated by diabetes mellitus, hypertension and detrimental blood lipid profiles. Most were able to lose weight while under close supervision. However, the majority regained their body fat (and weight) with the progression of time. An old saying that curing obesity has a success rate comparable to narcotic addiction seems to be true. It would appear that adults who do not want to become overweight or fat, exercise and monitor their food intake before they become obese. After human beings become grossly obese, it may be a little late to diet and exercise. Thus, it is likely that people must avoid becoming obese. This is a strange challenge for most humans who are designed to overeat and retain the calories in adipose tissue in preparation for possible periods of food deprivation. Human behavior has not adapted to an environment where food is usually present in overabundance. A new consciousness must be developed to protect humans from overeating. For many people this conscious behavior will be associated with a low grade of constant agony due to aggravating hunger. Nonetheless, Americans are now in a process of clearly identifying obesity with excessive caloric intake and a lack of exercise.

I am not sure physicians can be successful in treating morbid obesity without recommending drastic procedures like stomach surgery. The price patients pay to lose weight once they become fat is horrendous. From a historical point of view, it appears that avoiding obesity from birth and childhood will be more successful than treating obese adults. This should not be taken that I have overlooked the importance of genetics on body composition.

People who eat more calories than they need to maintain a reasonable body weight in keeping with their inheritance must accept the responsibility for overeating and predictable obesity. It is not the responsibility of a medical doctor; it is the personal responsibility of the patients (people) to take care of their bodies. I doubt that pushing doctors to promote good health is going to be worth the financial cost unless patients accept the responsibility to maintain a reasonable weight.

Chapter XIV. Weight Changes During Dietary Management

　　Starvation is clearly effective in reducing body weight. Both fat and lean body masses are lost during fasting. The loss of body weight continues as long as total starvation is ongoing or until death occurs. Although the overall effectiveness of total starvation as a tool for weight reduction was known to be excellent, we set out to reevaluate this technique as a method for the treatment of obesity. After a tremendous amount of work we learned, as did patient-volunteers, that starvation was not an effective way to approach the epidemic of obesity and impending diabetes mellitus. Nonetheless, the data are presented to augment knowledge so wise decisions can be made by advisors and patients regarding the loss of detrimental fat.

　　Figure 1 shows weight loss expressed as a percent of body weight per day in 10 obese men and women who volunteered to fast for 9-54 days. During the first week of starvation with a liberal intake of water and supplementary salt tablets, weight loss was accelerated due to diuresis. Large volumes of water were lost through urination. The retention of fluid with resulting boggy tissues and swelling of the legs, ankles and feet and other dependent structures during semi-starvation does not occur during total starvation. After about a week of starvation, with adequate water intake, weight loss becomes fairly constant at about *0.32% body weight* per day. This may be truly disappointing for obese people who desperately want to lose body fat. They pay a large price in time, discomfort and maybe money for weight loss. Figure 1 also shows how limited total starvation is as a method for weight reduction. In essence, it demonstrates the high caloric value of stored fat. Not much fat is needed to meet the metabolic requirements. Under certain circumstances this could be advantageous for survival.

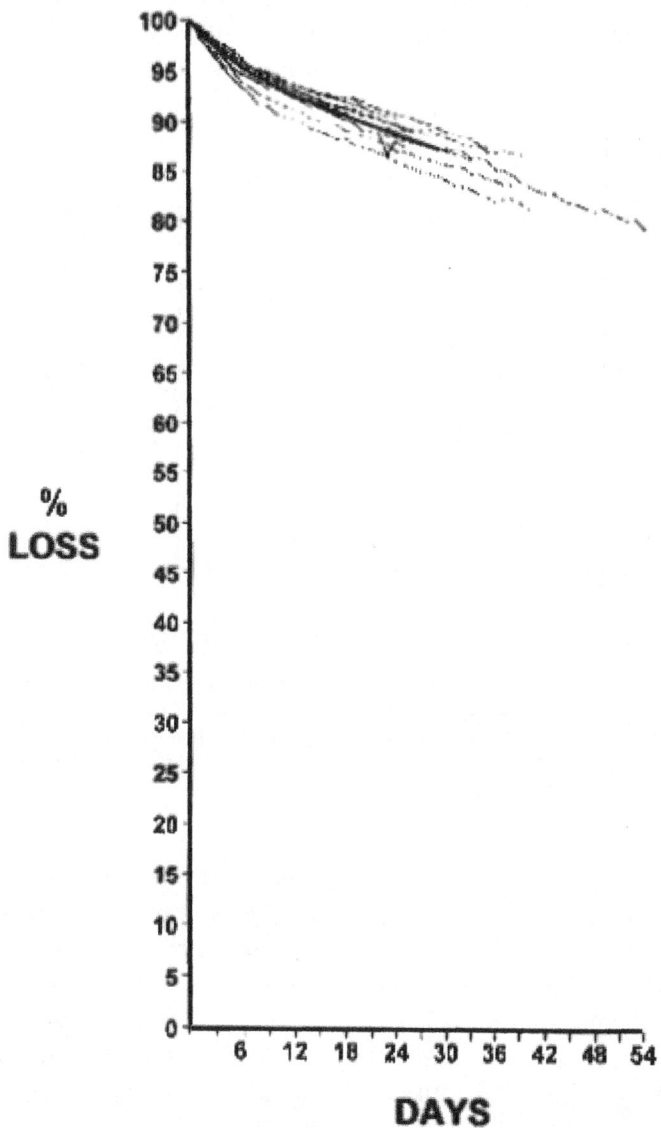

Figure 1. Weight loss, expressed as a percent of initial body weight, in 10 obese male and female volunteers who fasted for 9-54 days.

Once morbid obesity develops, the fat and lean body masses in men and women are approximately equal: 50% fat mass and 50% lean body mass. Figure 2 shows that among

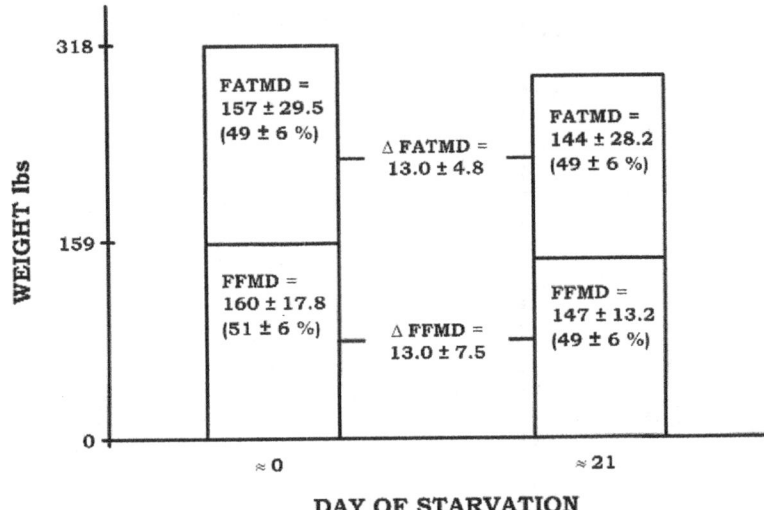

Figure 2. Body compositional changes measured by body densitometry are expressed as fat mass (FATMD) and fat-free mass (FFMD) near the beginning of starvation at about day 0 and after about 21 days of fasting. Weight losses in these compartments decreased in parallel.

morbidly obese individuals, initial weight loss during the first 21 days of total starvation causes comparable reduction in fat and lean body masses. The classic body compositional study was done by Keys *et al* when conscientious objectors to war volunteered to undergo 26 weeks of semi-starvation. The results showed that about as much lean body mass was lost as was fat mass during the 26 weeks of semi-starvation. Somehow these fundamental findings regarding the amount of lean body mass loss have remained "under the radar screen."

The percent of body weight loss can be put into perspective by considering a morbidly obese man [5' 11" tall with a weight of 308 lbs (140 kg)] who is living in a hospital and not engaged in a physical exercise program. He is

276

starving to lose weight. His resting metabolic rate (about 2300 Kcal/day) plus the energy requirements associated with the physical activities of cleaning, eating and walking (about 400 Kcal/day) total about 2700 calories per day. Fat has about 9 calories per gram and, after about a week of starvation, supplies about 93% of his total caloric requirements. Thus, 93% of 2700 calories per day is 2511 calories per day. This requires mobilization of approximately 0.6 pounds (279 grams) of fat per day. The remaining loss of tissue during this period of starvation is derived from lean body mass. This fat-free material is only 20% protein and 80% water. Its caloric value is about 0.8 Kcal/g wet weight. Thus, 7% of 2700 calories is 189 calories that are derived from lean body mass. This equates to about 0.5 pounds (236 grams) per day of lean body protein consumed. There is an additional small weight loss from fluids bathing the body tissues (interstitial fluids and blood).

The amount of weight lost in total starvation versus a diet containing 50% of the caloric requirements in the aforementioned case (about 1350 calories per day) is only twice as great. The cost of medical supervision in a hospital during total starvation is expensive. Weight reduction via diet should save money not only of cost of hospitalization but also on the cost of food. The problem with this reasoning is that many fat people cannot maintain a weight-losing diet. They simply cannot deny themselves the satiety or gratification that comes from consuming enough food to maintain their excessive body weight. Nonetheless, for most people, food restrictions are personal problems just like avoiding consumption of tobacco, alcohol or narcotic products. Medical help may facilitate individuals to reduce their fat mass, but acceptance of personal responsibility is required to achieve and maintain weight reduction. This comment also applies to patients who have undergone gastrointestinal surgery to reduce their body weight. I realize that these dogmatic statements are frowned upon by most obese humans, but the destruction induced by the obesity epidemic must be viewed realistically. The cost of treating diabetes mellitus, heart attacks, strokes, blindness and amputation of the lower extremities will be mind-boggling in the future.

Most of the patient-volunteers that we studied and discharged from the hospital after weight reduction were followed in the outpatient facilities. Initially most of the patient-volunteers retained salt and water while eating a low caloric diet of about 1200 calories per day, and they transiently gained weight. Their body compositions were similar to patients with congestive heart failure, with an abnormal accumulation of body fluids. However, after about two weeks of maintaining their prescribed hypocaloric intake, diuresis (water and salt loss through urination) occurred and weight reduction continued as would be expected on a diet deficient in calories. Our dietary recommendations stressed a relatively balanced content of carbohydrates, fats and proteins, emphasizing the consumption of fruits and vegetables, especially those low in caloric content like lettuce, cabbage, celery, broccoli, cucumbers, green beans, etc. (An unfortunate side-effect is that this diet causes gastrointestinal gases and a problem with flatus.) The success of continued weight loss was largely dependent upon whether or not the patients maintained the low caloric diet, continued to return to the outpatient facilities for monitoring, and maintained close personal relationships with the medical support team. However, the vast majority of patients progressively stopped returning to the outpatient clinic, and when they did, it appeared that they were regaining weight. Eventually, practically all of the patients were lost to follow-up, and I know that some (and I presume the majority) of them regained to their total body weight before the weight reduction program began. The failure to recognize and accept hunger as a natural consequence of semi-starvation for weight reduction may be the cause for "couch potatoes" to remain fat.

After being discharged from the hospital for weight reduction and followed in the outpatient facilities, the health status of almost all of the patients transiently improved. However, it should be noted that the subsequent comments are anecdotal in nature. Those with type 2 diabetes showed significant improvement in blood glucose concentrations. All patients with a significant weight reduction showed their heart pulse rates decreased and those with high blood pressure showed improvement. Mobility and agility increased, and joint pain in the lower extremities diminished. Fortunately, none of the obese patients who lost weight during starvation and returned to the outpatient clinic for follow-up developed peripheral nerve deficiencies. However, several of them consumed a daily multi-vitamin and daily mineral supplements.

Physicians often make recommendations for patients to lose weight. How strenuous or forceful should these recommendations be? As advisors, physicians must recognize that practically all dietary programs for weight reduction that are initially helpful subsequently fail. There are, however, very little data regarding the success rate of the vast majority of people who are engaged in weight reduction programs. There are no data regarding people who look into the mirror, step onto the scales and decide that they are overweight and are going to exercise and/or diet to lose excessive body fat. The success of this group, which composes the majority of U.S. citizens who don't seek physicians' help, is unknown except that epidemiological data demonstrate that Americans are increasing their body weights.

In spite of all of the hullabaloo, there are practically no currently available data published by reputable clinical investigators that define when a gain in weight is hazardous to the individual's health. More clinical research is warranted to understand the impact of weight gain and the accumulation of small or moderate amounts of body fat on health. It is known that heightened incidences of diseased states occur with obesity when body weight exceeds 25-30% over ideal body weight. Further, it is known that there is a sharp increase in mortality once an individual becomes morbidly obese (twice ideal body weight).

Does healthcare cost rise in parallel with obesity? If so, cost containment is patient-dependent.

Chapter XV. Alzheimer's Dementia

Clinical research is not a luxury; it is a necessity.

For more than four decades, I was a doctor engaged in practice, teaching, research and administrative activities. My greatest professional enjoyment came from being a clinical investigator. More recently, I began a new role as a son taking care of a demented, psychotic patient that I love. I became a different kind of caregiver, providing help for my mother who developed severe and progressive Alzheimer's dementia. It is agonizing to see an elderly parent die a few cells at a time. My mother often did not recognize me as her son.

It is important to protect and guard the dignity of a patient. However, it is also important to broadcast the humiliation and suffering Alzheimer's disease casts upon patients and their caregivers. My exposure of some of the following deeply personal experiences and expression of these events would have previously been unthinkable. I am seizing this opportunity to join with others in stressing the need for more research into the cause and alleviation of Alzheimer's disease.

When my mother entered her 80's her hearing and memory were good. At about 85 years old she asked me if I thought she had Alzheimer's disease. She also asked if she had schizophrenia. At the time I thought she was exaggerating her mental deficiencies and mental dysfunction. In retrospect, she had obviously been entertaining these possibilities and reading about these diseases. (It was interesting to learn later that Mother had told one of my brothers that her mother had become demented during her 80's. Bits of family history kept popping up.)

Mother's progressive degeneration of mental status became more evident and dangerous. She lost her memory. She had a regular physician overseeing her health care who prescribed Aricept. It did not help her memory or behavior.

She gradually began to say the same thing over and over. This perseveration became annoying, and her repetitive comment, "I'm afraid," was the usual and consistent statement she made. Her children tried to get her to live with one of them. She refused although she would leave the fire burning on her kitchen stove, and pots would burn and begin to melt. The children arranged for a home caregiver to visit her daily, but after a short time she would not open her door to let the help come into her home. At 87 years of age, she was placed in a large, complex, well designed assisted living quarters and nursing home. Mother pouted continuously until she was transferred to a small house where a licensed practical nurse with assistants oversaw 3 patients. My older brother, who lived nearby, visited Mother frequently in the caregiver's home, and my younger brother and I visited her periodically. After consultation, I recommended small doses of risperidone (Risperdal) for her inappropriate fears. However, the sedative effect of the medication was too great, and I thought she might fall and injure herself, so the antipsychotic medication was discontinued.

Mother's dementia and paranoia progressed along with loss of motor skills. Mumbling, agitation, and shuffling from chair to chair became devastating for her and her caregivers. Someone had to have a constant eye on her to keep her clean, fed, warm and free from injury. Although she was pleasant, this characteristic did not lessen the anxiety she created for the caregivers.

My mother's advanced Alzheimer's disease was complicated by a psychosis. This is not unusual. By definition, a psychosis is a mental disorder in which the patient may be harmful to self or others. If not guarded 24 hours a day she could easily fall and fracture bones, maybe her skull, if not a shoulder, hip or distal extremity. Nonetheless, some form of therapy was needed for her psychosis even though it may increase the likelihood that she would fall.

My wife, Paula, and I routinely traveled from Pennsylvania to New Mexico at about 3-6 month intervals to check on our elderly mothers, mine in Roswell and hers in

281

Farmington. We decided to visit them over the Christmas holidays of 2003.

Mother had been in the caregiver's home for five years and had been slowly deteriorating. Because it was late in the day when we arrived in Roswell, we decided not to visit Mother but instead went directly to my brother's home. He told me that he had noticed deterioration in Mother's hygiene and that the nurse had become more emotionally labile. He was eager to have my professional assessment.

Upon visiting Mother the next day, we found that she had undergone accelerated decay. She had a tongue tic (rapid movement of the tongue in and out of the mouth and licking the lips, interrupted by wiping the tongue with fingers or cloth) and kept spitting on the floor. She had become intermittently incontinent, and the caregiver was no longer able to keep Mother or the environment clean. She needed more attention. Mother's hygiene was unacceptable and her body was wasted. Her paranoia had become more evident. Communication was exceedingly difficult because of her near deafness and mental deficiencies. Caring for her was now demanding 24-hour awareness 7 days a week.

The practical nurse overseeing her care currently had only one patient, my mother. The reduced income she received from serving one patient instead of three was inadequate to have ancillary staff. The caregiver was demoralized and first cried and then became angry when criticized about my mother's poor personal hygiene and the unkempt housing facility. She would not accept criticism and had an explosive response to the suggestions that I offered her.

After empathizing and reasoning with her, the caregiver stopped crying and became somewhat receptive to my comments. I told her, as a physician, several techniques to help control Mother's incontinence. I also told her that I recognized she was exhausted and could not function without some time off during the week. I offered to give her additional money so she could hire help and have some free time to be away from giving care and cleaning the residence. Although she agreed to accept my proposal, she was clearly unstable and dysfunctional, and I knew that it was unlikely that she could regain equilibrium needed to be a health care provider for a demanding patient. She had not had a vacation in five years.

Since Paula's mother's birthday was December 25th, we arrived in Farmington on that date to celebrate Christmas/Birthday with her. It was our intent to stay a few days. However, when I called my brother from Farmington late on Christmas day, I learned that my mother's caregiver had asked him to come get my mother. I could not blame the caregiver. Paula and I decided to get Mother and take her to our home in Pennsylvania.

The next morning, December 26th, we packed up our car and headed back toward Roswell. I began to think that the task before us might be more difficult than I had previously recognized and decided to make notes as the process unfolded.

It was raining, which is unusual for this arid part of the nation. As we drove toward Cuba, New Mexico, and crossed the continental divide, the rain turned to snow and then to sleet. Further south toward Albuquerque we encountered a dust storm. The gusts of wind rocked the car and vision was modestly impaired. This situation augmented our anxieties already present about Mother's situation as we continued to travel southeast toward Roswell.

We removed Mother from the caregiver's home, packed her belongings and spent the night at my brother's home. The following morning we drove from Roswell to Albuquerque, checked in at the airport and returned the rental car. Mother did not walk without support, so getting her in and out of vehicles, restaurants, restrooms, through security and onto the plane was difficult in spite of the willingness of airline staff to help.

During the flight from Albuquerque to Baltimore-Washington International airport, Paula was seated between my mother and me. About mid-flight, Mother motioned toward me and said to Paula, "That's my son. I don't think he knows I'm here." She was sweet and tried her best to be cooperative.

We retrieved our car from the airport parking lot and drove about two hours to our home in Pennsylvania. Exhausted, we arrived near midnight. Having made no advance preparations for our "unexpected guest," we fed and cleaned Mother and prepared a bed for her. The nurse in Roswell had informed us that recently Mother had been pulling down her protective underwear (Depends) at night and urinating on the floor beside the bed. With great concern about the possibility of this occurring in our home, precautionary measures were taken. A plastic sheet was laid on the floor with several layers of towels and rugs placed on top of the plastic. The furniture was rearranged so if we were unaware of her getting out of bed, she could not wander out of the bedroom and down the hall. It was nearly 2:00 a.m. For an additional protective act, Paula got in bed with Mother and the first of many restless nights ensued.

Spending nights caring for an elderly patient with Alzheimer's disease is a major challenge. At 3:00 a.m. we both awoke and helped Mother to the toilet. Success. Again my wife got in bed with her, but later slept on the floor because of restless motions Mother made. They both "rested" until 7:00 a.m. when I heard them rustling. I got up and helped Mother to the bathroom. Again, success. Facing her, I held both of her hands and walked backwards as she followed me into her bedroom. I placed her in bed, covered her with blankets and encouraged my wife to go to bed in our bedroom. We all were up at 8:00 a.m. After Paula assumed responsibility I laid down for an hour of deeply sound sleep, the most restful hour of sleep I had experienced that night.

As a physician, I've always told nurses and other caregivers to get patients up in the morning and keep them awake so they will not stay awake and walk during the night, being a "sundowner." Therefore, since Mother had fallen back asleep, it was logical for me to go to her bedside at 9:30 and ask her to get up. She refused, saying she could not stand up. This dear 92 year old lady was utterly exhausted. I told her I would help her. She said, "I know you would, darling," the first "normal and sensible" response she had made recently.

After another hour of rest, a typical day of care for Mother began. We assisted her to the toilet to "wet." Since moving her up and down stairs was very difficult, she was escorted to a makeshift dining area in the second floor laundry room where I sat down with her. Paula brought breakfast up from the kitchen, and Mother spooned out and sipped all of the milk from the cereal prepared for her. She refused to drink juice or eat banana slices. However, she did take her crushed Synthroid (thyroid) medication. Eventually she swallowed the crushed Haldol pill recently prescribed to control her tongue tic.

I asked her if she liked being waited on. She answered, "It don't make no difference I guess."

Paula brought her additional toast with grape jelly. Then without encouragement, she suddenly began to drink the juice and eat the banana slices before humming and nodding off to sleep while still at the breakfast table.

I got her away from the table and into the bathroom to brush her teeth. Her breath smelled awful. Then I took her to the study, a room where I usually work. I got Mother to sit down in a large cushioned chair. She began to bounce up and down to gain the leverage she needed to stand up. Most of the time she fell back into the chair. Occasionally she would manage to rise and start shuffling from chair to chair via table to table. She would sometimes suddenly sit on the ottoman in front of the chair and lean back. I had to catch her so she would not fall backward and break her neck. At one- or two-hour intervals we would escort her to the toilet. Not much success from this preventive measure.

There were many chores that needed to be done but that day I lacked the intestinal fortitude to be physically or mentally active. In fact, it was difficult for me to do anything constructive. I wanted to go to bed, but I knew I could not go to sleep. A change in lifestyle was acutely being developed.

I wondered if Mother was ever going to nap or have a deep sleep. How can she stay awake and move around for so many hours without significant rest?

It took an hour to feed her a late lunch. We returned to the study. A few minutes of peace crept in, and I enjoyed watching news on television.

The day continued more of the same: constant motion, shuffling from one chair to another and pushing papers and books off the edge of tables. No naps for either caregiver. All three meals were poorly eaten. Today her appetite was poor. She pushed her food and drink back and said repeatedly, "That's enough."

About 8 p.m. we started getting her ready for bed. At 10-minute intervals she got up saying, "I got to wet." After putting her on the toilet for the third time she voided. I put her back in bed a half dozen times during the next 2 hours. She finally went to sleep and we temporarily collapsed. At 2:45 a.m. she got up and started wandering around in the hall. I put her down in bed and lay down with her. She was cold. Under blankets and in my arms her hands finally got warm. Near 5:00 a.m. she kept trying to get out of bed, but I restrained her until 8:00 a.m. My wife came to my assistance. We escorted Mother to the bathroom. Why she was not totally exhausted could not be explained. I got into my bed and slept lightly for a couple of hours.

Patients with senile dementia of the Alzheimer's type are not all the same. Age alone causes a fragile state. Different degrees of dementia superimposed on various levels of fragileness among 80-100 year old patients form a spectrum of disorders. Some simply sit and sleep (often with soiled buttock and pelvis) while others move continuously in an exaggerated state of anxiety. Sure, there are medicinal agents that help, but drugs are not very predictable in these degenerative patients. The drug dosages have to be adjusted to the patient's tolerance for the medication and the degree of brain damage

The second day it took about an hour to feed Mother breakfast, crush her thyroid and antipsychotic medications, mix them in applesauce, and get her to swallow them. Back to the toilet because she said she had to "wet." No success. Escorted her to the study where she sat down, got up, sat down, got up. She looked weary. We put her in bed for a nap. In 5 minutes she was up wandering the bedroom and hall. This recurred two more times over the next 15 minutes.

No person other than Mother has had the chance to perform daily ablutions. She totally consumes the attention of one or two people to feed her and keep her clean and warm.

It is interesting to note my own changes in response to my mother's weak, shuffling gait. I am standing up straight and taking firm, determined steps. None of that shuffling gait of the elderly for me. Being a caretaker of the frail is changing my gait.

Mother's tongue tic and spitting on the floor were clinical conditions that I had not seen before. Destruction of mid-brain nerves is associated with tongue tics. This neurodegenerative disorder responds to an old antipsychotic drug, Haldol. I started her on small doses of this drug to treat the tic and her fears.

Most of the 24 hours in the following days were consumed by subservient activities. I wonder if anyone has ever been productive during the period they served the needs of a patient with severe Alzheimer's dementia complicated by severe psychosis.

One afternoon, I decided to assist her in going down the stairs and sitting on the couch in the living room. As a medical doctor, I know that hallucinations are an integral part of schizophrenia. Nonetheless, I was set back by my mother's comments while sitting on the couch. Her tongue tic was rapid in spite of an increased Haldol dose given to her. Perseveration, stating repeatedly that she was afraid, developed, and she asked if I saw the people in the next room and was I afraid of them. She persisted and wanted to know if the "law" (cops) would prevent them from hurting her. (Although I am a retired physician, I have had limited experience in providing care for an elderly individual with paranoia and Alzheimer's disease.)

Damn. Do I need to up the dose of Haldol? One of the adverse side effects of Haldol is hallucinations. Which way do I go with the Haldol dose, up or down? Incidentally, Haldol is notorious for causing constipation.

I chuckled at myself for using the old generic anti-psychotic drug, haloperidol (Haldol) when the modern psychiatrists recommend Resperdol and Zyprexia. However, Haldol is cheap, and I believe it is as good as any anti-psychotic drug for a tongue tic.

Bladder and bowel activities began to dominate our thoughts. We would escort Mother to the toilet and sit her down until she would keep trying to get up. Then we would escort her to the study, to the eating table, or to the bed. One night after a brief period of putting her in bed, we heard her push the bedroom door closed. We jumped up and found her looking for a place to "wet" on the floor. We quickly walked her to the toilet, sat her down and waited and waited. No urination. We decided to walk her back to the bedroom and placed some old tuxedo suspenders on her so she could not lower her protective underwear and urinate on the floor. This maneuver was not successful. Somehow she later managed to bypass the suspenders and underwear. This bizarre behavior may relate to her childhood. She was reared in New Mexico on a ranch at the foothills of the Capitan Mountains. She spent some of her days in the fields and pastures watching sheep. Maybe she would lower or remove her underclothing and "wet" on the ground. Who knows?

After starting Haldol, Mother did not defecate for seven days. I gave her a laxative, Senna, and tightened the suspenders to hold her underwear up and over her buttock.

Mother was put in bed at 8:00 p.m. "Sweet, Jesus, be with us tonight." We got in bed at 9:30 and watched TV news briefly before turning out the light. I could not go to sleep. I got up at 11:00 p.m., midnight and 2:00 a.m. to check on Mother but did not take her to the toilet. My wife got up at 5:00 a.m. because Mother was out of bed and wandering. The absorptive pads on the floor beside the bed were filled with urine, and a small amount of feces was in the bed. Mother had once again managed to keep the

288

protective underwear dry. We cleaned her up and removed 3 wash- loads of bedding and bedside rugs. I got back in bed and dozed for about 2 hours.

There had to be a reasonable method for protecting the immediate environment from the consequences of her bizarre habit. We put sweat pants over the Depends, snapped them both into the tightly fitting suspenders, placed a sweat shirt on over the suspenders, and then put on top of that a thin cardigan which we buttoned in the back. With this combination in place, Mother could not circumvent the protective devices. And since she often complained about being cold, the multiple layers of clothing were actually welcomed by her.

We would soon learn that slow movements, deafness, hypothyroidism, unsteady gait, poor bowel function and/or incontinence were not the major problems. It was the florid psychosis that emerged as we provided her with food and warmth. It appeared as though we had energized her anguish rather than alleviated her suffering. Although she demonstrated no hostility, her behavior was, nonetheless, disruptive.

Watching a fragile elderly woman causes mental and physical fatigue. Being on continuous guard because she does unpredictable things -- getting up suddenly and sitting down on an ottoman and falling backwards which forces you to grab her quickly before she injures her back or breaks an extremity -- drained us. We began to seek help.

We hired a pleasant young Hispanic woman, Annabella, who had limited English but good common sense, to help us with Mother's care, thinking either Paula or I would be free to get other work done. The assistant would help with Mother about 8 hours a day, and we would care for her the remaining 16 hours a day.

On the eighth day we got up and began fixing breakfast. Our newly hired helper arrived. I crushed the Synthroid tablet, mixed it in applesauce and put it in Mother's mouth. I ordered a liquid form of Haldol from the drug store that could be added to fruit juice. The Haldol was added to apple juice and Mother drank the mix.

Another day for the caregivers was underway. It was punctuated by a massive defecation in the underwear and clothes. Three people initiated the clean-up including a soaking with a hand-held shower device. It took all of us to comfortably get Mother out of the tub/shower that was not designed for an elderly, fragile patient.

It's dead of winter and cold outside. However, our house needed fresh air and the windows were raised and in flowed the cold air.

When I was a practicing doctor and would walk down the hospital corridors where patients with fecal incontinence were housed, I complained about the odorous environs and stated that those quarters should have some fresh air. Hospital administrators, sitting in their palatial rooms, said that the heating cost was too great to allow the patient quarters fresh air.

Shortly after Annabella began to help with Mother she thought Annabella was "after her."

I bathed, shaved, got dressed and drove to Lititz, Pennsylvania, to evaluate the Lutheran chronic care facility. Thereafter, I visited three more nursing homes that had facilities and staff to care for elderly patients with Alzheimer's disease and psychosis.

The cost for care in an Alzheimer's Center varies, but in the Philadelphia region it is from $80,000-$120,000/year. The life expectancy after confinement for Alzheimer's disease is usually 2-5 years. Mother had already lived in a caregiver's home for 5 years. I began to wonder, "What does it take to qualify a patient for governmental financial assistance in a nursing home?"

One day after Annabella left, having helped with daily maintenance of Mother, Mother was brought to my study for me to watch her. She became irrepressible, moving up and down, bouncing from chair to ottoman and pouting when gently scolded. However, a rapid change occurred during the evening meal. First, her hearing seemed improved. She sat at the table and ate a reasonable amount of food and asked for more milk. She began to talk about her mother, Nancy Jane Roberts, and spoke about her brothers and sisters. This was a startling improvement in her distant memory. What on earth induced this sudden change, and was it mental improvement? This does not imply that she returned to normalcy, but she seemed to have acutely undergone some improvement. Maybe this is not unusual for patients suffering from Alzheimer's dementia.

Tonight is the 12th night we have given her care. I continued to keep a partial record of her activities. She has gotten out of bed to wander or to say, "I got to wet" four times between 8 and 9 p.m. Mother just got up again. When I scolded her she said, "Can't you just talk to me?" Believe it or not, I still have to do about 30 plus hours of paperwork per week. However, Paula and I have interrupted our usual routines of office work to take care of Mother. Maybe institutional care is necessary if Paula and I are going to do any meaningful work or have any relaxation.

Yesterday evening and night may have been the most uncomfortable ones spent to date. Mother was in perpetual motion in spite of increasing the Haldol dose to 2 mg three times daily. Admittedly this is a low dose but her face seems more fixed and her movements are more retarded. How can she continue to move nonstop? Her vision is obviously impaired. She searches to see things, but I do not know how much she sees. She is miserable and the two of us are equally, or more so, disturbed. Although we have a large, old 3-story home, since Mother's arrival we have lived primarily in one-half of the second floor -- two bedrooms, bathrooms, study, hallway and laundry room.

Tomorrow, Monday, I will start again looking for an affordable Alzheimer's center that will keep Mother well fed, clean and warm and protect her from injury.

After experiences during the past couple of weeks, it is easy to understand why some patients with Alzheimer's disease housed in centers sit on couches and chairs, over-sedated, smelling like urine. Treatment for Alzheimer's disease is a vexing problem. More in-depth, bold human research maneuvers need to be done to grasp the etiology of this devastating disease. Providing care for the elderly and demented is a daunting task.

Demented patients may place demands on caregivers that are excessive, depriving them of sleep and other forms of recuperation. Dementia may be associated with ungratefulness and cantankerous or aggressive behavior. Fortunately, Mother did not exhibit these traits. However she displayed disinhibition of behavior.

There may come a point where the 24-hour caregiver can no longer tolerate the stress. A facility that uses three shifts of workers to provide around-the-clock service seven days a week may need to be sought for relief.

After a demented patient violates every rule of civility and the caregiver is at the end of his or her tolerance, communication deteriorates. The question I have is, what happens to the personality of a caregiver who may have to use louder and more forceful language to get a patient to respond? Does this near-vile behavior become an integral part of the personality of the caregiver? Of course, a more docile behavior is needed. I'm looking at the cover of a book entitled, Choosing Civility, by P.M. Forni. He lists 25 rules of considerate conduct. I sure need his book to influence me.

I thought professional help was needed for Mother's management, and I telephoned Dr. Rita Reichard, a gerontologist. She suggested that we bring Mother for an evaluation the next morning.

We put Mother to bed at 8:30 p.m. I thought I heard her stirring and got up twice between 10:00 and 11:30. She was asleep in bed. We heard a noise at 1:00 a.m., got up, and found that Mother had fallen and was lying on the floor across the hall from her bedroom. I examined her and found no evidence of severe injury. We lifted her from the floor and placed her on the toilet. No success. Then she was put into bed. I got in bed with her because she was afraid and kept saying, "We got to get out of here." She began to move and raised up at 3:00 a.m. I removed her lower clothing and placed her on the toilet; she urinated. We redressed her and put her back in bed and covered her fully and carefully. Paula and I got into our bed and "rested" until 7:00 a.m. Then we started getting Mother ready to be seen by Dr.

Reichard who suggested we take her to the hospital emergency room for evaluation after the fall. We worked to get Mother down two flights of stairs and into the car and drove her to the hospital.

Mother went through registration, nurse's examination, emergency room doctor's examination, had blood drawn for analyses, and had an electrocardiogram and computerized tomography of the head. Mother was dehydrated. We sat in the ER examination room where IV fluids were administered while awaiting results from Mother's CT scan (which revealed no skull fracture) and other tests that revealed malnutrition.

Mother lay on a gurney half propped up and staring into space. That damn monitor dinged continuously in the background. Mother had a living will: do not resuscitate. She appeared to be frightened by the possibility that she was going to die but equally afraid she might live. She was hospitalized, rehydrated and transferred to a nursing home.

I've been in numerous nursing homes over the years as a practicing doctor, and I was somewhat aware of the physical plants and techniques employed by the nursing staffs. But being *somewhat aware* and being *highly aware* are clearly different perspectives. In sections where demented patients reside, the floors are level. The doors have warning systems if opened. The beds are low, and spongy cushions are placed on the floor beside the beds. The floors are linoleum so they can be readily cleaned. Patients may be placed in special devices for bathing/showering. Those with severe mental defects can be seated in wheelchairs with protective foam devices in front of them so they cannot fall. Patients are fed, and kept clean and warm. Food is prepared as solids, pureed or jelled. There are playful times, religious services, and some entertainment. The most important thing is that patients are watched around the clock, seven days a week. Medications, physical therapy, dental, and foot care (nails) are ordered as necessary by the physician responsible for overseeing the patient's care. The environment is safe but financially costly and can be emotionally draining for all personnel and family members.

I visited my mother most days of the week and tried to cheer her up. She slowly deteriorated. She suffered two episodes of mini-strokes and could no longer verbalize her thoughts. Her paranoia was mostly replaced by facial frowns and mutters of anger. She had been in this nursing home for about 20 months. I began to wonder if the visits did anyone any good. However, two days before her 94th birthday, I realized that the visits were well worthwhile. While sitting at a table in a wheelchair with her arms flexed on her abdomen and her legs flexed, I reached for her hand and told her that I would take her home. I said, "I'll take you back to Roswell." She looked at me, and I put my mouth close to her ear and asked, "Do you understand what I'm saying?" She shook her head up and down for "yes". That was the last conversation I had with her. The next day when I visited the nursing home she was lying in bed on her side with her arms folded in front of her and her lower extremities flexed. She was in a classic fetal position. She was unresponsive to gentle physical stimulation and did not answer to voice questions. Her eyes were shut, and she did not appear to identify with the environment. Her skin felt warm, and her heart rate was 120 beats per minute and irregular. When I returned the next day, she was again in the fetal position and unresponsive to my voice or gentle nudging. She was breathing 40 times a minute and her skin was warm and clammy. I knew she was dying. The look on her face was bland; she never frowned nor smiled. After awhile I left her and returned to my home. On August 25, 2005, her 94th birthday, the phone rang at 1:15 a.m. The nurse said her color was bluish (cyanotic), and she had mottled lower extremities. She was receiving oxygen by facemask. Paula and I rapidly dressed and drove to the nursing home. When we arrived she was lying on her back, her eyes closed. Her skin was moist and warm, and her joints were flexible. She was not breathing, and no heartbeat could be detected. God bless her soul. Until she had become demented, she had been a kind and considerate woman, willing to share her bounty with many people.

I couldn't help but think that the ravages of dementia had robbed Mother of nine years of her life. A woman so willing to help others had become dependent upon others, requiring a tremendous amount of essential support to stay clean, fed and comfortable. In spite of the effort we had devoted to her, I feel that we were relatively ineffective in offering her comfort. Dementia is a horrible disease.

Clinical Investigation

There is a genetic predisposition for the development of Alzheimer's disease, but probably at least two types of this neurodegenerative disease exist: early onset and late onset. Early onset accounts for about 5% of the cases and is referred to as familial Alzheimer's disease. Late onset is much more prevalent and accounts for the other 95% of the patients. Both early and late onset Alzheimer's disease have specific brain lesions, tangles of fibers inside the nerve cells and amorphous plaques outside the nerve cells. The latter is composed primarily of pleated sheets of protein termed beta-amyloid. (These intracellular neurofibrillar tangles and extracellular amyloid plaques, found primarily on postmortem examinations, are the pathological hallmarks of Alzheimer's disease.)

The early onset Alzheimer's disease has an abnormal gene on chromosome 21. (Down's syndrome has an extra chromosome 21 and the same kind of plaques that brain tissue from Alzheimer's patients have.) The mutations in this gene are associated with increased amyloid deposition in the brain. Amyloid is derived from a precursor protein that is extruded from nerve cells. Amyloid collects in the extracellular spaces and is associated with death of adjacent nerve cells. The later onset Alzheimer's disease exhibits this same process of amyloid accumulation in brain with nerve cell death, but late onset Alzheimer's disease also has an additional risk factor for developing this neurodegenerative disease. Late onset Alzheimer's disease has an apolipoprotein (apoE) embedded in the surface of spherical lipoprotein particles that carry lipids (fats) in the bloodstream. Specifically, apoE functions to transport cholesterol, a water-insoluble compound, in the blood. One of the types of apoE is ε4, and its presence increases the risk of developing Alzheimer's disease several-fold. One group of investigators has put forth a strong contingency that the presence of apoE genotype in combination with a bacterial infection, specifically Chlamydia pneumoniae, promotes the severe brain deterioration of Alzheimer's disease.

The role of infection in neurologic diseases has recently been heightened with the discovery of chronic herpes brain infections, post-polio syndrome, HIV and AIDS, Lyme disease organism in brain, and prions in mad-cow disease, which are transmittable to human beings. The reports of Brian J. Balin, Ph.D. and coworkers are convincing that a bacterium, Chlamydia pneumoniae, invades the brain and induces the pathologic changes that characterize Alzheimer's disease. However, widespread confirmation of this possibility is lacking. Other investigators are focusing more on genetic variety of early onset Alzheimer's. Their work shows that mutation on chromosome 21 is responsible for the destruction that characterizes Alzheimer's disease. These researchers believe that outgrowths from the nerves are clipped off from the cell wall. This cellularly derived material contains a precursor protein of amyloid. This precursor undergoes breakdown and it is the remnant material that accumulates and becomes the amyloid neurofibrillary material deposited in the brain.

There are several research centers in the USA where Alzheimer's disease is the major focus of inquiry. The neurofibrillary tangles in Alzheimer's disease are about twice the size of red blood cells. A compound, the Pittsburgh compound, has been developed that can be given intravenously that will travel to the brain, cross the blood-brain barrier and stick to the amyloid plaques in the brain. Highly specialized imaging techniques (positron emission tomography: PET) display the Alzheimer's lesions with the Pittsburgh compound stuck to the amyloid plaques. When the compound leaves the brain, it pulls the amyloid material with it, effectively removing the material that kills nerve cells. Reversal of the dementia has not been demonstrated.

A vaccine against Alzheimer's disease has also been developed, but during clinical trials patients had an adverse reaction. A dangerous inflammation of the brain developed. Further use of the vaccine in people with early-onset Alzheimer's disease is in abeyance.

There is another possibility for the death of nerve cells in patients with Alzheimer's disease. Body organs are composed of cells that contain genes which program death as well as function. Thus, cells have genes that are internal time clocks. When the time for survival runs out, the cell dies. There is little inflammatory response with migrating scavenger cells to clean up the debris or cause swelling and pain. The dead cells slowly disappear and their natural function is lost. This process is known as apoptosis. Maybe those with Alzheimer's disease have an accelerated program for nerve cell death: programmed apoptosis. If so, genes that cause programmed cell death should be identified and regulated by medicinal agents.

Alzheimer's disease has become an epidemic as Americans age. It is estimated that after 85 years one-half of the survivors will develop Alzheimer's dementia. This disease has to be cured. The cause must be defined by molecular and genetic pathology. Treatment must be developed. At present, Alzheimer's disease is defined by symptoms, by description of behavior or functional activities. It is not defined by the cause of the disease.

The families of patients and the general public must recognize that research studies that may carry a significant risk to humans must be done. Americans must stop frivolous medical malpractice lawsuits. Our society should be encouraging clinical investigations to probe this dastardly disease rather than making it practically impossible to do research on human beings.

There is, however, a much more prevalent problem with this recommendation: capable clinical investigators willing to undertake needed studies have become an endangered species. Young individuals who have completed 4 years of college, 4 years of medical school, 3-5 years of residency training, and sometimes an additional 2-3 years of fellowship, who have old clothes and cars are usually deep in debt. Their spouses, children and other family members are often reluctant to tolerate another few years of highly specialized training, with an inadequate annual salary, in order to gain knowledge necessary to become an established investigator. Further, after all this effort to become a clinical investigator, the chances of receiving a federal grant to continue the research effort are only about 25%. This creates a lot of insecurity for young doctors who want to make patient oriented research their career. Therefore, it is not surprising why the number of applicants and the number of grants awarded to young, would-be clinical investigators have fallen precipitously over the last two decades.

Contrast the lack of today's clinical investigators researching Alzheimer's disease with the rise of clinical research during the 1950-1970's. In 1959 half of the patients who were brought to the hospital emergency room in diabetic (ketoacidotic) coma died. Basic scientists and clinical investigators were stimulated to develop methods for evaluating and treating the severely compromised patients. Responses to therapy were designed and measured. Today, if the same patient population is brought to the emergency room only 2-3% die, and those who die have complicating diseases like a stroke, pneumonia or heart attack. Clinical investigators took on the task and resolved the dilemma of diabetic coma and developed useful treatment.

The success medical doctors have had in resuscitating patients dying in diabetic ketoacidosis has not been extended to patients slowly dying with Alzheimer's dementia. There are many reasons for this lack of success. The one that I want to emphasize is the progressive, dangerous decline in the number of individuals who are willing to devote their lives to becoming physician-scientists or clinical investigators. These doctors devote most of their working hours to gaining new information regarding normal mechanisms for maintaining health and contrast their findings with disease states. They use scientific methods to seek new knowledge. The data collected are open to scrutiny by others. Their results and interpretations should be confirmed. The physician-scientists usually work in interdisciplinary groups which have no boundaries between basic science and clinical science. The doctors who investigate human beings usually have a medical degree, M.D. It is this group of physician-scientists that is disappearing from America. If they become extinct, all aspects of health care will be in great jeopardy. Their scientific medical minds shore up the entire medical profession. Yet these valuable professionals are dwindling in number. Many years are required to become a qualified physician-scientist who can interphase the basic techniques with patients' diseases. The probability of getting a grant with enough money to execute the studies is low, and the grants are for a short period of time. The salaries of clinical scientists are low in spite of their enormous contributions. The rigors of developing a hypothesis that can be tested in human beings and getting protocols through the scientific review and human welfare review committees are exasperating. Having enough protected time so the physician-scientists can pursue research rather than phone in a prescription, see a patient, teach a class, make rounds with residents, or run the outpatient clinics is an unlikely possibility. The few remaining clinical investigators are often disgruntled and serve as poor role models for young protégés. This is in part due to third parties that create the frustrations associated with trying to do investigator-initiated research and make a reasonable living. Ironically, patients hold clinical investigators in high regard and develop deep-seated appreciation for the effort put forth on their behalf as patients. Most patients are willing to sacrifice and work with physician-scientists to solve their health problem or promote their health or the health of others. However, sometimes family members are ready to sue if research efforts fail or result in detrimental outcomes.

The thrill that emanates from a discovery that allows a clinical investigator to understand a normal or diseased process that benefits humans is gigantic: to understand how human beings survive under a given circumstance and how to help dying patients is exhilarating. Clinical investigators employ their knowledge to help people; they are anxious to share knowledge.

We must encourage more physician-scientists to undertake bold maneuvers to discover the causes and methods of treating the various types of Alzheimer's disease.

Bring the excitement of gaining knowledge back to clinical investigation. Remove the blockades. Encourage capable physician-scientists to aggressively pursue inquiry into Alzheimer's disease by providing financial resources, laboratory space, and dedicated time. Create a spirit of satisfaction and a sense of accomplishment from alleviating human suffering associated with Alzheimer's disease.

Why haven't a few clinical investigators with imagination and moxie studied Alzheimer's disease the way the researchers of old studied and defined how to treat diabetic ketoacidosis, replace hips and knees, or revascularize the heart?

How did we as a nation with the most highly trained physician-scientists let the incidence of Alzheimer's disease progress to epidemic levels among people 85 years and older without significant clinical investigators defining and treating this horrendous disease?

Who has biopsied the brain looking for fungi, bacterial, viral or prion traces in patients with family histories of Alzheimer's disease and early manifestation of mental dysfunction? Who has defined mode of inheritance or genes responsible for disease development? Has adequate attention been given to the possibility (likelihood) that Alzheimer's disease is a natural genetically programmed system of neural cell death via apoptosis? Are there environmental factors responsible for the predisposition of Alzheimer's disease to occur? Are clinical researchers afraid to do any aggressive studies because mishaps will occur, and they will be sued by some family member coupled with a trial lawyer? Get on with studying this horrific disease. Mishaps are sure to occur. Nonetheless, finding some form of successful treatment would be rewarding for countless patients and caregivers.

Not only are patients with Alzheimer's disease severely disabled, so are the caregivers of patients with Alzheimer's disease.

Chapter XVI. Obscure Side of a Clinical Investigator

After my first year of medical school, my immediate family needed more money for living expenses. So, during the summer break, I went to work for a pathologist as a technician in a laboratory where numerous kinds of measurements were made on urine, blood, bacteria (for infections), and on tissue fragments (biopsies) to uncover diseases. Quite frankly, I soon learned that I was inadequately prepared to perform such a broad array of laboratory work. Therefore, I confined myself to doing those analyses in which I had previously gained an element of expertise. During the second year of medical school, I began to work at the Beth Israel Hospital in a Denver suburb. There, well-qualified laboratory technicians were extremely helpful and generous with their time. They taught me additional techniques including simple x-ray procedures, e.g. chest x-rays, and making electrocardiogram tracings. After I became familiar with the laboratory techniques and staff operations of the hospital, during the school year I worked in the hospital from noon on Saturdays until 8:00 a.m. Monday mornings every other weekend. Somehow during my travels through life I failed to express my gratitude to those who oversaw my training and paid me for work done at Beth Israel Hospital.

After graduating from the University of Colorado School of Medicine, I was awarded an internship on the coveted Osler Medical Service at Johns Hopkins University Hospital. In addition to my training, I was one of the medical residents paid to do physical examinations on the entering class of medical students. The enthusiasm I encountered from these students was stimulating and enjoyable.

I passed the board examinations for a Maryland medical license and worked during my brief summer vacation time in Ocean City, Maryland, providing primarily emergency health care for patients who had developed acute illnesses or injuries during their jaunt at the beach. It was amazing how grateful a patient would be when I put his/her dislocated shoulder back in place or removed a large piece of glass or wooden splinter from the foot. However, I was somewhat surprised when he/she skipped town without paying the medical bill or providing a home address where a bill for medical services could be sent. I worked part of each day and provided emergency care for a population of about 100,000 every-other night. I spent the night going from "house-to-house" or "trekking back to the office" to help people in need. In those days, portable telephones were not available. After I finished giving service to a patient in his/her "home" I would call my wife who was answering emergency calls from our apartment near the beach. She would usually be frantic, urging me to get to the next emergency as fast as possible because she was convinced that someone was dying. I would arrive at the next patient's dwelling, and sure enough, the patient was acutely ill, but not dying. I would perform a service or give advice or an injection of medication to stop the vomiting, diarrhea or pain and hustle to the next patient. This was my first experience at learning that patients had an inalienable right to "free care" day or night.

Upon completion of my residency training, I was awarded a fellowship at Harvard's Joslin Research Laboratories. The chair of medicine at the affiliated Peter Bent Brigham Hospital, Dr. George Thorn, insisted that fellows doing clinical research spend at least 20 percent of their time seeing patients in the outpatient department. This was designed to assure that medical fellows kept abreast with their clinical skills. In addition, I took a side job, first working one night a week at the Harvard University Health Services facility. There, I met Harvard students working part-time at the medical facility to enhance their incomes. The student employees and students and staff from Harvard and Radcliffe were delightful and exhilarating individuals. Their array of knowledge and vocabulary were fascinating. Later during my fellowship training, one morning per week I arrived at work extra early, gathered blood and urine samples, attended to the medical and mental needs of the

303

volunteers undergoing starvation studies on the clinical research center, and then quickly dashed downtown Boston to the New England Life Insurance Company to serve as a physician. I was impressed by the organizational formats presented at New England Life and considered giving up my research and academic pursuits to become a full-time member of the company's professional staff. Also during my fellowship I had the opportunity to work on Cape Cod in the emergency room of Falmouth Hospital. A small house was provided for doctors in training who came to work during their summer vacation. I labored 12 hours on and 12 hours off 7 days a week during my vacation time, providing care to many people who suddenly became ill while on vacation. They were marvelous patients. In addition, I made enough money to make the effort worthwhile, and my family enjoyed the wonderful atmosphere on the beach. This time remains dear to my heart. During my second summer doing this work I met the affable and intellectually curious surgical resident, Dr. George Blackburn, who became a lifelong friend. He had the best organized mind in dealing with medical emergencies of any individual I have ever met. His interest in nutrition peaked during our summer discussions, and he went on to become an international star in clinical nutrition and surgery.

After I was recruited to Temple University School of Medicine in 1968, I met a resident who later became a fellow in clinical cardiology. He had the most facile ability of anyone I ever encountered to pass catheters into and through arteries supplying blood to organs and into and through veins draining these organs. His clinical abilities were augmented by his innate talents. He was most helpful to my team when we engaged in catheterizing the arterial supply and venous drainage of organs (e.g. liver). As an aside, he ran a private medical office to deliver health care to a deprived and poor patient population in a ghetto of Philadelphia. I began to work there from 5-10 p.m. one evening a week to supplement my income. There was a strange but obvious appreciation given by the patients for medical service provided at this clinic. An elderly black man and his family lived across the street from the outpatient clinic. During the winter he watched from inside his house for my arrival and departure from the clinic, and in the summer when the days were long and warm, he watched from his front porch. He made sure that the young aggressive black males brought no physical harm to me or my car as I entered and left the ghetto area. Many of the patients had diseases that I could not handle in the ghetto clinic, so I referred the adults to Temple University Hospital and the children to St. Christopher's Hospital. This job experience also taught me how to deliver health care in an efficient manner. I took that talent back to the Temple outpatient diabetic clinic and restructured it so it was converted from a money-losing clinic into a money-making clinical operation with improved patient care.

I remember well picking pieces of glass out of the feet of an elderly white woman who had run through an open lot, cutting her bare feet with glass fragments from broken bottles strewn everywhere. I asked her why on earth she ran through this area and cut the soles of her feet so seriously. She replied, "Doc, you would have run through that glass strewn area too if you were caught in the crossfire of two rival gangs shooting at each other." I also remember pulling teeth, a job I did not like because I thought a good dentist could save those teeth. I gave information to unmarried young women regarding planned parenthood. I prescribed birth control medications for children. For example, I told a 13 year old girl that she needed her mother's approval for a prescription. She quickly replied, "I do not want to have *another* child." She got the prescription for "the pill." A young male neighbor who had a propensity for catching venereal diseases had an interesting and engaging personality. I wonder what happened to him as he grew older. A small Hispanic man who had been beaten up by his larger Caucasian wife needed his eyebrow stitched together. I saw my first case of Peutz-Jeghers syndrome, a young woman with pigmented spots on her lips and such severe bleeding from her intestine that she had lost two-thirds of her blood volume. The most beautiful 16 year old mulatto I have ever seen was brought to the clinic by her mother because girls at school were attacking her; I hoped that she could get an education to benefit her life. There were so many more patients who were dear to me, but eventually that clinic closed as the environment continued to decay and families left the area.

I went to work in the ghetto clinic primarily to supplement my income, but I got a lot more out of it than money.

Chapter XVII. Changing Environment of Medical Practice

There are about 800,000 medical doctors providing health care to approximately 296 million Americans. Each practicing doctor needs about 4-5 people to help him/her with the practice. About one-half of these helpers are handling "paper work." Outside the doctors' offices, over 4 million clerks handle the paper work for "third party payers" responsible for payment or rejection of bills related to medical service. Thus, there are about 10 helpers per doctor doing mostly paper work. What an unbelievable waste of money. The healthcare system is in a hell of a mess.

Leaders at academic medical centers have several responsibilities. They must advocate excellence in education and training. They must insist on the highest quality of education, research and patient care. It is difficult to fulfill these requirements without having experience as a medical doctor, but taking care of patients is time consuming. Therefore, people who do not take care of patients have the time needed to emerge as administrators of healthcare programs. However, they are deficient in knowledge related to education, research and patient care. On the other hand, practicing doctors often have inadequate knowledge pertaining to finance and organization.

In other chapters, I have touched upon the deterioration of investigator-initiated clinical research in the USA. Here, I describe the changes being pushed by financial managers and politicians who do not take care of patients but who deliver strong and enforceable fiats.

This chapter is written for a broad audience because I believe it will be social forces that ultimately determine the environment in which healthcare service, education and research are provided and advanced. In this chapter, I focus on health care in a large university-controlled hospital. Citizens of the USA have provided tax money and philanthropic support for medical leaders to build the most advanced biotechnical healthcare system in the world. In a democracy, adequately informed people from all races and broad socioeconomic, educational and employment backgrounds have the potential to generate the most powerful forces known to modulate their society, including the medical practice within its confines.

The impetus for this presentation was the recognized need of the medical professions to communicate better with the general public. It was primarily written to augment the people's trust and support for all aspects of medical care. People must believe their healthcare providers and have faith in their medical institution. In addition, I ask the public to recognize that in the valuable long-term alliances between patients and doctors, both parties must benefit from the relationship and be fair to each other.

Unfortunately, doctors were not prepared to deal with the revolution that occurred in the medical marketplace during the past one to two decades. They were overwhelmed by gradual but progressive forces that were foreign to them. They did not abrogate or surrender professional or fiscal responsibilities for healthcare delivery; they were simply not prepared to handle new societal demands, an increasingly complex relationship with third party payers, and a burgeoning morass of federal and state regulations. Doctors were slow to recognize the changes in their external environment and were not sensitive to the concept that cost of medical care rather than quality emerged as the major determining force in healthcare delivery, and that patients or purchasers of health care have some characteristics of simple customers in a commercial deal. Doctors are individuals dedicated to the healing profession and did not view patients as customers looking for bargains but as human beings needing help.

The gap that occurred between doctors and patients and the marketplace was a predictable phenomenon. The body of knowledge that must be understood by doctors to practice state-of-the-art medicine, coupled with ever-increasing patient expectations in the face of dwindling resources to pay for the latest and best conceived healthcare services, created a frustrating dilemma for both patients and doctors. Neither patient nor doctor possessed the understanding, adaptability, and tolerance needed to cope with the changes triggered by revolutionary technological advances. Over-taxed doctors, who acquired new responsibilities for coordinating the proliferating specialties and subspecialties, produced a healthcare system that was not fully integrated. Patients are unwilling to pay for medical advice, and this problem is going to get worse with the lack of generalists being trained in the USA.

Modern medicine is linked to the accelerating accumulation of knowledge, which has never been orderly. Some chaos must be accepted as part of the information explosion. The environment is unstable, and disorder prevails because each new change leads to another change. Society in general, and doctors in particular, will remain in an unpredictable state of flux as long as the knowledge base continues to expand. It is a mistake to think that physicians can adapt in synchrony with the constantly changing base of knowledge. Only partial, transient, artful solutions for the ever-evolving problems of healthcare delivery can be expected.

Doctors are in the process of assuming more fiscal responsibility for patient care. By contracting with insurance companies to provide health care for a given rate, physicians have accepted the insurance risk for their services. This creates an untenable situation where the patient's care is pitted against the doctor's financial interests. These are awesome challenges because, in the last half of the previous century, the medical enterprise has outgrown concepts on how to deliver cost-effective, universal health care. Doctors have not capitulated or given way to forces they can no longer resist, but their confidence to formulate suitable remedies in a quickly changing clinical environment is compromised. This loss of professional confidence in the face of miraculous cures for human disease creates a bizarre paradox.

The inappropriate, hostile, deficient environment generated by unsustainable, low reimbursement rates and third party denial of payments for hospital and physician services, coupled with impossible expectations of patients, have created medical care chaos.

The first and foremost issue is that doctors and medical center personnel must maintain public trust. The morality of doctors as well as the ethical behavior of leaders and trustees at academic medical centers should be above reproach.

The following is paraphrased and extracted from *The Pharos*, the journal for the honor medical society, Alpha Omega Alpha. The messages and aspirations apply to all doctors practicing medicine:

"Doctors must be ready to act. They must be deeply and sincerely committed to the scholarly application of biomedical scientific information to improve the physical and mental states of people. They should be dedicated to optimizing the health and welfare of their patients and society. Further, they should encourage a never-ending search or research of knowledge, influence and teach colleagues to recognize and appreciate their responsibilities to individual patients and to society.

Doctors should openly promote (seek) colleagues who have demonstrated a desire 1) to influence the performance of others who want to excel in providing wise, honest, and compassionate health care to people; 2) to foster doctoring through professionalism by placing the concerns and welfare of the patients and society first in the mind of the physicians-surgeons; 3) to bring good cheer and charisma to patients; 4) to pay homage to good health; 5) to pledge to work for the good of the patient, which can only be done if the state-of-the-art or the best information available is employed in a humane manner for maximizing the well and healing the sick; 6) to use psychic and physical energies to gather information and master the art of healing; 7) to consider and be tolerant of the idiosyncrasies of patients; and 8) to influence proactive behavior among health care providers.

Civilized cultures of human beings define, honor, and seek high standards of behavior. Medical doctors should put forth conscious efforts toward laudable goals in providing outstanding health care."

As beneficiaries of physicians' expertise and dedication, patients should be appreciative and willing to pay for services. Neither physicians nor patients should take advantage of the other.

When unscrupulous profiteers are limiting patients' access to state-of-the-art health care, there has never been a more opportune time for reflections and actions from the physicians-surgeons to serve as exemplary leaders to design and deliver excellent health care for people at affordable costs.

The medical institutions must 1) get intellectual support from the business, law and computer schools, 2) obtain financial investment from the universities to modernize medical education, and 3) revolt against any bureaucratic annoyances that impair health care for patients and frustrate doctors. A gathering of social planners, clergy, industrialists, legislators and visionaries is needed to initiate corrective actions for the health care profession.

Leaders of American medicine have to be role models, not only in moral conduct but also in managing people, communicating ideas, augmenting resources and promoting progress in education, research and patient care. They need to develop model administrations characterized by honesty and cooperation and to allow medical students and junior trainees learn how to organize to augment health services. They need to let leaders from all ranks be part of the decision-making. Profiteers should not be allowed the opportunity to dictate policies. Medical leaders should join forces with businessmen, clergy, community leaders and politicians. (Collectively, these elements of society are synergistic in improving the welfare of people.) The doctors and medical centers should have the legal right to sue because of arbitrary and capricious decisions affecting any aspect of their operations. Medical doctors and institutions need the same protection that other democratic individuals and institutions have.

Changes in the practice of medicine require education of doctors and students alike. Education costs money! Philanthropy and public funds are essential to promote education and change in the environment where people's healthcare needs are not met. We must all be cognizant that no physician-surgeon is more costly to society than a poorly trained doctor.

Doctors must have compensated time to practice medicine, conduct research, and engage in educational endeavors to maintain the skills necessary to provide high quality health care. Doctors engaged in teaching must provide exemplary medical service and display professionalism if they are to serve as role models. Further, the environment must be appropriate. One cannot teach good judgment and cost efficient healthcare delivery without practicing medicine. Trainees are taught how to resuscitate a patient dying from either diabetic (ketoacidosis) coma or a heart attack by serving patients under the guidance of skilled clinicians. Surgical judgments and talents are passed to the students, residents, fellows and colleagues in active operating rooms. One learns how to deliver a baby by participating in the birth process. Patient care is an integral part of education and training, and the clinical doctors must have access to large patient populations in order to teach others how to practice the various disciplines that are essential for providing good health care.

Business principles must be introduced early in training doctors: how to provide the best outcome for the best price; how to negotiate and collaborate; and how to develop common goals and unite to obtain objectives. Other components include exposing current distribution of monies spent on health care, i.e. hospital, pharmacy, physician,

312

profit, etc.; development of outpatient and/or inpatient practice services, and methods for closing the gap on billing and collecting for services rendered; and how to maximize computer techniques. Management of outpatient and inpatient shared computer data should be learned as well as how to record, document, transcribe and store medical notes; finally, enculturate how to be innovative. Other mandatory topics are the determination of the number of individuals who should work in subspecialty groups or group practices, and how to staff offices and keep medical records; how to refer patients to consultants and how to respond as a consultant; and how to promote efficiency and encourage relaxation and to demonstrate the joys of "doctoring."

Perspectives from practicing physicians may be helpful to people to use their political powers to promote realigning reimbursements for health care. We are convinced that reimbursement rates should be centered around real and current problems facing practitioners. In the 1960's, when we were fresh out of our training to serve patients, the diagnostic methods and treatment options were much more limited. An hour for an initial visit and 15 minutes for a follow-up visit were sufficient times to evaluate and initiate therapy and make follow-up recommendations. This may not be true today because patients now survive medical insults that killed them 30-40 years ago. Further, the technological advances and therapeutic modalities have increased exponentially during the last 30-40 years. What has not increased is time allotted to providing medical services to decompensated patients.

The complexity of healthcare delivery has become astronomical because multiple diseases, numerous drugs, chronic complications and monumental bureaucratic regulations modify or rob time needed to provide good care to patients. Nonetheless, the first and most important question remains: How can a doctor serve patients? Therefore, it is appropriate to ask how does a doctor evaluate patients, make recommendations including referral to other doctors, e.g. surgeon, renew prescriptions, maintain an awareness of the various kinds of equipment and resources

313

available (e.g. for diabetic patient: glucose reflectance meter, blood glucose test-tapes, syringes, pens for dialing insulin dose, etc.) via resource manuals, and provide lists of phone numbers and addresses for medical organizations to help patients keep informed?

The second issue relates to maintaining a prepared mind. How does the doctor select the appropriate journals to read and attend meetings to stay abreast of medical knowledge?

The third concern relates to the business issues: no profit margin, no professional mission. How does a clinician learn about practical business issues? What are the third party reimbursement rates? How is a group practice formed, and how is overhead shared? How does one bill for services honestly and properly? How has electronic billing worked? What kind of medical records are needed? How does the physician close the loop of treating the patient, billing and collecting for service? What alliances with third party payers should be sought and which ones should be avoided? Most importantly, how were the decision powers usurped from doctors and can these professional strengths be regained? Let medical needs, rather than financial concerns, determine what care should be delivered.

Fourth, consider the work, time and knowledge needed to provide health care for modern day patients. What kinds of problems are doctors faced with when providing medical consultation? Can the physician complete a new patient consult in 45-60 minutes and provide a follow-up treatment plan in 15-20 minutes? As doctors, we feel these time frames are usually too short to accomplish the tasks that need to be done for many patients with complicated diseases.

When we were medical students, interns, residents and fellows in the late '50s and early '60s, patients with numerous diseases and medications were rarely seen because most of them died before they developed so many complications. For today's subspecialists who provide outpatient health care for adults, a patient may have numerous compounding diseases, e.g. diabetes mellitus, high blood pressure, elevated blood cholesterol values, abnormal blood flow to the heart, legs and brain, kidney failure, visional impairment, etc. The average complex patient requires about 10 powerful and expensive medications. The clinician needs a firm grasp on the interplay among many diseases and medications. Knowledge garnered from different medical specialties is needed to provide good health care for most patients. For a medical consultant to obtain a history, do a physical examination, make tentative diagnoses, and develop treatment plans occasionally requires over two hours for the initial visit. Appropriate reimbursement for time, knowledge and office expenses should be paid.

The discharge summary of a typical patient released from the hospital may suggest a relatively smooth and well organized course, but the activity actually involved in his/her healthcare delivery by the consultants may have been rushed and disorderly. Perhaps it was distressful for both the patient and family and all of his/her healthcare providers because the environment for healthcare delivery has changed drastically in the last 10-15 years. "Too much of the allotted time is spent on 'paperwork' and too little time is spent on dealing with the patient."

In the 1980's when we as practitioners were working in university hospital environments and were asked for a consultation on a patient, often a resident or fellow in training saw the patient first, obtained the history, did the physical and developed a therapeutic plan for the patient who was usually in his/her assigned bed when one of us arrived for a complete overview. However, as private practitioners in today's world of rush, rush, rush, when we arrive at the patient's assigned location in the hospital, the patient may be undergoing urgent radiographic examination, or having cardiac catheterization studies or another procedure done somewhere in the hospital. Therefore, the consultant must find the patient, either present in his/her assigned bed or in one of many hospital laboratories located on different floors and different wings of the hospital before advice can be given. The historical, physical and laboratory data should be synthesized before therapeutic recommendations are quickly initiated while the patient is resting on a gurney or an x-ray, scanning or catheterization table. A complete bedside history and physical examination may out of necessity be delayed. Hopefully, a learned colleague will be able to convey to us his/her concerns about the status of the patient. There may be a helpful nurse, nurse practitioner or physician assistant assigned to the patient who will be able to communicate the urgency of the medical problems while we personally dig further into the situation. We enjoyed interpreting, teaching and demonstrating clinical medicine to students, residents, fellows and colleagues, but now we may not encounter young inquisitive members of the healthcare team. Third party payers have squeezed out the time needed to interact at a slower, more reasonable and intellectual pace. It is a privilege to serve patients, but for former professors it is disheartening to not encounter a student, house officer or fellow. Teaching has been devastated by this assembly-line, high-tech corporate style of providing health care.

After the initial encounter the doctor must interpret the clinical course and laboratory data. On the front-line, the physician cannot always remember all of the best procedures or recommendations that need to be done or made immediately. Time allotted to the decision-making processes is short. The consultant must recognize the importance of the care team: physicians, nurses, technicians, clerks, dieticians and others. The consultant should think through the patient's welfare to change orders, to communicate with other team members, and to be humanistic, kind and considerate. Simultaneously, he/she must recognize that one must move to the next task in an orderly manner. Oh, and by the way, the consultant must not forget to document the visit and every detail, pertinent or not to managing the case. These include the dates of the intended contributions, and eventually, the codes for services rendered so a reduced (or denied) reimbursement payment can be used for malpractice insurance and personnel and office expenses in order to continue the practice of medicine.

About 68% of physicians make coding errors because the system for selecting the appropriate code needed to bill for service rendered is extraordinarily difficult and complex. No fraud is intended for the vast majority of coding errors.

316

However, third party payers can use quantitative codes (numbers) to deny paying for quality patient care.

Serious issues are related to satisfying the hospital's requirements for managing patients' illnesses.

- Have safety requirements been satisfied?
- Have the diseases been documented?
- Are the verbal orders signed?
- Was the discharge timely?
- Were follow-up arrangements after discharge provided?

Health care in the USA costs too much, but cost containment levied on hospitals and doctors by third party payers after insurance stockholders and some drug industry profiteers have extracted their portion of the healthcare dollar, has brought harsh challenges for survival in the unfriendly marketplace for patients, hospitals and doctors.

The prospective payment system for reimbursing hospitals for services was developed in 1983. The federal government passed legislation for Medicare expenses where payment was connected to one of 467 diagnosis-related groups (DRG). If the costs for the care of a patient were less than the DRG payment, the hospital could keep the difference as profit. On the other hand, if the costs were higher than the DRG payment, the hospital would suffer a loss. DRG promoted rapid patient throughput, curtailing length of hospital stay. Thus, financial success or survival depends on moving more patients through hospitals quickly. Furthermore, in an attempt to seek greater functional efficiencies, the work forces were reduced. In the hospitals, more low paid employees were hired to measure vital signs, transport patients, dump food trays at bedside, and clean up the debris, all under the guise of increasing throughput and maintaining hospital economical viability. However, it has become increasingly difficult to move a progressively aging patient population through hospitals faster. Costly diagnostic technology and therapeutic techniques and devices continue to emerge in the industry. Moreover, the patients currently hospitalized are generally more decompensated than they were 15-30 years ago because the patients are selected from people whose treatment as

317

outpatients failed. Furthermore, patients' expectations have risen.

Some hospitals have attractive entrances and palatial administrative offices. However, it is not surprising that much of the physical plants at medical centers where patients are housed are outdated for current clinical care. Moreover, the housing for patients and the work environment for doctors are often inadequate. Usually, one or two patients are crowded into rooms too small for comfort and equipment: beds, monitoring devices, intravenous infusion apparatus, cardiac monitoring devices, food tables, and yes, television sets. No quietness or privacy is possible. Most of the hospitals in the northeast are old, antiquated buildings with inadequate power supplies, and due to the cost of heating and cooling, they are poorly ventilated. The malodorous stench from feces permeates the rooms and hallways and foul smells persist for hours. At the nurses' stations, computers to convey laboratory data are crammed on top of desks, shelves, or whatever. No place exists for the physicians to sit down and review the patients' medical records.

Increasing operational efficiencies by redesigning complex procedures may create more hazardous situations than cutting operational costs.

In this complex, overcrowded, noisy, impersonal, rushed hospital environment, is there any doubt why significant medical mistakes are made? In fact, many hospitals, nurses and physicians have been strangled by inappropriately low reimbursement for services, and time has been extracted from patient care to do the bureaucratic paper work. Patient service, medical education and research in the USA are in the process of changing from one of the best systems in the world to a more compromised corporate structure. This situation prompts questions and comments.

- Why is the USA the only large, industrialized nation in the world which allows investors the opportunity to make profit from sick people without doing anything but buying stock in a medical insurance company?

318

- Why does only 10 cents of the healthcare dollar spent on patients who have diseases like diabetes mellitus go to the physician for health services?
- What third party reimburses healthcare costs at a level where quality health care can be consistently provided?
- Where are the monies for investment to develop the needed, functional informatic systems to help in the care of patients and reduce costs?
- Has greed been accentuated or has civility been introduced and promulgated in the medical center? Is the greater good for patients being pursued?
- Have collegiality, cooperation, unity and communication been maximized among healthcare providers?
- Is there fair use of current management and billing codes, and who is responsible for introducing complex billing systems that functionally prevent reimbursement for healthcare services? Are such people directly engaged in the practice of medicine, having face-to-face time with patients, or are some individuals entangled in a scheme to cheat for profit?
- Where have most of the master clinicians gone that used to take a history, perform an examination and recommend evidence-based care? Have their arts been lost?

The value of medical education is so low that the public is unwilling to pay for it. Healthcare expectations for advancements are extraordinarily high, but the attitude toward paying for services as well as for training and education of subsequent practitioners has been mean and brutal. Most state governments and federal agencies have not increased financial support for medical education during the past 10-20 years. In fact, the federal government's balanced budget act enacted in 1997 reduced monies for educating residents. Further, grant funds from the National Institutes of Health pay for only 70-90% of the total costs associated with research projects.

- Is there any wonder why the educational institutions are collapsing?

319

- Who is going to pay for teaching students bio-ethics, humanity and legal medicine, informatics, biometrics, sociology, epidemiology and business?
- The practice of medicine occurs at the "front line," the precipice of medical events. How does the CEO of a medical center direct investments to deliver state-of-the-art medical services in a hospital if he/she does not understand the importance of time to listen to and examine patients, or the importance of having a quiet place to sit and write or dictate a progress or consultation note after reviewing the patient and the data in the medical record or on the computer screen?
- Where is the room to discuss a patient's diagnosis, investigational studies and therapeutic plan?
- Why are members of the nursing staff being reduced, and are there sophisticated assistants to oversee the patients' progress and eliminate mistakes that could cause death?
- In essence, have the investments been made in hospital personnel, equipment and space to provide the best health care possible for the best price or has the money gone to profiteers?

At healthcare centers the first evidence of time restrictions (poverty) is the loss of scholarship. Research activities fade or disappear. With a further crunch on money and time, teaching is compromised; learning is no longer fostered. Next, physicians stop adequate communications with patients, and finally, physicians stop taking the time to communicate with each other. Health care deteriorates with the loss of each of these functions.

Of course the gap between basic science knowledge and clinical application is widening, but the greater societal threat to USA health care is loss of morale among healthcare providers. When doctors feel they have lost control of their professional lives, it is doubtful that they can provide optimal, compassionate health care to others. In a soft voice, we cry, "People, institutional leaders and congressmen, please be careful." The single biggest problem with health care in the USA is that those who know very little or nothing about medicine want to regulate healthcare delivery. The impact of the deterioration of the medical marketplace and unwarranted litigation are threatening the quality of medical care in the USA. These have become critical social issues that must be resolved to protect the welfare and health of our fine citizens. There is no place for greedy profiteers in American medicine, be they insurance and pharmaceutical companies, lawyers, stockholders or egregiously overpaid physicians and hospital administrators.

Recently it has been publicized that many lethal mistakes occur in hospitals. Before federal bureaucracy begins to deliver more fiats (rules) to correct these terrible mishaps, maybe the pace or throughput of patients in hospitals needs to be slowed down, permitting time to think and exercise judgment. Don't add more useless, time-consuming paper work responsibilities to further overburden healthcare providers.

People should not be expected to pay more money for health care. Nonetheless, solutions to some of the aforementioned can be generated. Citizens should insist that more financial aid be given to educational and developmental issues, but profit for investors in third party payers should be eliminated. Take the proceeds from third party payers and use the money to train better doctors, educate medical center workforce, increase space per patient and update information-computer systems. Support impartial systems that update doctors continuously on the practice of medicine. Do not expect drug companies and equipment manufacturers to provide unbiased information. In addition, recognize that more intellectual resources and financial investments are needed from the universities' schools of law, computer sciences, public relations and business. A magnetic force is needed to recruit social planners, clergy, business titans, legislators, biomedical statesmen and visionaries required to initiate corrective actions for the healthcare profession to better serve mankind. The greatest reward in life is appreciation. Hopefully the public will maintain appreciation for quality health care and regenerate a more humanistic environment for the practice of medicine.

I predict that it will be the new and young breed of medical scholars and practitioners that will salvage and reshape health care for Americans.

Chapter XVIII. Reflections

Friends and cohorts were generous in their behavior toward Paula, the children and me. Maybe it was natural for us to aim for medical school when we were young. The medical profession prepared individuals to make a comfortable living and eventually to give back to people some of the blessings received. Little did we know how hard and long the road to success was going to be. Further, we did not realize how fragile success was. Nonetheless, I am still interested in promoting the health and welfare of patients, especially those with obesity, diabetes, hypertension and abnormal blood fat content. This interest in patients causes me to frequently reflect upon health care in America.

There is no question that clinical investigators should be studying the benefits of functional magnetic images of body parts, stem cell transplantation, and methods to control spontaneous programmed cell death (apoptosis). In addition, simple reassessment of medications whose patent restrictions have expired needs to be evaluated along with the new drugs for the control of obesity. However, the most important thing to do for weight reduction is to eat fewer calories.

Over the years I have reflected on healthcare delivery and the role that the physician-scientist-teachers and scholars should play in formulating a mission statement for doctors in America. The following two paragraphs were extracted from an item I recently wrote for the AΩA journal, *The Pharos*, and only slightly modified from what was written in Chapter XVII.

"Members of the Honor Medical Society, Alpha Omega Alpha, shall be deeply and sincerely committed to the scholarly application of medical scientific information to improve the physical and mental states of people. They shall be dedicated to optimizing the health and welfare of their patients and society. They will struggle to share information, serve as mentors, teach junior and senior colleagues to be the most effective and efficacious medical servants possible, maintain an open mind, and be a ready recipient of new information. Further, they shall encourage a never-ending search or research of knowledge, influence and teach colleagues to recognize and appreciate their responsibilities to individual patients and to society, and enculturate humanity in its broadest context.

The Society shall seek members who have demonstrated academic excellence and desire to influence the performance of others who want to excel in providing wise, honest and compassionate health care to people; to foster doctoring through professionalism by placing the concerns and welfare of the patients and society first in the mind of the physicians-surgeons; to bring good cheer and charisma to patients; to pay homage to good health; to pledge to work for the good of the patient which can only be done if the 'state-of-the-art' or the best information available is employed in a humane manner for maximizing the well and healing the sick."

The foregoing "sermon" causes me to reflect on my own behavior and attitudes. Although I stopped the practice of medicine several years ago, old patients continue to ask my medical opinions regarding personal or family medical problems. While lying in bed one night, unable to sleep, I expressed to my wife that I was dreading a meeting the following day with a former patient. I anticipated the "consultation" would be undesirable. My wife offered no sympathy. She simply said, "Why don't you read what you wrote in *The Pharos* regarding behavior and attitudes that a physician should have?" I did not go to sleep, but I did stop complaining!

Medical professionals are good people but their personalities, like human beings in general, are mixtures of "good and not so good."

I recently had a dream: On the second floor of a busy medical school in a room off of the main corridor, basic scientists and physician-scientists were coming toward me to express their interest in clinical issues that needed to be

324

investigated to gain understanding of a disease and possibly to develop new approaches for therapy. Their interest not only intrigued me but also created a flash of optimism. How could this be? A renewed interest of people actually desirous of studying abnormalities in human beings to resolve their maladies. Good Heavens! This is the soul of medicine: alleviate human suffering. And in my dream the enthusiasm from bright capable physicians and scientists was genuine, maybe a little Quixotic, but genuine.

After I got out of bed, reality crept into my thoughts. I briefly reflected on my last few years in academic medical centers. As a clinical investigator, I had tried to maintain grant support and fought for the money needed to educate students, residents, fellows, faculty members and other support staff. I failed, and my experiences lacked adequate personal and financial rewards. I "walked away from the table" and suffered a functional death as an academic leader. However, my thought-processes about universities continue to reverberate in my mind.

The president of a university should have an enlarged vision of the academic institution, and his/her authority should be viewed as judicial for the benefit of all of the colleges. The president must be cautious about inflicting his attitudes and philosophies on the entire university community. A dictator can suppress the fluidity of academia, the intellectual enthusiasm, the art of discovery, and the very joy of being part of a university community.

Temple University Medical Center was the site of most of my professional activities. It was financially limited from its beginning. It suffered through one struggle after another. The hospital and the outpatient clinics served mostly an indigent patient population: 80% of the patient care income came from Medicaid and Medicare recipients. Medicaid reimbursement for health care in Pennsylvania is among the lowest in the nation. A practice plan to generate faculty salary based upon performance and to pay for operating expenses was developed in the 1970's. A medical dean's tax was placed upon this source of revenue. This source of income helped the medical school's administration pay for faculty recruitment and promote research programs. However, the president of the university also placed a tax on the clinical income generated by the practice plan. The medical school teaching and research programs were already suffering. I saw the decline in academic excellence at the university. Some of the school's leaders stated that Temple's School of Medicine could not afford to be engaged in research. The school's rankings in grant money from the National Institutes of Health to support research fell from about 34th in the mid 1970's to about 75th in the mid 1980's.

I sought an opportunity to leave Temple University Medical School and Hospital. I jumped "out of the frying pan and into a fire." I thought an opportunity to become Professor and Chair of Medicine at Southern Illinois University, a fledgling medical school with alleged resources to generate a research-intense institution, would provide me a chance to build an academic medical center that was moving toward goals I thought were important: research that promoted education and patient care.

I wanted to go to a university where I could have a major impact on advancing its research programs and its teaching and patient care activities. I wanted to look back some day and see that I had made a difference, a good difference, leaving a well-marked trail for others to follow. It did not work out like that.

In a state-supported medical school where the state legislators and school administrators declare their desires by fiats rather than democratic options that a medical school cannot afford research, they have knowingly or unknowingly slammed the door on advancing patient care and blindly limited medical education. Nonetheless, the faculty, managers, nurses, secretaries, fellows, residents and students at Southern Illinois University had the strongest work ethic I ever encountered. They were good people. An example of their devotion to the welfare of others can be illustrated by their behavior during the flooding of the Mississippi River in 1993. On Saturday mornings I met with the residents to discuss the medical conditions of the patients hospitalized in the previous 24 hours and any patient under their care that needed special attention. The residents who had been on service the day before and throughout the night without sleep were joined by most of the other residents who had Saturday afternoon and night off-duty. They got into their cars, drove to the edge of the Mississippi River flood area and volunteered to work in the makeshift medical emergency rooms to treat the people who were working and injured along the river. They were noble in their effort to relieve the suffering of people, sick in the flood zone, removing splinters, covering blisters, wrapping sprains, and if needed, packing and carrying sandbags.

When I arrived in Springfield, Illinois, the town-gown phenomenon (the separation between the practicing physicians in town and the academic physicians/surgeons) was the most evident cleavage in healthcare delivery that I had ever encountered. That split was largely resolved over the next six years. The private practicing doctors joined the medical school faculty's efforts to educate the students and residents and promote good health care. Considerable maturation and understanding developed between both parties.

With reasonable state support, the academic medical center could have become all it desired and deserved to be as an intellectual institution. However, state funding for the medical school remained flat for 10 years. There were not enough resources available to become reasonably competitive for national research grants. It became blatantly obvious to me that an insightful visionary cannot move an academic institution forward without money, a lot of money. Financial resources must come from local and state coffers and philanthropists before an institution can obtain federal support.

Probably a sizeable number of clinical investigators have ended their productive careers by accepting administrative positions filled with good intentions and promises but devoid of substance. What happened at Southern Illinois University School of Medicine is similar to what has happened across America in other medical schools. The general public and legislature have the inappropriate

327

attitude that free health care is an inalienable right. This is silly. Health care has cost. No one has the right to take free of charge from others to meet his/her needs.

Maybe our work in clinical research was not as influential or important as I thought it was. Nonetheless, the work in clinical investigation gave me a lot of satisfaction. I believe we did something to help physician-scientists understand human body metabolism. Such knowledge should have promoted their ability to improve the treatment of patients.

In reviewing the data from my efforts as a clinical investigator, it was obvious that the "path to understanding" how the body maintained a supply of fuels to meet the metabolic requirements of various organs, e.g. brain, liver, kidney and muscle, "was not a straight line."

As I browsed through my old research notebooks looking for information to help me write this book, it became grossly evident that my colleagues and I completed many more research protocols than we published. For me, unfortunately, synthesizing the data in an intelligent manner and submitting them for peer review were steps that I too often failed to take. However, many of the research protocols were done on patients who volunteered for studies. The results of studies were inclusive. Some of the patients were extremely sick and the research studies were done to find a therapeutic tool to benefit their care; however, some of the efforts were in vain.

Young clinical scientists must be stimulated to tackle medical diseases in a manner that was most useful in 1960-1980 before trial lawyers, insurance executives and well-meaning legislators handicapped medical progress.

In every physician's career there are periods or patients from which they learn a lot about the medical sciences: patients have pertinent messages. Outpatient and bedside learning rises and falls every 20-30 years. No one knows why this occurs. William Osler enshrined bedside teaching at Johns Hopkins Hospital from 1888 to 1912. Interestingly, the research protocol developed for the starvation study was based on laboratory techniques to delineate body metabolism. Some of the information provided from bedside observations was initially handled in a superficial manner and came into full light many years after the laboratory measurements were published. It takes a combination of medical scientific data and compassionate and time consuming patient care observations to advance medical understanding and delivery.

Very definitive research protocols are designed to study similar patients under identical circumstances. However, no two volunteers or patients provide identical results.

Laboratory data cannot supplant the dialogue between a patient-volunteer and the clinical investigator.

A battery of laboratory determinations done in research facilities does not reduce the immediate need of the clinical investigator to oversee the patient-volunteer's medical needs/welfare. Observing starving volunteers was an intense process. Constant personal care was demanded to avoid oversight of impending danger.

To understand the hunger pains and agony experienced by starving patient-volunteers the clinicians must take the time needed to listen and observe these people. A quick walk-by-the-bedside evaluation is inadequate to learn the patient-volunteers' deep-seated feelings. An engaging conversation between the patient-volunteer and the physician-clinical scientist reveals evidence not recorded on the charts, displaying weight, blood pressure, pulse, temperature, etc. Assuming the responsibility to watch over another human being generates a powerful, protective force. Brief glimpses of the patient-volunteer do not portray the human being under study.

As I reminisced over my career in clinical research I could not help recalling all of the reasonable but farfetched ideas presented to me regarding the possible outcomes of research proposals. Over the three or four decades that I worked as a clinical investigator, I learned that "good research ideas are worth about ten cents a dozen." It is the execution of a hypothesis and publishing the research results in a top peer reviewed scientific journal that counts, not an

329

idea. Asking questions regarding human biology is easy, but answering them with verifiable data is hard, if not nearly impossible, because clinical investigators who initiate research projects are a disappearing species.

Glossary

abdomen – the belly, the portion of the trunk below the chest

acid base balance – a condition in which the net rate of acid or alkali production by the body is balanced by net rate of acid or alkali excretion from the body, resulting in a stable concentration of H^+ (hydrogen ions) in the body fluids

adenosine triphosphate (ATP) – a triply phosphorylated organic compound that functions as "energy currency" for organisms

alanine – key gluconeogenic amino acid that transports nitrogen from other amino acids to the liver, and whose carbon skeleton is used to synthesize glucose

alpha ketoanalogues – used in this text to mean an amino acid in which its nitrogen has been replaced by oxygen

amine – an organic compound that may be a derivation of ammonia (NH_3)

amino acid – an organic acid carrying an amino group (-NH_2); the building block compound of proteins

anabolism – any constructive process by which simple substances are converted by living cells into more complex compounds

anaplerosis – the addition or replacement of compounds or materials (anions) to a metabolic cycle to maintain its function (balance). The replacement of materials equals the quantity of materials removed from a cycle.

anastamosis – a communication between two vessels created by surgery so the blood in one vessel can flow into the blood of another vessel

anion – a negatively charged ion

aorta – the main artery of the circulation system

arteriole – a small artery

artery – a blood vessel that carries blood away from the heart

basal – at the base level

blood flow rate – the quantity of blood that flows per unit time

caloric requirements – the amount of heat (energy) required or generated by the body under different circumstances

calorie – the quantity of energy, in the form of heat, required to raise the temperature of one gram of pure water one degree (from 14.5 to 15.5° C)

calorimeter – a device used to measure heat produced or absorbed (by the body)

capillary – a tiny blood vessel with walls one cell thick across which exchange of materials between blood and tissues occurs

carbohydrate – any of a class of organic compounds composed of carbon, hydrogen and oxygen in a ratio of about two hydrogens and one oxygen for each carbon

carboxyl group – the –COOH group characteristic of organic acids

catabolism – any destructive process by which complex substances are converted by living cells into more simple compounds

catalyst – a chemical substance that accelerates a reaction, but it is not permanently changed or consumed by the reaction

cataplerosis – the removal or drainage of anions (compounds or materials) from a cycle to maintain its function. Anaplerosis must equal cataplerosis in order to maintain a balance in a cyclic process.

cation – a positively charged ion

deamination – removal of an amino group

diffusion – the movement of dissolved or suspended particles through a liquid or gaseous material

endocrine – pertaining to ductless glands that produce hormones

energy – the capacity for activity or work

enzyme – a protein produced in a cell that greatly accelerates a reaction

extraction – the process or act of pulling or drawing out something

fat mass – the whitish-yellow tissue that furnishes a reserve supply of fuel; serves to smooth and round out bodily contours; forms soft pads between various organs

flux rates – the rate of passage of materials, fuels, oxygen, etc., through the bloodstream or body

fuel homeostasis – the maintenance of a constant supply of fuels, usually for energy production

fuels – substances used to produce energy

gas – the state of matter in which a substance has neither definite volume nor definite shape

glucagon – a hormone produced by the alpha-islet cells of the pancreas that works in opposition to insulin and promotes mobilization of protein, glycogen and fat

gluconeogenesis – the formation of glucose from molecules not themselves carbohydrates. However, the term "gluconeogenesis" is generally used in a broader context and implies new glucose formation from whatever the source, including lactate, pyruvate and glycerol.

glucose – a six-carbon sugar that plays a crucial role in providing fuel for the body

glutamate – an amino acid; transports the carbon skeleton of glutamine from the liver to the muscle by traveling primarily in red blood cells

glutamine – the primary amino acid in the bloodstream and the amino acid that transports nitrogen from other amino acids to the kidney for ammonia and glucose formation

glycerol – a three-carbon component of fat which serves as a docking site for long-chain fatty acids in adipose tissue and other lipid storing cells; a compound that the liver converts into glucose for recycling to intracellular lipid deposits

glycogen – a polysaccharide that serves as the principal storage form of glucose

glycolysis – anaerobic catabolism of carbohydrates (primarily glucose) to pyruvic acid

gram – a metric unit of weight equal to one thousandth of a kilogram

hepatic – pertaining to the liver

histology – the structure and arrangement of the tissues of organs; microscopic anatomy

homeostasis – a tendency to stability in the body; for fuels, the maintenance of steady-state

hormone – a control chemical secreted in one part of the body that affects other parts of the body

hybrid – a cross between two genetic types, used in this text to mean an intellectual concept of an equal mixture of men and women body parts to reflect an average

insulin – a hormone produced by the β–islet cells of the pancreas that helps to regulate glucose (carbohydrate), fat and protein metabolism

ketogenesis – the synthesis of acetoacetate and beta-hydroxybutyrate and the generation of acetone from the spontaneous decomposition of acetoacetate

ketone bodies – three- and four-carbon compounds that are water-soluble and synthesized primarily from long chain fatty acids; valuable fuels for tissues that require water-soluble fuels; primarily beta-hydroxybutyrate, acetoacetate and acetone.

ketosis – a condition in which ketone bodies are prevalent in the body fluids

kilogram – a unit of mass (weight); one kilogram equals 2.2 pounds

kinetic analysis – analyzing the motions of reactions, such as measuring the movement of a fuel through the body

lactate – a three-carbon chemical compound usually derived from glucose and in equilibrium with pyruvate, both of which are converted into glucose primarily by the liver and recycled to the peripheral tissues as glucose for utilization

lean body mass – a mass consisting of protein and water and devoid of fat. It is a conceptualized mass of bodily tissues composed primarily of muscle and organs other than adipose tissue.

mentor – a loyal advisor (of Odysseus) entrusted with the care, education and advice to a student or younger colleague

meter – a basic unit of linear measure in the metric system, approximately equivalent to 39.4 inches

mitochondrium – subcellular organelle (little organ) in which aerobic respiration takes place; the site where most of the energy is released from fuels

nephron – the functional unit of a vertebrate kidney

nutrient – a food substrate usable in metabolism as a source of energy or of building material

organ – a body part composed of tissues grouped together into a structural and functional unit

oxidation – the energy-releasing process involving the removal of electrons in a substance and oxygen generally receiving the electrons

pH – the negative of the common logarithm of the hydronium ion concentration of a solution; in essence, the concentration of the hydrogen; an indication of how acid or alkaline is a water solution, pH 7 is neutral, lower = acidic, higher = alkaline

physiology – the study of the life processes and functions of organisms or the body

plasma – blood minus the cells and platelets

polymer – a large molecule consisting of a chain of small molecules bonded together by condensation or similar reaction

portal system – a blood circuit in which two beds of capillaries are connected by a vein (e.g. hepatic portal system, renal portal system)

pound – a unit of mass (weight); one pound equals 0.45 kilograms

precursor – a forerunner; a substance from which another substance is formed

product – a substance that is formed by a chemical change

production – something is being produced or is being formed or synthesized

propanediol – a three-carbon compound largely derived from acetone which, in the context of this book, can be converted and used to synthesize glucose

protein – a long polypeptide chain

proteolytic – protein-digesting

pyruvate – a three-carbon compound derived mostly from glucose and in equilibrium with lactate produced in cells and transported to the liver in the blood for conversion into glucose for recycling as pyruvate (and lactate)

quantity – something that has magnitude, size or amount

radioactive tracer – a radioactive atom that is incorporated into a substance so that movement of the substance can be followed by a radiation detector

radioimmunoassay – a technique used to measure material in biologic fuels by employing radioactive immune globulin to attack the material of interest and separating the labeled complex

release – the addition of a compound into a body part, usually the contribution of a fuel or other compound to the blood, urine or feces

scientific method – a logical approach to solving problems by observing and collecting data, formulating hypotheses, testing hypotheses, and formulating theories that are supported by data

statistics – numerical facts pertaining to a body of things; the science which deals with the collection and tabulation of such facts

substrate – a substance acted upon by an enzyme; something usually converted into another compound

tracer techniques – identification of a compound and following its behavior through a biologic system using an isotope, usually a radioactive material

triglyceride – a compound consisting of three molecules of fatty acid attached (esterified) to glycerol; it is a neutral fat stored in animal adipose tissue; it releases free fatty acid and glycerol into the blood after being broken down

uptake – the removal of a compound from a body part, usually the extraction of a material from the gut, blood or urine

variceal – an enlarged or tortuous vein, artery or lymphatic vessel

vein – a vessel through which blood passes from various organs or parts back to the heart

vitamins – a group of organic micronutrients, present in minute quantities in natural foodstuffs, that are essential to normal metabolism

Made in the USA
Monee, IL
07 July 2026

56552247R00193